NURSING IN TODAY'S WORLD

Challenges, Issues, and Trends

D1302222

Janice Rider Ellis, R.N., M.N.

Professor of Nursing
Shoreline Community College
Seattle, Washington

Celia Love Hartley, R.N., M.N.

Director of Nursing Education
Shoreline Community College
Seattle, Washington

with illustrations by
Kari Berger, B.A.

Bainbridge Island, Washington

Nursing in Today's World

Challenges, Issues, and Trends

Third Edition

J.B. Lippincott Company
Philadelphia
London   Mexico City   New York
St. Louis   São Paulo   Sydney

Sponsoring Editor: Diana Intenzo
Editorial Assistant: Mary Murphy
Manuscript Editor: Barbara Hodgson
Indexer: Angela Holt
Cover Designer: Stephen Cymerman
Design Coordinator: Michelle Gerdes
Production Manager: Carol A. Florence
Production Editor: Rosanne Hallowell
Compositor: Digitype, Inc.
Text Printer/Binder: R.R. Donnelley & Sons Company, Inc.
Cover Printer: New England Book Company

6 5

Ellis, Janice Rider.
    Nursing in today's world.

    Includes bibliographies and index.
        1. Nursing—United States.   I. Hartley, Celia Love.
II. Title.   [DNLM: 1. Nursing—United States.
WY 16 E47n]
RT4.E42   1988   610.73   87-22554
ISBN 0-397-54696-3 (pbk.)

Preface

By far the largest segment of the educational preparation of any student pursuing a nursing career is spent developing a theoretical foundation for and applying the clinical aspects of care. The rapidly increasing body of nursing knowledge and the new technologies that have reshaped nursing practice demand that the new graduate have a sound understanding of nursing theory that will guide the performance of the many psychomotor skills that comprise the art and science of nursing. Another essential aspect of professional education exists, however — a nonclinical dimension. It would be as foolish for a student to plunge into the practice of nursing without some understanding of nursing's history and evolution as a profession as to begin care for a patient without an understanding of the patient's problems and condition. To fill the role demanded of today's nurse, it is critical that the student understand the development, heritage, and history of nursing as a profession; the many studies that have helped us to know more about ourselves and our profession, its struggles, controversies, and victories; and the battles that are yet to be waged and won. It is also important for the student to be aware of the many issues to which there are no ready solutions and the questions that are likely to remain unanswered, or that can be answered only on an individual basis. It is for this aspect of nursing that *Nursing in Today's World* is written.

Students need to gain an understanding of how nursing relates to society as a whole. What impact does nursing have on society and, conversely, what impact does society have on the practice of nursing? What are the effects of legal, ethical, bioethical, legislative, and political concerns? What type of image does the public hold of nurses and nursing? How should this image be changed?

Students can benefit additionally from information that will help them into the nursing profession. This includes knowledge of opportunities in nursing as well as the specifics of applying and interviewing for positions, anticipating conflicts that may occur in their professional roles, and understanding the organizations that represent nursing. The student with this preparation will be better able to practice nursing as it exists today and influence the development of future nursing practice.

We have written this book as an introduction to that task. It is our hope that it will assist you with your course in "Issues," "Trends," or "Professional Adjustments," or with such material integrated into other courses. Each chapter is preceded by a list of general objectives designed to guide you to an understanding of the information that follows. Additional bibliographic references at the end of each chapter lend direction to each of you seeking a more in-depth exploration of a given topic.

We recognize that many of the topics presented in the context of the book have enough subject matter to fill an entire textbook or, in cases such as bioethical issues, an entire encyclopedia. Our express purpose is to provide you with an overview of basic information necessary to move into the nursing role, while at the same time stimulating a desire for further reading. Changes in our society occur so rapidly that many of our most heavily and heatedly debated issues are history by the time they can be placed in a textbook. While time adds perspective, day-to-day reading of newspapers and periodicals is vital to remain currently informed; thus, we encourage students using this book to read additional materials to be completely up to date.

With each edition we have tried to make this book more responsive to your needs. The aspect of the book receiving the widest range of comments has been the illustrations. Some have been critical of the illustrations, finding them inappropriate for a text about the profession of nursing. But more overwhelmingly readers, especially the students, have responded positively. Therefore, we have chosen to continue with the cartoon-type illustrations, through which we hope the student will gain a varied visual introduction to nursing issues. We hope that you, like us, will be able to find humor, as well as gratification, in your involvement in nursing.

In accomplishing our task, many thanks are in order and we hesitate for fear of omitting anyone. Certainly we need to acknowledge the support of our colleagues at Shoreline Community College who continue to bring new issues to our attention, and the unfailing effort of a special librarian, Patricia Kelley, who would go to all ends to find a particular reference. As we worked at perfecting the content of the third edition, we were especially appreciative of the comments of fellow educators throughout the United States who have used our text and offered enthusiastic support and constructive criticism of the content.

Your continued suggestions and recommendations will be valued. We are thankful for the emotional support provided by our respective husbands, Ivan and Gordon, and our families, who have allowed us to put the book first when necessary. And last, but not least, we thank the editors of the J.B. Lippincott Company for their help with this text.

Janice Rider Ellis, R.N., M.N.
Celia Love Hartley, R.N., M.N.

Contents

UNIT II
Legal and Ethical Accountability for Practice

4 *Credentials for Nursing Practice*   *109*

5 *Legal Responsibilities for Practice*   *137*

Unit I
Understanding the Development of Nursing as a Profession

1 | # Nursing as a Developing Profession

Objectives

After completing this chapter, you should be able to

1. State a definition of nursing.
2. Identify reasons the profession has had difficulty defining nursing.
3. List the formal characteristics of a profession.
4. Describe the health care practices in the early civilizations of Egypt, Babylon, Palestine, India, China, Greece, and Rome.
5. Discuss the three major historical images of the nurse.
6. Describe how each of these historical images has influenced the development of nursing as a profession.
7. Explain the significance of the "Dark Ages of Nursing" to the development of the nursing profession.
8. State the name and location of the first hospital founded in the United States.
9. Identify the early nursing schools in America.
10. Discuss the contribution of Florence Nightingale to the development of nursing as a profession.
11. Discuss factors that have affected the image of nursing today.
12. List at least three studies about nursing and explain their significance.

What is nursing? How has it emerged as a profession? Is it a profession? Is nursing an art or a science? Does it possess a unique body of knowledge? Is the nurse a professional? If so, what education is required for professional standing? Should there be different levels of educational preparation for nursing? If so, what is the scope of practice of the graduates prepared by the various educational programs? What is the position of the nurse in relation to other members of the health care team? What is the exclusive role of the nurse? What forces have had a hand in the development of that role? What is the future of that role? These are only some of the questions that are asked about nurses and nursing today. Many remain unanswered. Some of the answers that are given are debated by nurses, health care providers, and the public as health care consumers. One can be certain that if we as nurses cannot find solutions to some of the controversies facing our profession, others will remedy our problems for us—and perhaps not to our liking.

This chapter exposes you to some of the issues that surround nursing today. Will nursing be your occupation, or your profession? Is there a difference? As the nurse of tomorrow, you can help to shape a response to some of these issues.

NURSING DEFINED

Defining nursing is difficult. Nurses themselves cannot agree on a single definition. This may be due in part to nursing's historical background. Some nurses are not interested in such discussions of definitions and would say, "A nurse is a nurse is a nurse." However, the advancing technology in the health fields, the varying areas of specialization, the different routes to educational preparation, and the variety of practice settings force nurses to provide some answers for themselves as well as for the public. To state that you are a registered nurse says little about what you do. It conveys nothing about where you are employed or about your educational background. The words *nurse* and *nursing* have been applied to a wide variety of health care activities in many different settings performed by many variously educated people.

Technological advances have also affected the definition of nursing. This is reflected in the comments made by a colleague after looking in her late-1950s medical–surgical nursing textbook to see how nurses at that time managed the care of a patient with an aortic aneurysm. She found that nurses did not usually manage such patients because these patients seldom lived long enough to require any nursing care. Today such patients are in intensive care units. They are making a good, although cautious, recovery after careful diagnosis that perhaps requires angioaortograms, ultrasonography, or tomography; delicate surgery to excise and repair the distension of the artery; and specialized critical care nursing. "A nurse is a nurse is a nurse" no longer accurately reflects the role of the person who may care for this patient, the skills needed to fulfill the expected behaviors, or the diversity that exists within the profession.

Nurses in many positions have been required to assume ever greater levels of responsibility. Paradoxically, they have not always been given the official authority, autonomy, or recognition that would be expected to accompany those responsibilities.

Beginning with the simplest definition, a nurse is a person who nourishes, fosters, and protects, a person who is prepared to care for the sick, injured, and aged. In this sense *nurse* is used as a noun and is derived from the Latin *nutrix*, which means "nursing mother." An

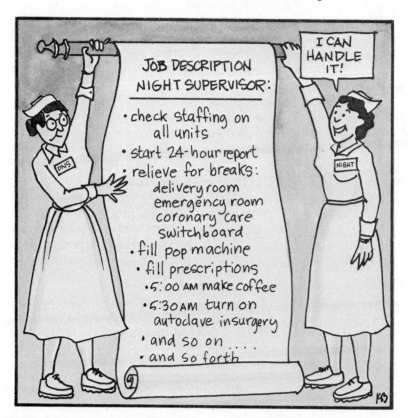

Figure 1–1. The word *nursing* has been applied to a wide variety of activities, but nurses of today would take exception to many of them.

early use of the word was associated with the meaning of a woman who suckled a child, usually not her own—a wet nurse. Dictionary definitions of nurse also include such words as "suckles or nourishes," "to take care of a child or children," "to bring up; rear." In this way *nurse* is used as a verb, deriving from the Latin *nutrire*, which means "to suckle and nourish." With such an origin it is understandable that people generally have associated nursing with women.

References to "the nurse" can be found in the Talmud and in the Old Testament, although the role of this person is not clearly stated. It was probably more similar to that of the wet nurse than to that of someone who tended the sick. Slowly, over the centuries, the word nurse has evolved to refer to a person who cares for the sick. It is more than just a coincidence that the development of nursing as a profession has been inextricably tied to the role that women occupied in society at that given time. People who functioned in the capacity of the nurse were undoubtedly more concerned about carrying out the responsibilities of the role than about defining the role.

Florence Nightingale, in her *Notes on Nursing: What It Is, and What It Is Not*, described the nurse's role as one that would "put the patient in the best condition for nature to act upon him."[1]

More recent definitions include that of Sister M. Olivia Gowan, who described nursing as an art and science that involves the whole patient —body, mind, and spirit— and that promotes his spiritual, mental, and physical health and stresses health education and health preservation as well as ministration to the sick.[2] Dorothy Johnson defined nursing as a discipline that focuses on direct service to individuals and groups of people, with the ultimate goals of promoting and maintaining optimal health using nursing care through the nursing process.[3]

In 1958 Virginia Henderson was asked by the nursing service committee of the International Council of Nurses to describe her concept of basic nursing. Hers is one of the most widely accepted definitions of nursing:

> The unique function of the nurse is to assist the individual, sick or well, in the performance of those activities contributing to health or its recovery (or to peaceful death) that he would perform unaided if he had the necessary strength, will or knowledge. And to do this in such a way as to help him gain independence as rapidly as possible.[4]

Certainly many would agree with the American Nurses' Association (ANA) position paper that the "essential components of professional nursing practice include care, cure, and coordination."[5] Others would concur that it is both an art and a science: an art in the sense that it is composed of skills that require expertness and proficiency for their execution, and a science in the sense that it requires systematized knowledge derived from observation, study, and research carried on in such a way that they will determine the principles for what is being studied.

In 1980 the ANA, through their Social Policy Statement, provided yet another definition of nursing: "Nursing is the diagnosis and treatment of human responses to actual or potential health problems."[6] That definition is having widespread effect and is being realized in the language used in some of our nursing diagnoses today.

In 1982 the National Council of State Boards of Nursing (NCSBN) developed a Model Nurse Practice Act. The single most important part of any nurse practice act is the legal definition of nursing practice. This is necessary because it provides the foundation for education, licensure, scope of practice of the profession, and, when necessary, the basis for corrective actions against the nurse who violates the practice act. The committee that developed the act had difficulty arriving at a precise and succinct definition. It found a lack of consensus within the literature and the profession. The committee was looking for a definition that would clearly differentiate nursing from the practice of any other health discipline. It was looking for terms that would describe the essential elements unique to nursing but that would be broad enough to include all levels of nurses who should be licensed to practice. In reaching for these goals the committee found that the term nursing was not differentiating or limiting, and therefore did not use it in the definition. As a working alternative the NCSBN incorporated currently accepted concepts of the nursing process and proposed that the practice of nursing be defined around these.[7]

CHARACTERISTICS OF A PROFESSION

Since the 1950s some nursing leaders have been primarily concerned about providing an explicit definition of nursing, whereas others have examined, challenged, and defended nursing's standing as a profession. Certainly at the time nursing and nursing education were evolving in the United States, no one asked if nursing qualified as a profession. As a matter of fact, there is evidence, as cited by Strauss, that from an early date the word profession was associated with nursing. He gives as an example a magazine article titled "A New Profession for Women" that appeared in 1882. The article described nursing reform and carried with it a picture of Isabel Hampton.[8] Strauss also refers to writings of Lizabeth Price, published in 1892, in which nursing was discussed as a profession.[9]

Over the years reference to nursing as a profession has become common, and the nurse practice acts of some states include this language. Before we can continue a discussion of whether the term profession should be applied to nursing, we need to find an acceptable definition of profession.

Assume for a moment that you are a student in one of our classes, and we ask you to name some ways of earning a living that you would categorize as professions. It would not be long before we would have a sizeable list started on our chalkboard or overhead projector. If you were to respond as many of our students have, you would quickly volunteer "physician," "attorney," "clergyman," "teacher." Others would add "nurse," "physical therapist," "psychologist," "pharmacist," and "certified public accountant." As the list grows, our interpretation of the word profession would become less clear and more ambiguous. For example, if we were to say "musician," would you think of opera stars Joan Sutherland and Placido Domingo, or would you think of popular singers such as Phil Collins or Madonna? If we were to say "actor," would you think of performers like Lord Laurence Olivier and Katharine Hepburn, or would you think of Meryl Streep and Dustin Hoffman? Is there a difference? When we list "engineer," do you think of an electrical engineer, who gains entry into a career only after completing 4 years of college, or do you think of the so-called sanitary engineer, who picks up your garbage? Does expertise in a particular sport represent professionalism? Are John Elway and Martina Navratilova as professional as one might consider Robert K. Jarvik or Jonas Salk to be? At this point we are beginning to confuse the words profession and professional. Do they have separate meanings? Is it possible to enter a profession and not be professional, or, conversely, can one be professional but not operate within a profession? These are the kinds of questions with which nursing is struggling. Although we may be involved in a word game played often in our society, you will begin to understand the need to spell out some of the characteristics of a profession, if only for academic purposes.

Profession has several dictionary definitions. The two that apply in this context state that it is (1) a vocation or occupation that requires advanced training in a specialized field, and that often involves intensive academic preparation, such as medicine, law, theology, engineering, and teaching; and (2) the body of people who are engaged in any such calling or occupation. It is to the first definition that sociologists have referred when developing a list of characteristics of a profession. Nurses have added their own expectations to this list.

One of the first persons to identify characteristics of a profession was Flexner, in 1915. His classic criteria include the following:

- The activities of the work group must be intellectual.
- The activities, because they are based on knowledge, can be learned.
- The work activities must be practical, as opposed to academic or theoretical.
- The profession must have teachable techniques, which are the work of professional education.
- There must be a strong internal organization of members of the work group.
- Altruism, a desire to provide for the good of society, must be the workers' motivating force.[10]

By the 1950s nurses were becoming concerned about the application of various criteria to nursing. In 1945 Bixler and Bixler identified seven criteria for a profession and compared nursing's progress toward meeting these criteria.[11] The criteria they set forth state that a profession

1. Uses in its practice a well-defined and well-organized body of specialized knowledge that is on the intellectual level of higher learning.
2. Constantly enlarges the body of knowledge it uses and improves its techniques of education and service by the use of the scientific method.
3. Entrusts the education of its practitioners to institutions of higher education.
4. Applies its body of knowledge in practical services, which are vital to human and social welfare.
5. Functions autonomously in the formulation of professional policy and in the control of professional activity thereby.
6. Attracts people of intellectual and personal qualities, who exalt service above personal gain and who recognize their chosen occupation as a lifework.
7. Strives to compensate its practitioners by providing freedom of action, opportunity for continuous professional growth, and economic security.

Pavalko, writing in 1971, developed a continuum model to determine how professionalized a particular work group might be. His eight criteria included

1. The extent to which the work is based on a systematic body of theory and abstract knowledge.
2. The basic social value of the work performed.
3. The amount and length of education required to attain the specialization.
4. The motivation for the work, which emphasizes the ideal of service to the public.
5. The freedom of a group to regulate and control its own work behavior (autonomy).
6. The sense of commitment the members have toward work as a lifetime or at least a long-term pursuit rather than as a stepping-stone to another profession.
7. The degree to which members of a work group share a common identity and possess a distinctive subculture.
8. The existence within the group of a code of ethics.[12]

Some critics challenge that nursing falls short of meeting these criteria. A major claim is that nursing has no "body of specialized knowledge" that belongs uniquely to nursing. Critics state that nursing borrows from biological sciences, social sciences, and medical science, and then combines the various skills and concepts to call it "nursing." Although there is some truth to the statement, this amalgamation and synthesis of some areas with application to another may be one of the unique qualities of nursing. Nursing researchers are also working to help develop an organized body of knowledge that is unique to nursing. Even simple tasks, such as the length of time required to get an accurate reading on a rectal thermometer, are being researched and recorded. Other nurses are working to advance the standing of nursing through the development of a code of ethics, standards of practice, and peer review.

Some of the criteria are subject to question and challenge. For example, is there a conflict between altruism and professionalism? Are nurses lowering the standards of nursing as a profession when they engage in collective bargaining (see Chapter 9)? When the material needs of the nurse come into conflict with the general needs of society, what is the solution?

Many of the subjects mentioned above are discussed in greater detail in later sections of this book. After reading and discussing the various sections, you can decide for yourself whether nursing is moving

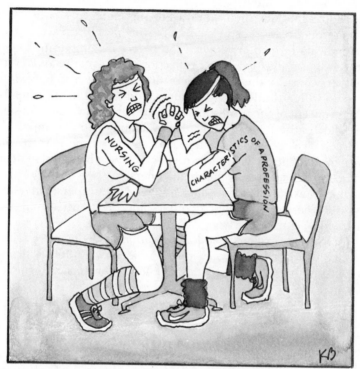

Figure 1–2. Giving professional status to nursing is sometimes challenged.

aggressively toward becoming a profession, or whether it remains in the realm of an occupation.

Let us now focus on the second dictionary definition of the word profession (*i.e.*, "the body of people who are engaged in any such calling). That definition adds to our confusion. The practice of nursing involves many activities that may be performed by many care givers. These people include nurse aides, orderlies, practical nurses, and registered nurses prepared for entry into nursing through any of several educational avenues (see Chapter 2). Each of these care givers is contributing to nursing as a profession. To meet the nursing needs of the public, it is essential that care givers function at various levels of practice, but there is a difference in looking at the practice of nursing in its totality and at the practice of *professional* nursing.

A popular view of a profession involves the approach a person has to an occupation. Most *professionals* are seriously concerned about their occupation, strive for excellence in performance, and demonstrate a sense of ethics and responsibility in relationship to their occupation.

Such people consider their work a lifelong endeavor, rather than a stepping-stone to another field of employment. They place a positive value on being termed *professional* and perceive being termed *nonprofessional* or *technical* as an adverse reflection on their status and position.

Others consider the attributes of professionalism to have a great deal to do with attitude, dress, conduct, and deportment. Often built into this concept of the professional are the personal values and stereotypes held by the person doing the evaluating. For example, some would perceive the "truly professional" nurse as the person who is dressed in a starched white uniform and cap, whose hair is off her collar, and whose shoes are freshly polished. Others may perceive the "professional nurse" as the one who is open and kind in interpersonal relationships, who focuses on the needs of others, and who is tactful and skillful in interview techniques.

In at least one instance, federal legislation has helped to establish a list of characteristics of a professional. Public Law 93-360, which governs collective bargaining activities, defines the professional employee as follows:

(a) any employee engaged in work (i) predominantly intellectual and varied in character as opposed to routine mental, manual, mechanical, or physical work; (ii) involving the consistent exercise of discretion and judgment in its performance; (iii) of such a character that the output produced or the result accomplished cannot be standardized in relation to a given period of time; (iv) requiring knowledge of an advanced type in a field of science or learning customarily acquired by a prolonged course of specialized intellectual instruction and study in an institution of higher learning or a hospital, as distinguished from a general academic education or from an apprenticeship or from training in the performance of routine mental, manual, or physical processes; or

(b) any employee, who (i) has completed the courses of specialized intellectual instruction and study described in clause (iv) of paragraph (a), and (ii) is performing related work under the supervision of a professional person to qualify himself to become a professional employee as defined in paragraph (a).[13]

As you can see, the sociological and legal definitions are much more restrictive than the popular view of the term *professional*. One of the difficulties is the communication block that results from people using the term in different ways. When one person is using a restrictive, sociological definition and the other person responds from a standpoint of personal belief and feeling, agreement is almost impossible.

Debate over the use of the terms profession and professional in nursing is prevalent. One can better understand the debate if one knows something about the historical development of the field of nursing.

HISTORICAL PERSPECTIVES

Muriel Uprichard identifies three heritages from the past that tend to inhibit the progress of nursing. They are "the folk image of the nurse brought forward from primitive times, the religious image of the nurse inherited from the medieval period, and the servant image of the nurse created by the Protestant-capitalist ethic of the 16th to 19th century."[14] Whether they impeded progress, certainly these concepts of the nurse have had an impact.

The Folk Image of the Nurse

Since the time of the first mother, women have carried the major responsibility for the nourishing and the nurturing of children and for caring for elderly and aging members of the family. It is difficult, however, when examining the pages of history, to pinpoint a particular time or place for the beginnings of nursing as we know it. It is reasonable to assume that early tribes and civilizations had needs for health care. It is also reasonable to assume that within those tribes and civilizations, there would come forth people who demonstrated adeptness and special interests in meeting the needs of the sick, the injured, and those bearing children. The education of these people was largely by trial and error, advancing those methods that appeared successful, and by the sharing of information with one another. Superstition and magic played no small part in the treatment rendered; folklore abounded, and a close relationship existed between religion and the healing arts.

Nursing skills primarily evolved from intuition. For example, during the process of planning a diet for the family, the wise woman noticed that eating certain foods resulted in episodes of diarrhea and vomiting, whereas eating other herbs, roots, and leaves had a soothing effect on the body. Families developed recipes that were handed down from generation to generation.

Most of the writing about early health care makes almost no mention of nursing or nurses. In primitive societies illness and suffering were thought to result from some evil spirit that may have been inflicted on a person as a punishment or curse for failing to do as the gods wanted. The role of healer was fulfilled by medicine men and witch doctors who "cured" by driving out evil spirits. Medicine and magic tended to be confused. Ritualistic ceremonies designed to drive away evil spirits eventually developed into religious rites, and the medicine man of some societies was replaced by a priest. Because of strong beliefs in the occult, an infinite variety of superstitions about illness was developed. Some of the superstitions still persist. Each primitive society had its own curative agents, taboos, and practices, some more advanced than others. These practices were shared as countries warred and conquered one another, with the more effective medical practices surviving. As one might anticipate, some ancient civilizations advanced more than others, but absent from most cultures was a sound theory of disease.

Ancient Cultures

Egypt. The oldest medical records so far discovered and deciphered are those from Egypt, with one early papyrus dating back to the sixteenth century before the Christian era. Ancient Egyptians, who settled along the Nile (while other cultures were settling along the Indus, Euphrates, and Tigris rivers), developed community planning that helped to avoid public health problems, especially those related to disease transmitted through water sources. Egypt is credited with being one of the healthiest of ancient countries, perhaps because of the progress it made in the fields of hygiene and sanitation. Strict rules were developed around such things as cleanliness, food, drink, exercise, and sexual relations. The Egyptians also established a "house of death," which was located at a site away from civilization. People in the early cultures classified more than 700 drugs and developed the art of embalming. Their skill in bandaging was carried over for history to observe in the mummies. It is also believed that they were skilled in dentistry, often filling teeth with gold. The oldest known medical books came from this society. The books outlined surgical techniques and methods of birth control, described disease processes, and suggested remedies. Out of this culture came the first physician known to history, Imhotep (2900–2800 B.C.). He was recognized as a surgeon, an architect, a temple priest, a scribe, and a magician.

Babylonia. Babylonia, like Egypt, was located in an area known as the Fertile Crescent and the Cradle of Civilization. The area was so named because of its well-watered soil and warm climate, a combination that was favorable to the establishment of civilizations. The life-style of the Babylonians was entirely different from that of the Egyptians. Each city was a complete community in itself, governed by a divine ruler and a priest-king. It was believed that illness was the punishment for sinning and for displeasing the gods. A cure was brought about by purifying the body, usually by incantations and the use of herbs. Temples, in which the purification occurred, became centers of medical care.

The Babylonians were skilled mathematicians and astronomers. It is not surprising, therefore, that many of their beliefs were based on nature study and the potency of numbers, and on observations of the movement of stars and planets. Horoscopes were cast in terms of a person's birth and the position of the planets on that occasion. The Babylonians were fond of the number seven, which still holds a high place in the superstitions of various cultures. From this culture developed the famous Code of Hammurabi (Hammurabi was then the king of Babylonia) in 1900 B.C. (The principal source of this code is a stone monument found in 1901 and preserved today in the Louvre, in Paris.) The Code may represent the first sliding scale for fee payment by dividing the public into three classes. Those classified as "gentlemen" might expect to pay their surgeons in silver coins rather than in goods or services. A surgeon who bungled an operation on a "gentleman" carried heavy obligations, since the surgeon might have his hands cut off if the surgery went poorly. This makes the malpractice rates absorbed by physicians today seem more palatable.

Palestine. The Hebrews made their home in the area called Palestine, adjacent to Egypt. Primarily an agricultural society, the country was ruled by kings. The Hebrews are credited with more democratic sharing of knowledge than any of the other ancient civilizations. Through the leadership of Moses, the adopted son of the Egyptian pharaoh's daughter, the Hebrews developed the Mosaic Code, which represented an organized method of disease prevention. The Code emphasized isolation of persons with communicable diseases and differentiated clean from unclean. Bible scriptures such as Leviticus 7:16-19 and 19:5-8, which forbade that meat be eaten past the third day after the animal was slaughtered, were no doubt written because of the warm climate and the lack of refrigeration. The Hebrew culture recognized one God who had all power over life and death. From this belief evolved the role of the priest as supervisor of medical practices relating to cleansing and purification. Priest-physicians took on the function of health inspectors.

India. Located in the southern part of the Far East, India was essentially isolated by mountains from other parts of the world. The earliest cultures of India were Hindu. Sources of information about health practices come from the *Vedas*, the sacred book of the Hindus dating back as far as 1200 B.C. Medicine, as described in these books, apparently included major and minor surgery, children's diseases, and diseases of the nervous and urinary systems. Their surgery may have been the most highly developed of any ancient culture. Later Buddhism was to replace Hinduism as the major religion of early India. During the Buddhist period, India is credited with an advanced understanding of disease prevention, hygiene and sanitation, medicine, and surgery. The importance of prenatal care to both mother and baby seemed well understood and practiced. In disregarding the caste system of the Hindus, Buddhism made education and the right to peace possible for everyone. Public hospitals were constructed during this time, and some vital statistics were collected. The early hospitals were staffed with nurses whose qualifications were similar to those expected of today's practical nurse, except that the Indian nurses were all men. When Buddhism fell, the hospitals were abolished.

China. The ancient Chinese followed the teachings of Confucius, who sought to relieve the country's oppression by reviving ancient customs. Patriarchal rule dominated, and emphasis was placed on the value of the family as a unit. Ancestor worship attained great importance. Woman's role was seen as being vastly inferior to man's, her major value being determined by the number of sons she could produce. Early Chinese established the philosophy of the yang and the yin. The *yang* represented the active, positive, masculine force of the universe, and the *yin* represented the passive, negative, feminine force. These two forces were always contrasted with and complementary to each other. Health practices focused on prevention and good health resulted from a balance between the *yang* and the *yin*.

The Chinese also developed acupuncture skills that are still being practiced today. No faith was placed in the patient's history as a diagnostic tool, and diagnosis was made on the basis of a complicated pulse theory. The Chinese had elaborate *materia medica*, and many of the drugs they used, such as ephedrine, are used in modern medicine.

Greece. The ancient Greek culture is remembered in part for its worship of gods and goddesses, and for the emphasis that was placed on healthy bodies. (Remember that the Greeks started the Olympic games.) In Greek mythology, Asklepios, son of Apollo, was the chief healer. He is usually represented as carrying a staff, to show that he traveled from place to place, around which is entwined a serpent, representing wisdom and immortality. (Some persons believe that when the army medical services fashioned the caduceus, the symbol of the medical profession, the staff and serpent that were incorporated into the symbol came from this legendry.)

Exquisite temples, located on beautiful sites, were built as shrines to Asklepios and became social and intellectual centers as well as places to obtain cures. The curative process usually began with animal sacrifice and continued through various purifying processes. It is rather surprising that from this Greek society, so heavily steeped in mythology, animal sacrifice, and faith in the power of the gods, was to come the Father of Medicine. Hippocrates was born about 400 B.C. on the island of Cos. He stressed a natural cause for disease, treated the whole patient in a patient-centered approach to care, and introduced the scientific method of solving patient problems. He also taught the necessity of accurate observations and careful record keeping. Hippocrates did not attribute ill health to an infliction by the gods, but rather believed that health depended on equilibrium existing between mind and body, and the environment. From this evolved the humoral theory of disease, which has lasted for centuries.

His early writings speak to almost all branches of medicine. Many early physicians were also from Greece, although they often practiced their skills in Rome after Greece was conquered by the Roman Empire. Galen, Asklepiades, and Pedanim Dioscorides were all Greek physicians who worked in Rome.

Rome. The medical advancements of the ancient Romans fell short of those of the Greeks. Medical practices were often borrowed from the countries the Romans conquered and the physicians from those countries were made slaves who provided medical services to the Romans. The Romans clung to gods, superstition, and herbs when faced with disease, although hygiene and sanitation were fairly well developed. Many homes were equipped with baths, and cleanliness was valued. The role of women was considerably different from that in other ancient cultures. Women were allowed to hold property, appear in public, and campaign publicly for causes they felt should be advanced, and they could entertain guests and sit with them at the table.

Although the ancient cultures developed medicine as a science and profession, they showed little evidence of establishing a foundation for nursing. With the possible exceptions of the male attendants of the early Buddhist culture in India and the midwives, who had an established role in several cultures, nursing, as we think of it, did not exist. It was not until the early Christian period that nursing was to take root.

The Religious Image of the Nurse

The first continuity in the history of nursing began with Christianity. Christ's teachings admonished people to love and care for their neighbors. With the establishment of churches in the Christian era, groups were organized as orders whose primary concern was to care for the sick, the poor, orphans, widows, the aged, slaves, and prisoners, all done in the name of charity and Christian love. Christ's precepts placed women and men on a parity, and the early church made both men and women deacons, with equal rank. Unmarried women had opportunities for service that were never imagined earlier.

Of particular significance in the history of nursing are the deaconesses in the Eastern churches. These women, who were required to be unmarried or widowed but once, were often widows or daughters of Roman officials, and thus had breeding, culture, wealth, and position. These dedicated young women practiced *works of mercy* that included feeding the hungry, clothing the naked, visiting the imprisoned, sheltering the homeless, caring for the sick, and burying the dead. The deaconesses were the early counterparts to the community health nurses of today. When they entered homes to distribute food and medicine, they carried a basket, which would later become the visiting nurse bag of today. No discussion of nursing history would be complete without mentioning Phoebe, who is often referred to as the first deaconess and the visiting nurse. She carried Paul's letters and cared for him and many others. In the Epistle to the Romans, dated about A.D. 58, reference is made to Phoebe and to her work.

Not clearly distinguished from the deaconesses were the widows and the virgins. The members of the *Order of Widows* had not necessarily been married. It seems that the title was used to designate respect for age. If married, a member was required to be widowed only once, and vows were taken never to remarry. The *Order of Virgins* emphasized virginity as essential to purity of life, and Virgins ranked equal to the clergy. These three groups — deaconesses, widows, and virgins — shared many common characteristics and carried out similar responsibilities. Because these women often visited the sick in their homes, they are sometimes recognized as the earliest organized group of public health nurses. The movement peaked in Constantinople about A.D. 400, when a staff of 40 deaconesses lived and worked under the direction of Olympia, a powerful and deeply religious deaconess. The influence of the deaconess order diminished in the fifth and sixth centuries, when church decrees removed clerical duties and rank from the deaconess.

Although the position of deaconess originated in the Eastern Church, it spread west to Gaul and Ireland. In Rome women who served in comparable positions were known as *matrons*. Active during the fourth and fifth centuries, these women held independent positions and had great wealth, which they contributed to charity and to nursing. Among these Christian converts were three women who contributed significantly to nursing.

St. Marcella

St. Marcella established the first monastery for women in her own beautiful and palatial home, which became a center for Christian study and teaching. It was here that St. Jerome worked on translations of the Bible while teaching Christian principles. Marcella herself was regarded as an authority on difficult scriptural passages. Her home was later invaded by warriors who expected to find valuables stored there. When they found little more than a bare building, they whipped Marcella, hoping that she would reveal the hiding places of riches. After the assault she is said to have fled to a nearby church, where she died.

Fabiola

Fabiola is said to have studied at Marcella's home. She was reputably a beautiful woman from a great and wealthy Roman family; however, she was unhappy in her first marriage and so divorced her husband and remarried. She converted to Christianity and, after the death of her second husband, began her career of charity. On becoming a Christian, Fabiola realized that her new beliefs made marriage after divorce a sin. She publicly acknowledged this, committed her life to charitable work, and in A.D. 380 built the first public hospital in Rome. Here she cared for the sick and poor that she gathered from the streets and highways, personally washing and treating wounds and sores that repulsed others. St. Jerome tells of some of her work and her attributes in his writings. She died about 399, and scores of Romans are said to have attended her funeral to show their respect for her.

St. Paula

St. Paula was also a scholar of Marcella. Widowed, learned, and wealthy, she is said to have assisted St. Jerome in the translation of the writings of the prophets. St. Paula traveled to Palestine and devoted a fortune to the establishment of hospitals and inns for pilgrims traveling to Jerusalem. In Bethlehem she organized a monastery, built hospitals for the sick, and developed hospices for pilgrims, where tired travelers and the ill were cared for. Some credit her with being the first to teach nursing as an art rather than as a service.

The Role of the Monastic Orders

Also developing during this time were the monastic orders. Through them young men and women were able to follow careers of their choice while living a Christian life. One of the earliest organizations for men in nursing, the *Parabolani* brotherhood, was established at this time. Responding to needs created by the Black Plague, this group reportedly organized a hospital and traveled throughout Rome caring for the sick. The order of Benedictines, which still exists, was founded during this period. Such famous monastic nurses as St. Brigid, St. Scholastica (a twin sister of St. Benedict), and St. Hilda were founding schools, tending to the sick, and giving to the poor. The monasteries played a large role in the preservation of culture and learning as well as in offering refuge to the persecuted, care to the sick, and education to the uneducated. The learning of the classical period would have been lost when the empire fell were it not for the monks and monasteries. During this period (approximately A.D. 50 to 800) the first hospitals also were established. These hospitals, located outside the monastery walls, are still standing. There were more than 700 hospitals in England by the middle of the sixteenth century. The Hotel Dieu in Lyons was established in 542 and the Hotel Dieu in Paris, around 650. The Hotel Dieu in Paris was staffed by the first order specifically devoted to nursing, the Augustinian Sisters. The Santo Spirito Hospital in Rome, the largest medieval hospital, was established by papal order in 717.

The Crusades, which swept northern Europe, were to last for almost 200 years (1096–1291). The deaconess movement, suppressed by the Western churches, became all but extinct. Military nursing orders evolved as a result of the Crusades. The Knights Hospitallers of St. John was one such order. It was organized to staff two hospitals that were located in Jerusalem. The knights, organized as a nursing order, at times were required to defend the hospital and its patients. For this reason they wore a suit of armor under their habits. On the habit was the Maltese cross. The same cross was to be used later on a badge designed for the Nightingale School. The badge became the forerunner of the nursing pin as we know it today. The symbolism of the pin dates back to the sixteenth century, when the privilege of wearing a coat of arms was limited to noblemen who served their kings with distinction. As centuries passed the privilege was extended to schools and to craft guilds, and the symbols of wisdom, strength, courage, and faith appeared on buttons, badges, and shields. The pins of many schools of nursing are fashioned after a cross of some kind.

Secular orders of nurses also came into existence at this time in history. Operating much like the monastic orders, members of this group could terminate their vocations at any time and were not bound to the vows of monastic life. Examples of the secular orders include the Order of Antonines (1095); the Beguines of Flanders, Belgium (1184); the Misericordia (1244); and the Alexian Brothers, founded during the bubonic plague epidemic of 1348. The only nursing education offered to these dedicated people was in the form of an apprenticeship; a new-comer to the organization would be assigned to a more experienced person and would learn from that person.

The inquiring student is encouraged to seek greater depth of knowledge about the orders, their purposes and goals, and the lives of those who devoted their energies to the care of the sick and the poor by consulting the nursing references given at the end of this chapter.

The Servant Image of the Nurse

The Middle Ages were followed by the Renaissance (occurring from the fourteenth through the sixteenth centuries) and the Reformation. During the Renaissance, also known as the Age of Discovery, a new impetus was given to education, but not to medical education, which was still caught up in the humoral theory of disease, or to nursing education, which was all but nonexistent.

The Reformation, a religious movement that started with the work of Martin Luther, began in Germany in 1517. It resulted in a revolt against the supremacy of the pope and the formation of Protestant churches across Europe. Monasteries were closed, religious orders were dissolved, and the work of women in these orders became almost extinct.

Also associated with the Reformation was a change in the role of women. The Protestant Church, which stood for freedom of religion and thought, did not allow much freedom for women. Once revered by the church and encouraged toward charitable activities, women of the Reformation were deemed subordinate to men. Their role was within the confines of the home; their duties were those of bearing children and caring for the home. Work in hospitals no longer appealed to women of high birth. Hospital care was relegated to "uncommon" women, a group comprising prisoners, prostitutes, and drunks.

Women faced with earning their own living were forced to work as domestic servants and although nursing was considered a domestic service, it was not a desirable one. Pay was poor; the hours were long; the work was strenuous. The nurse was considered the most menial of servants. Thus developed what may be called the "Dark Ages of Nursing."

The image of nurses and nursing during this time was described by Charles Dickens through the characters of Sairey Gamp and Betsy Prig in his book *Martin Chuzzlewit*.

> She was a fat old woman, this Mrs. Gamp, with a husky voice and a moist eye, which she had a remarkable power of turning up, and only showing the

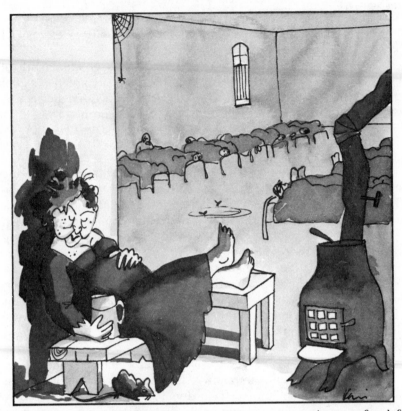

Figure 1–3. From the Middle Ages to the 19th century, nursing was often left to "uncommon women."

white of it. Having very little neck, it cost her some trouble to look over herself, if one may say so, at those to whom she talked. She wore a very rusty black gown, rather the worse for snuff, and a shawl and bonnet to correspond. . . . The face of Mrs. Gamp—the nose in particular—was somewhat red and swollen, and it was difficult to enjoy her society without becoming conscious of a smell of spirits. Like most persons who have attained to great eminence in their profession, she took to hers very kindly; insomuch, that setting aside her natural predilections as a woman, she went to a lying-in or a laying-out with equal zest and relish.[15]

Mrs. Prig was of the Gamp build, but not so fat; and her voice was deeper and more like a man's. She had also a beard.[16]

The sixteenth and seventeenth centuries found Europe devastated by famine, plague, filth, and horror. In England, for example, King Henry VIII had effectively eliminated organized monastic relief provided to orphans and other displaced persons. Throughout Europe vagrancy and begging abounded, and those caught begging were often severely punished by being branded, beaten, or chained to galleys of boats, where they served as oarsmen. Knowledge of hygiene was insufficient; the poor suffered the most. Social reform was inevitable. Several nursing groups were organized. These groups gave money, time, and service to the sick and the poor, visiting them in their homes and ministering to their needs. Such groups include the Order of the Visitation of Mary, St. Vincent de Paul, and, in 1633, the Sisters of Charity. The last group became an outstanding secular nursing order. They developed an educational program for the intelligent young women they recruited that included experience in a hospital as well as visiting in the homes. Receiving help, counsel, and encouragement from St. Vincent de Paul, the Sisters expanded their services to include caring for abandoned children. In 1640 St. Vincent established the Hospital for Foundlings.

The Beginning of Change

Countries remaining Catholic escaped some of the disorganization caused by the Reformation. During the 1500s the Spanish and the Portuguese began traveling to the New World. In 1521 Cortes conquered the capital of the Aztec civilization in Mexico and renamed that capital Mexico City. Early colonists to the area included members of Catholic religious orders, who became the doctors, nurses, and teachers of the new land. In 1524 the first hospital on the American continent, the Hospital of Immaculate Conception, was built in Mexico City. Mission colleges were founded. The first medical school in America was founded in 1578 at the University of Mexico.

Farther north Jacques Cartier sailed up the St. Lawrence River in 1535 and established French settlements in Nova Scotia. In 1639 three Augustinian Sisters arrived in Quebec to staff the Hotel Dieu. Jeanne Mance, who had been educated at an Ursuline Convent, arrived in Montreal in 1641 to care for the Iroquois Indians and the colonists. The Ursuline Sisters of Quebec are credited with attempting to organize the first training for nurses on this continent. They taught the Indian women of the area to care for their sick.

The first hospital founded in what was to become the United States was started in Philadelphia, at the urging of Benjamin Franklin, in 1751. Franklin believed that the public had a duty to provide care to the poor, friendless, sick, and insane. A bill was passed that year authorizing the establishment of the Pennsylvania Hospital.[17]

In Europe outstanding men of medicine began to make vital and valuable contributions to medical knowledge. William Harvey (1578–1657), who became known as the Father of Modern Medicine, theorized first about circulation of the blood. Anton van Leeuwenhoek

(1632–1723) used a microscope to delineate bacteria and protozoa. Later Rene Laennec (1781–1826) described the pathology of tuberculosis; Ignatz Semmelweis (1818–1865) explained the relationship between handwashing, or the lack of it, and puerperal fever; Louis Pasteur (1822–1895) discovered anaerobic bacteria and the process of pasteurization; and Joseph Lister (1827–1912) developed aseptic technique.

Among lay persons influencing social change during this time was a young minister in Kaiserwerth, Germany, Theodore Fliedner (1800–1864). With the assistance of his first wife, Friederike, Fliedner revived the deaconess movement by establishing a training institute for deaconesses at Kaiserwerth in 1836. During a fund-raising tour through Holland and England, Pastor Fliedner met Mrs. Elizabeth Fry of England, who had brought about reform at Newgate Prison in England. Greatly impressed with Mrs. Fry's accomplishments, the Fliedners followed her example and first worked with women prisoners in Kaiserwerth. Later they opened a small hospital for the sick, and Gertrude Reichardt, the daughter of a physician, was recruited as their first deaconess. The endeavors at Kaiserwerth included care of the sick, visitations and parochial work, and teaching. A course in nursing was developed that included lectures by physicians. No small part was played by Friederike, who helped bring Theodore's visionary plans to fruition and who was herself much dedicated to the deaconess movement. While away from home promoting deaconess activities, she learned that one of her children had died. A second child died shortly after her return, and she herself died in 1842, after the birth of a premature infant. Pastor Fliedner was also assisted in his work by his second wife, Caroline Bertheau, who had had some nursing experience before her marriage. In 1849 Pastor Fliedner journeyed to the United States, where he helped to establish the first Motherhouse of Kaiserwerth Deaconesses in Pittsburgh, Pennsylvania.

In England, at about the same time, Elizabeth Fry (1780–1845) organized the Institute of Nursing Sisters, often called the Fry Sisters, a secular group. To follow were the Sisters of Mercy, a Roman Catholic group formed by Catherine McAuley (1787–1841), and another Catholic group called the Irish Sisters of Charity, formed by Mary Aikenhead (1787–1858).

THE NIGHTINGALE INFLUENCE

The three images discussed above all influenced the development of nursing, but in the latter half of the eighteenth century one woman changed the form and direction of nursing and succeeded in establishing it as a respected field of endeavor. This outstanding woman was Florence Nightingale.

Born May 12, 1820, the second daughter of a wealthy family, she was named after the city in which she was born, Florence, Italy. Because of her family's high social and economic standing, she was cultured, well traveled, and educated. Through the influential people she met, she was expected to select a desirable mate, marry, and take her place in society. Florence Nightingale had other ideas. She wanted to become a nurse. To her family this was unthinkable. She continued to travel with her family and their friends. In her travels she met Mr. and Mrs. Sidney Herbert, who were becoming interested in hospital reform. Miss Nightingale began collecting information on public health and hospitals and soon became recognized as an important authority on the subject.

Through friends she learned about Pastor Fliedner's institute at Kaiserwerth. Because it was a religious institution under the auspices of the church, she could go there, although she could not go to English hospitals. In 1851 she spent 3 months studying at Kaiserwerth.

In 1853 she started working with a committee that supervised an "Establishment for Gentlewomen During Illness." She eventually was appointed superintendent of the establishment. As her knowledge of hospitals and nursing reform grew, she was consulted by both reformers and physicians who were beginning to see the need for "trained" nurses. Still her family objected to her activities.

When the Crimean War broke out, war correspondents wrote about the abominable manner in which the sick and wounded soldiers were cared for by the British Army. Florence Nightingale, by then a recognized authority on hospitals and care, wrote to her friend Sir Sidney Herbert, who was then secretary of war, and offered to take a group of nurses to Crimea. At the same time he had written a letter requesting her assistance in resolving this national crisis. Their letters crossed in the mail. Her achievements in Crimea were so outstanding, although they seriously affected her own health, that she was later recognized in 1907 by the Queen of England, who awarded her the Order of Merit.

In 1856 she returned to England, her health broken. Much has been written of her "illness," many suggesting it was, to a large degree, a neurosis. She retreated to her bedroom, and for the next 43 years conducted her business from her secluded apartment.

Throughout her lifetime Florence Nightingale wrote extensively about hospitals, sanitation, health and health statistics, and especially about nursing and nursing education. She crusaded for and brought about great reform in nursing education.

In 1860 she devoted her efforts to the creation of a school of nursing that was financed by the Nightingale Fund. Among the basic principles on which Miss Nightingale established her school were the following:

- The nurses should be trained in teaching hospitals associated with medical schools and organized for that purpose.
- The nurses would be carefully selected and should reside in nurses' houses that would be fit to form discipline and character.
- The school matron would have final authority over the curriculum, living, and all other aspects of the school.
- The curriculum would include both theoretical material and practical experience.
- Teachers would be paid for their instruction.
- Records would be kept on the students, who would be required to attend lectures, take quizzes, write papers, and keep diaries.

In many other ways Florence Nightingale advanced nursing as a profession. She believed that nurses should spend their time caring for patients, not cleaning; that nurses must continue learning throughout their lifetime and not become "stagnant"; that nurses should be intelligent and should use that intelligence to improve conditions for the patient; and that nursing leaders should have social standing. She had a vision of what nursing could and should be.

Florence Nightingale died in her sleep at the age of 90. The week of her birth is now honored as National Hospital Week. The enthusiastic student is encouraged to learn more about this fascinating lady in Cecil Woodham–Smith's book *Florence Nightingale*.

After the establishment of the Nightingale School in England, nursing programs flourished, and the Nightingale system spread to other countries, including the United States. It was extended to America in 1849 when Pastor Fliedner arrived in Pittsburgh with four deaconesses. They assumed responsibility for the Pittsburgh Infirmary, which was the first Protestant hospital in the United States. The hospital is now called Passavant Hospital. Since that time, nursing education has grown in the United States.

The Civil War broke out in the United States in 1861. Although social reform was on its way, nursing was still in an embryonic, unorganized stage. Responding to the nursing needs created by the war, women volunteered to help, and after a brief training course, they performed nursing duties. Dorothea Dix, already well known for her concern for the mentally ill, was appointed superintendent of women nurses for the

Union army. Clara Barton, who served as a volunteer with the 6th Massachusetts Regiment, later founded the American Red Cross. Black nurses, such as Harriet Tubman and Susie Taylor, carried out nursing duties for the Union army while supporting antislavery activities for the blacks. Mary Ann (Mother) Bickerdyke challenged the work of lazy, corrupt medical officers. Jane Stuart Woolsey and her sisters Georgeanna and Abby championed for standards of selection and training for nurses of the Union nurse corps. The Woolseys continued their efforts to establish sound nurse training schools after the Civil War. Students who want to learn more about the nurses of the Civil War should explore the writings of Walt Whitman, who was a nurse during this time, and Louisa May Alcott. Both wrote poignantly about nursing and war conditions of this period.

EARLY SCHOOLS IN AMERICA

The popularity of Florence Nightingale in England and the conditions exposed during the Civil War provided the impetus necessary to heighten the interest in nursing education in the United States. In 1869 the American Medical Association established a committee to study the issue. The New England Hospital for Women and Children established a one-year program to train nurses in 1872, and by 1873 three additional schools were opened: the Bellevue Training School in New York City, the Connecticut Training School, and the Boston Training School. The evolution of nursing education in the United States is fully discussed in Chapter 2.

THE IMAGE OF NURSING TODAY

During the late 1970s and early 1980s a great deal of time and energy was invested in studying the image of nursing. Much of this work was done by Beatrice and Phillip Kalisch, who have written prolifically about the topic. Much of their writing deals with segments of an overall study of the image of the nurse in various forms of the mass media, including radio, movies, television, newspapers, magazines, and novels. Kalisch and Kalisch believe that popular attitudes and assumptions about nurses and what nurses contribute to a patient's welfare can influence the future of nursing to a large extent. It is their contention that since the 1970s, the popular image of the nurse has not only failed to reflect changing professional conditions, but also assumed derogatory traits that have undermined public confidence in and respect for the professional nurse. Nurses should be concerned about negative or incorrect images because such images can influence the attitudes of patients, policymakers, and politicians. Negative attitudes about nursing may also turn away many capable prospective nurses, who will choose another career that offers greater appeal in stature, status, and salary.

In studying nurses on television (the single most important source of information in the country), Kalisch and Kalisch found that nurses often had no substantive role in the television stories. Often the nurse was part of the hospital background scenery for the physician characters, whose careers were viewed as more important and who scored high on such attributes as ambition, intelligence, rationality, aggression, self-confidence, and altruism. When nurses were singled out, most of the

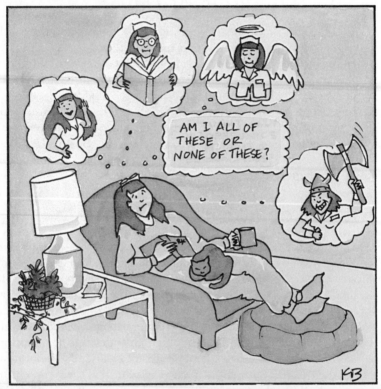

Figure 1–4. Nurses should be concerned about negative or incorrect images because these are sure to influence the attitudes of patients, policy-makers, and politicians.

attention was directed toward solving the nurse's personal problems, as opposed to portraying her role as a nurse. The nurse frequently was portrayed as the "handmaiden" to the physician and scored high on such attributes as obedience, permissiveness, conformity, flexibility, and serenity. It is interesting to note that nurses ranked lower than physicians on such items as humanism, self-sacrifice, duty, and family concern, all of which are values traditionally ascribed to nurses.[18]

Kalisch and Kalisch found a rise and fall in the image of nurses in motion pictures, with the high point occurring during the war years of the 1940s and the low point occurring in the 1970s, when the nursing profession was denigrated and satirized in many films. This latter fact will have an impact on the attitudes of prospective nurses because the largest proportion of moviegoers each year are adolescents. The earlier, positive images of nurses usually came from films that were biographies of outstanding nurses such as Sister Kenny, who worked with polio patients, or Edith Cavell, a World War I heroine who was shot by the Germans for helping Allied soldiers escape from occupied Belgium. For a time the nurse-detective was a popular theme in films; such nurses were portrayed as being intelligent, perceptive, confident, sophisticated, composed, tough, and assertive. During the 1970s, however, nurses in films often were portrayed as being malevolent and sadistic (*e.g.*, the roles of Nurse Ratched in *One Flew Over the Cuckoo's Nest* and Nurse Diesel in *High Anxiety*). This was the lowest point in the history of films for the nurse figure with regard to such values as duty, self-sacrifice, achievement, integrity, virtue, intelligence, rationality, and kindness. Few films centered on the individual achievement or personal autonomy of the nurse. When compared with the physician's role, nursing was seen as less important.[19]

In studying the image of nursing in novels, Kalisch and Kalisch analyzed 207 books. As was true of the review of films and television, they found that the nurse in the novel was almost always female, usually single, childless, white, and under the age of 35.

Because nurses almost always have been depicted in novels as women, emphasis has also been on traditional female roles (*i.e.*, wife, mistress, mother). Three nurse stereotypes have resulted: (1) the nurse as man's companion, (2) the nurse as man's destroyer, and (3) the nurse as man's mother or the mother of his children. The man of the novel was often a physician. Novelists of the 1970s and 1980s have, as was seen in movies, often maligned their nurse characters, ignoring the nurses' professional motivations and health care perspectives.[20]

Muff has analyzed feminine myths and stereotypes and has elaborated on nursing stereotypes. In looking at books about nurses written for school-age children (*e.g.*, Cherry Ames, Sue Barton, Kathy Martin, and Penny Scott) she has made the following conclusions. Nursing is described as glamorous; medicine and nursing are imbued with a sense of mystery and elitism; nursing is simplistic; nurses move from job to job; and nurses are subservient and deferential, following orders, running errands, and idolizing the physicians for whom they work. All of the nurses in these books were educated in hospital-based diploma programs in which the hard-earned "R.N." was finally won after hours of hospital service, although the Martin and Scott series were both written in the 1960s.[21]

Muff has also examined the role of the nurse as it is captured in the romance novel. In many instances appearances (*e.g.*, color and condition of the hair) were most important, and the nurse was portrayed as a "pure" girl, dressed in white, whose main aim was to get a man, usually the doctor. Those women who were not looking for husbands were in nursing for altruistic reasons, and duty and self-sacrifice were glamorized. Muff also found that the image of the nurse as found in the novel generally could be classified into one of the following categories: ministering angels, handmaidens, battle-axes, fools, and whores. She also stated that the stereotypes of nursing presented by television and films usually would fit one of these categories. When reviewing the nurse image on get-well cards, she had to add a new category, that of "token torturer."[22]

Only newspapers and news magazines tended toward realism rather than fantasy. News articles tended to cover information about the nursing shortage, including some reasons for it, for example, working conditions, salaries, benefits, and hardships. Articles also provided information about new nursing roles, or special features, such as nurses in Viet Nam.[23]

Although some might argue that nursing has better things to do than worry about how the nurse is revealed in the media, a consistently misrepresented image can negatively affect the way the public thinks about nurses. Misrepresentation of nursing may be responsible, to some degree, for the nationwide decline of applicants to nursing programs during the late 1970s and early 1980s. This decline will have an effect on the nation's health care industry, and therefore nurses have begun measures to help correct their image in the public's eye. In 1981 the National League for Nursing (NLN) prepared a videotape, titled "Nursing: A Career for All Reasons," that attempted to attract and recruit ambitious and intelligent men and women into nursing. The NLN also formed the Task Force on Nursing's Public Image in 1982. Nurses are organizing as groups to make their force felt politically.

Individual nurses are responding to television advertisements or programs that portray nurses and nursing in a negative light with letters and telephone calls. In instances where a product was involved, a boycott on the purchase of that item has proved to be a fairly effective way to bring about a change.

STUDIES FOR AND ABOUT NURSING

As schools of nursing grew in number, the quality of many of the schools and their graduates often suffered, and many of Florence Nightingale's admonitions regarding nursing education were forgotten. Nurses, doctors, friends, and critics of nursing became concerned about the inadequate preparation being offered. Before the problem could be corrected, it was necessary to learn more about the programs, how nurses were being used in the employment market, and the problems that resulted. To accomplish this, studies about nursing and nurses were initiated.

Although we recognize that many students in nursing are not turned on by studies, especially those conducted years ago, the development of nursing as a profession has been affected by them, and it seems important that a few of the significant studies be discussed. Although the first studies were not begun until the early 1900s, the number of studies since the 1950s is voluminous. It is impossible to pick up any professional publication and not find mention of some new study in progress. In an effort to classify and catalog references to these studies, Virginia Henderson has prepared *A Nursing Studies Index*. In 1952 a group of nurses, under the sponsorship of the Association of Collegiate Schools of Nursing, launched a new journal called *Nursing Research*, which was designed to disseminate information about nursing research.

Early Studies

One of the earliest studies was carried out under the guidance of M. Adelaide Nutting in 1912. It was published by the U.S. Bureau of Education and was titled *The Educational Status of Nursing*. The study investigated what and how students were being taught at the time and under what conditions students were living. Although it did not receive the attention it probably deserved, it began to establish nursing as a profession and led the way to later studies.

The Winslow–Goldmark Report, sometimes simply called the Goldmark Report, was to follow in 1923. This was also referred to as *The Study of Nursing and Nursing Education in the United States*.[24] The report focused on the preparation of public health nurses, teachers, administrators, clinical learning experiences of students, and the financing of schools. Subsequently, the Yale University School of Nursing was established.

A three-part study, sponsored by the Committee on the Grading of Nursing Schools, followed in the years 1928 to 1934. The first part, which was socioeconomic in nature and titled "Nurses, Patients, and Pocketbooks," attempted to determine if there was a shortage of nurses in the United States; the second part, an "Activity Analysis of Nursing," looked at nurses' activities that could be used as a basis for improving the curricula in nursing schools; part three, "Nursing Schools Today and Tomorrow," described the schools of the period and made recommendations for professional schools.

The last of the early studies that we will mention was not really a study but often is referred to as one because of its far-reaching effects. *A Curriculum Guide for Schools of Nursing*, published in 1937, was a revised version of earlier publications. It outlined the curricula for a 3-year course, emphasizing sound educational teaching procedures. It was read and followed by many schools that were operating programs at that time.

Midcentury Studies

By the 1950s studies about nurses and nursing were numerous and dealt with many aspects of the profession. Only a few of those studies will be mentioned here.

Of particular significance was a study published in 1948 titled *Nursing for the Future*. Conducted by Esther Lucille Brown, the study is also known as the Brown report. Funded by the Carnegie Foundation, the study was done to determine society's need for nursing, and recommendations were made for higher education for nurses. It prompted serious examination of professional education and pointed out weaknesses in the existing educational programs. The investigators recommended that basic schools of nursing be placed in universities and colleges, and encouraged the recruitment of large numbers of men and members of minority groups into nursing schools. This report set the stage for studies of nursing education that followed in the 1950s and 1960s.

The Ginzberg report was published the same year. This study reviewed problems centering around the current and prospective shortage of nurses. The conclusions and recommendations were published in a book entitled *A Program for the Nursing Profession*. The study recommended that nursing teams consisting of 4-year professional nurses,

2-year registered nurses, and 1-year practical nurses be developed. Some of these conclusions are not far from where we are now.

In 1958 a study entitled *Twenty Thousand Nurses Tell Their Story* was published. It was part of a 5-year research project that was conceived by the ANA and financially supported by nurses throughout the country. The report was prepared by Everett C. Hughes, a professor of sociology at the University of Chicago. The study looked at nurses, what they were doing, their attitudes toward their jobs, and their job satisfaction. As a result, nurses learned a great deal about themselves.

Another significant study was initiated by Mildred Montag in 1952. This study on *Community College Education for Nursing* resulted in the creation of associate degree education (see Chapter 2).

Significant Studies of the 1960s and 1970s

In 1961 the surgeon general of the U.S. Public Health Service appointed a 25-member panel called the Consultant Group of Nursing. This group was to advise him on nursing needs and identify the role of the federal government in assessing nursing services to the nation. In 1963 this group presented a report titled "Toward Quality in Nursing," which recommended a national investigation of nursing education that would place emphasis on the criteria for high-quality patient care.

After publication of this report, the ANA and the NLN appropriated funds and established a joint committee to study ways to conduct and finance such a national inquiry. The committee decided that there was a need to "examine not only the changing practice and educational patterns in nursing today but also the probable requirements in professional nursing over the next several decades."[25] W. Allen Wallis, president of the University of Rochester, agreed to head the study. Financing was obtained from the American Nurses Foundation, the Kellogg Foundation, the Avalon Foundation, and an anonymous benefactor. A National Commission for the Study of Nursing and Nursing Education (NCSNNE) was set up as an independent agency and functioned as a self-directing group. The commissioners, 12 in all, were chosen for their broad knowledge of nursing, for their skills in related disciplines, or for their competencies in relevant fields. It was emphasized that no commissioner should represent a particular interest group or position. In August 1967, at the first meeting of the Commission, Jerome P. Lysaught was appointed director to conduct the planning and operation of the inquiry.

The study focused on the supply and demand for nurses, nursing roles and functions, nursing education, and nursing as a career. The Commission found it necessary not only to examine these key concerns, but also to relate these issues to the social system that provides care to the public.

The final report of the Commission, entitled *An Abstract for Action*, was published in 1970. It included 58 specific recommendations and concluded with four central recommendations. It also listed three basic priorities: (1) increased research in both the practice and education of nurses, (2) enhanced educational systems and curricula based on research, and (3) increased financial support for nurses and for nursing.

The four general recommendations were as follows:

1. That the Federal Division of Nursing, the National Center for Health Services Research and Development, other governmental agencies, and private foundations appropriate grant funds or research contracts to investigate the impact of nursing practice on the quality, effectiveness, and economy of health care.

2. That the same agencies and foundations appropriate research funds and research contracts for basic and applied research into the nursing curriculum, articulation of educational systems, instructional methodologies, and facilities design so that the most functional, effective, and economic approaches are taken in the education and development of future nurses.

3. That each state have, or create, a master planning committee that will take nursing education under its purview, such committees to include representatives of nursing, education, other health professions, and the public, to recommend specific guidelines, means for implementation, and deadlines to ensure that nursing education is positioned in the mainstream of American educational patterns.

4. That federal, regional, state, and local governments adopt measures for the increased support of nursing research and education. Priority should be given to construction grants, institutional grants, advanced traineeships, and research grants and contracts. Further, we recommend that private funds and foundations support nursing research and educational innovations where such activities are not publicly aided. We believe that a useful guide for the beginnings of such a financial aid program would be in the amounts and distribution of funds authorized by Congress for fiscal 1970, with proportional increases from other public and private agencies.[26]

In 1973 a progress report from the NCSNNE concerning the status of the implementation of the recommendations of the original report was published under the title *From Abstract into Action*. The Commission believed that it was imperative that nursing achieve the goals established in the recommendations so that nursing could emerge as a full profession and in the interest of optimal health care for this country.

Studies of the 1980s

One of the major studies of nursing conducted in the 1980s was that of the National Commission on Nursing. This group was composed of a forum of 30 commissioners from disciplines such as nursing, hospital management, business, government, education, and medicine, all of whom were concerned about the current nursing-related problems in the health care system, especially the apparent shortage of nurses. The Commission was sponsored by the American Hospital Association, Hospital Research and Educational Trust, and the American Hospital Supply Corporation. Its chairman was H. Robert Cathcart. The group began its work in September of 1980 and had seven charges, which were as follows:

1. Analyze the internal and external forces that influence the environment of nurses at work.
2. Identify the effects of professional nursing issues on nursing practice in health care agencies.
3. Assess the professional characteristics of nurses in relation to the organizational structure of health care agencies.
4. Explore the motivation and incentives for nursing education and nursing practice.
5. Analyze the relationship among education, nursing practice, and professional interaction in the health care agency.
6. Develop a platform of issues to be dealt with in the commission activities.
7. Plan methods to enhance the professional status and top management role of the nurse through:
   • research to define status and role,
   • publication of information to describe or explain status and role in relation to health care, and
   • demonstration projects to provide models for problem resolution, development, and reshaping of relationships and structures in health care agencies.[27]

Moving from these charges, the Commission began systematically to examine and evaluate data sources. Journal articles, state studies, and policy documents were reviewed. A series of public hearings held in six major cities across the nation provided the opportunity for input about nursing issues from each region of the country. Two open forums also were held. After the hearings the Commission conducted an *Inventory of Innovative Programs and Projects.*

The highlights of these findings, along with the Commission's recommendations and future action plans, were published in the initial report of the group in September 1981. The final recommendations were published in 1983. Although the findings and recommendations are too lengthy to be included in this chapter in their entirety, it is important to mention the five major categories of issues identified by the study. They are as follows:

1. The status and image of nursing, which includes changes in the nursing role
2. The interface of nursing education and practice, including models for education to prepare for practice
3. The effective management of the nursing resource, including such factors as job satisfaction, recruitment, and retention
4. The relationship among nursing, medical staff, and hospital administration, including nursing's participation in decision making
5. The maturing of nursing as a self-determining profession, including defining and determining the nature and scope of practice, the role of nursing leadership, increasing decision making in nursing practice, and the need for unity in the nursing profession.[28]

A series of publications that explore the work of the National Commission on Nursing is available from the Hospital Research and Educational Trust, 840 N. Lake Drive, Chicago, Illinois. The publication *New Directions in Nursing* deals with nursing practice, credentialing, licensure, accreditation, and education.

Many of these issues are discussed in other sections of this book. A number of the issues are not new to nursing; most of them will not be completely resolved in the next decade. Thus you as a new graduate will have the opportunity to influence the outcome.

Many of the Commission's findings were no surprise to people who are involved with nursing. Included was information that indicated that physicians and health care administrators often did not understand the role of nurses in patient care and that traditional and outdated images of nurses (including Victorian stereotypes and traditional male-female relationships) impeded acceptance of current roles. Some physicians and administrators perceived nurses as being overeducated, and they did not support an increase in the nurse's authority to make decisions concerning health care.

The findings that individuals and nursing groups have not unified in defining fundamental, professional goals for nursing, and that nursing, as a profession, lacks cohesiveness and a clear understanding of its role and direction were no revelations to many seasoned nurses. Nor were these same people astonished to learn of the numerous and diverse associations that represent nursing but lack any arrangement to determine common goals for nursing education, practice, and credentialing. The disagreement and confusion about educational preparation for nurses and the controversy about entry into practice were identified as further blocks to the advancement of the profession. Clearly there is a need for a system of nursing education that promotes realistic expectations, provides appropriate support for practice and advancement, and includes educational mobility in nursing.

The National Commission on Nursing has accomplished much in terms of gathering data about nursing and identifying nursing-related issues. It is hoped that individual nurses, institutions, and nursing organizations can work together to resolve some of the problems.

Following on the footsteps of the National Commission of Nursing was the National Commission on Nursing Implementation Project, which began in 1985. Funded by the W. K. Kellogg Foundation for three years, the project was cosponsored by the NLN, the ANA, the American Organization of Nurse Executives, and the American Association of Colleges of Nursing. Administered by the American Nurses' Foundation, it had as its purpose to provide leadership in seeking consensus about the appropriate education and credentialing for basic nursing practice, effective models for the delivery of nursing care, and the means for developing and testing nursing knowledge. The focus of this project was to lay the groundwork and take action wherever possible to support effective, high-quality nursing care delivery in the immediate and long-range future.

The results of another study of nursing were released January 27, 1983. This 2-year study, mandated under the 1979 Nurse Training Amendments, was conducted by the Institute of Medicine Committee on Nursing and Nursing Education and was funded by the Department of Health and Human Services at a cost of $1.6 million. The objectives of the study were

> to offer advice on the shape of future federal support of nursing education, to identify why more nurses do not work in medically underserved areas, to find out if — and why — nurses do not stay in the profession, and to recom-

mend public and private measures for improving the supply and effective use of nursing resources.[29]

The Institute of Medicine study made 21 specific recommendations to Congress, and these will most likely influence future congressional policy and funding decisions when such decisions relate to nursing. The study found that the shortage of nurses of the 1960s and 1970s had largely disappeared and that federal support of nursing education should focus on graduate study. The first recommendation of the study was that the federal government discontinue efforts to increase the supply of "generalist nurses."

Some nurse leaders have expressed concern over the statements about the nurse shortage. They believe that current economic conditions have brought more nurses back into the work market as a primary wage earner in the family, and a decline in the demand for health services because of the inability to pay has distorted current figures. The nurse leaders are also concerned that improved economic conditions could release a pent up demand for care and once again will result in a serious shortage of nurses if the nurse supply is not maintained at a high level. The report recognized shortages that occur unevenly throughout the nation in different geographical areas and in different health care settings, especially those serving the geriatric or the economically disadvantaged patient.

It is interesting to note that in the early 1980s, two major studies of nursing were conducted: one, sponsored by the American Hospital Association, concerned the shortage of nurses and the second, conducted by the federal government, concluded that no shortage existed (if it ever had). The fact that two significant study groups could have opposing views of the supply of nurses could in itself represent an important issue in nursing.

CONCLUSION

There are two major trends that will shape the direction of nursing. Education for nursing has moved progressively into the mainstream of education in postsecondary settings and away from vocational apprenticeship-type preparation. There has been a move toward more research in nursing as a theoretical foundation for nursing education and practice.

However, after all our discussion, we return to our initial questions and restate that there are no clear-cut answers for many of the other concerns. The definition of nursing is continuing to evolve. The differences over the use of the words *profession* and *professional* continue to exist.

Nurses have been delivering health care for many years in the best way they are able without waiting for definitive answers to questions about nursing. Perhaps part of the strength of nursing is that whatever our personal philosophical concerns, we continue to see the patient, or client, as the appropriate focus for our major efforts.

REFERENCES

1. Nightingale F: Notes on Nursing: What It Is, and What It Is Not. *In* Seymer LR: Selected Writings of Florence Nightingale, p 214. New York, Macmillan, 1954
2. Gowan Sister MO: Proceedings of the Workshop on Administration of Collegiate Programs in Nursing, June 12–24, 1944, p 10. Washington, Catholic University Press of America, 1946
3. Johnson D: The nature of a science of nursing. Nurs Outlook 7:293, 1959
4. Henderson V: The Nature of Nursing, p 15. New York, Macmillan, 1966
5. American Nurses' Association's First Position on Education for Nursing. Am J Nurs 65:107, Dec 1965
6. American Nurses' Association. Nursing: A Social Policy Statement, p 9. Kansas City, MO, American Nurses' Association, 1980
7. Pavelka M: Definition of nursing practice. Issues 3:2, Summer 1982
8. Strauss A: The structure and ideology of American nursing: An interpretation. *In* Davis J (ed): The Nursing Profession, p 67. New York, John Wiley & Sons, 1966
9. Strauss A: The structure and ideology of American nursing: An interpretation. *In* Davis J (ed): The Nursing Profession, p 91. New York, John Wiley & Sons, 1966
10. Quoted in Bernhard LA, Walsh M: Leadership: The Key to the Professionalization of Nursing, p 1. New York, McGraw-Hill, 1981
11. Bixler GK, Bixler RW: The professional status of nursing. Am J Nurs 45:730, Sep 1945
12. Pavalko RM: Sociology of Occupations and Professions. Itasca, IL, Peacock Publishers, 1971
13. Labor Management Relations Act (1947), as amended by Public Laws 86–257 (1959) and 93–360 (1974), Section 2
14. Uprichard M: Ferment in nursing. *In* Auld E, Birum LH: The Challenge of Nursing, p 24. St Louis, CV Mosby, 1973
15. Dickens C: Martin Chuzzlewit. *In* The Works of Charles Dickens, Vol II, p 318. New York, Books Inc, 1936
16. Dickens C: Martin Chuzzlewit. *In* The Works of Charles Dickens, Vol II, p 417. New York, Books Inc, 1936
17. Kalisch PA, Kalisch BJ: The Advance of American Nursing, 2nd ed, p 29. Boston, Little, Brown, 1986

18. Kalisch PA, Kalisch BJ: Nurses on prime-time television. Am J Nurs 82:264, Feb 1982
19. Kalisch PA, Kalisch BJ: The image of the nurse in motion pictures. Am J Nurs 82:605, Apr 1982
20. Kalisch PA, Kalisch BJ: The image of nurses in novels. Am J Nurs 82:1220, Aug 1982
21. Muff J: Handmaiden, battle ax, whore. *In* Muff J (ed): Socialization, Sexism and Stereotyping, p 122. St Louis, CV Mosby, 1982
22. Muff J: Handmaiden, battle ax, whore. *In* Muff J (ed): Socialization, Sexism and Stereotyping, pp 126–144. St Louis, CV Mosby, 1982
23. Muff J: Handmaiden, battle ax, whore. *In* Muff J (ed): Socialization, Sexism and Stereotyping, pp 142–143. St Louis, CV Mosby, 1982
24. Winslow–Goldman Report: The Study of Nursing and Nursing Education in the United States. New York, Macmillan, 1923
25. National Commission for the Study of Nursing and Nursing Education: Summary report and recommendations. Am J Nurs 70:279, Feb 1970
26. National Commission for the Study of Nursing and Nursing Education: Summary, report and recommendations. Am J Nurs 70:285, Feb 1970
27. National Commission on Nursing: Initial Report and Preliminary Recommendations: p 1. Chicago, Hospital Research and Educational Trust, 1981
28. National Commission on Nursing: Initial Report and Preliminary Recommendations, p 5. Chicago, Hospital Research and Educational Trust, 1981
29. I.O.M. study sees need for funds in graduate, specialty areas. Am J Nurs 83:343, 344, 454, Mar 1983

FURTHER READINGS

Baker N: Nurses as news. Nursing & Health Care 3:132–133, Mar 1982
Bullough VL et al: The Emergence of Modern Nursing. New York, Macmillan, 1969
Christy T: Entry into practice: A recurring issue in nursing history. Am J Nurs 80:485–488, Mar 1980
Christy T: Equal rights for women: Voices from the past. Am J Nurs 71:288–293, Feb 1971
Christy T: First fifty years. Am J Nurs 71:1778–1784, Sep 1971
Christy T: Portrait of a leader: Lavinia Lloyd Dock. Nurs Outlook 17:72–75, Jun 1969
Christy T: Portrait of a leader: M. Adelaide Nutting. Nurs Outlook 17:20–24, Jan 1969
Christy T: Portrait of a leader: Isabel Hampton Robb. Nurs Outlook 17:26–29, Mar 1969
Christy T: Portrait of a leader: Isabel Maitland Stewart. Nurs Outlook 17:44–48, Oct 1969
Cowden P: Dissatisfaction and the changing meaning and purpose of the nurse's work. Nurs Forum 17(2):202–209, 1978

Curran CR: Shaping an image of competence and caring. Nursing & Health Care 6:371–373, Sep 1985

Dolan JA: Nursing in Society: A Historical Perspective, ed 14. Philadelphia, WB Saunders, 1978

Donahue MP: Nursing: An Illustrated History. St. Louis, CV Mosby, 1985

Fuller SS: Holistic man and the science and practice of nursing. Nurs Outlook 26:700–704, Nov 1978

Gamer M: The ideology of professionalism. Nurs Outlook 27:108–111, Feb 1979

Griffin GJ, Griffin JK: Jensen's History and Trends of Professional Nursing, ed 7. St Louis, CV Mosby, 1973

Ingles T: The physician's view of the evolving nursing profession. Nurs Forum 15(2):123–164, 1976

Kalisch BJ, Kalisch PA: The nurse-detective in American movies. Nursing & Health Care 3:146–153, Mar 1982

Kalisch BJ, Kalisch PA: Heroine out of focus: Media images of Florence Nightingale: Part I: Popular biographies and stage productions. Nursing & Health Care 4:181–187, Apr 1983

Kalisch BJ, Kalisch PA, Scobey M: Reflections on a television image. Nursing & Health Care 2:248–255, May 1981

New Directions in Nursing. Chicago, Hospital Research and Educational Trust, 1986

Parsons M: The profession in a class by itself. Nurs Outlook 34:270–275, Nov/Dec 1986

Roberts MM: American Nursing: History and Interpretation. New York, Macmillan, 1954

Schirger MJ: Introspection: A prerequisite for emancipation. Nurs Forum 17(3):317–328, 1978

Selected Writings of Florence Nightingale. Compiled by Seymer LR. New York, Macmillan, 1954

Sleeper R et al: Issues in Health Care: The Edna A. Fagan Health Care Lecture Series, pp 1–71. National League for Nursing, Publication No. 14–1599, Div of Nursing, 1976

Woodham–Smith C: Florence Nightingale. New York, McGraw-Hill, 1951

Educational Preparation for Nursing

2

Objectives

After completing this chapter, you should be able to

1. Describe the educational preparation and role of the **licensed practical nurse**.
2. Compare and contrast the three major educational avenues to becoming a **registered nurse**.
3. Explain the concept of the external degree.
4. Identify the purposes of other forms of nursing education: registered nurse baccalaureate programs, master's preparation, doctoral studies, and nondegree programs.
5. Discuss what is meant by **articulated** programs.
6. Define the **continuing education unit** and discuss the purpose of that unit.
7. Present the major points in support of mandatory continuing education and the major points in support of voluntary continuing education.

It would be less confusing if nursing, like many other professions, had one major avenue to educational preparation; however, the development of nursing as a profession has resulted in three major educational routes that prepare graduates to write the National Council Licensure Examination (NCLEX) for registered nursing. Although this circumstance has offered various alternatives and opportunities to the prospective student, it has resulted in much confusion. The health care consumer is often unable to put meaning and interpretation to the vast array of initials (*e.g.*, RN, CRN, MN, or DNS) that can now follow a nurse's name. The employer has difficulty discriminating among the different types of graduates who, at least initially, enter the hospital work environment with similar behaviors. The educator is charged with the responsibility of graduating a "safe" practitioner but lacks clear direction as to how the professional preparation provided by the various educational routes should differ in purpose, design, and structure. This situation has also provided a springboard for much discussion, debate, and, in some instances, dissension among nurses, educators, and interested lay persons regarding aspects of each program as they relate to professional nursing practice.

The three avenues preparing men and women for registered nursing are the hospital-based diploma programs, the baccalaureate programs located in four-year colleges and universities, and the two-year associate degree programs primarily found in junior and community colleges. To further cloud the issue, we are now seeing students begin their nursing education in programs that culminate in a master's degree, and one program exists in which a student can earn a doctorate before being eligible to write the state licensing examination for registered nursing.

A fourth program, that of preparing the practical nurse, is also an option to the person seeking a health career, although it is considered vocational training, and graduates write a separate licensing examination.

PRACTICAL NURSE EDUCATION

Although licensed practical nurses (LPNs), or licensed vocational nurses (LVNs) as they are titled in California and Texas, are not considered within the realm of professional nursing, it seems prudent to discuss the education and role of these health care providers. Controls on licensing of practical nurses and on the accreditation of curricula of practical nurse programs have been slower in evolving than in professional nursing, but by and large they do exist in some form today.

The practical nurse is no newcomer to the health care delivery system. In the past the practical nurse was the family friend or community citizen who was called to the home in emergencies. This person, usually self-taught, learned by experience which things were effective and which were not. She would perform basic care procedures such as bathing, and also would cook for the family and do light housekeeping duties. When many states adopted licensure laws governing the practice of practical nursing, a large number of people who had been functioning in this capacity were granted a license by waiver, thereby never really having any formal training. However, attrition brought about by time and retirement are removing most of these people from nursing practice.

The first program to offer formal preparation for practical nursing was started through the YWCA in Brooklyn, New York, around 1892. It was known as the Ballard School, after Miss Lucinda Ballard, who provided the funding to operate the school. The course of study was approximately 3 months long. The students, called "attendants," were trained to care for invalids, the elderly, and children in a home setting.

Although the YWCA may seem to many of us to be a strange place for a practical nurse program, we need to remember that in the late 1890s and early 1900s, young women traveled from their homes to large cities seeking new careers and a better life. Many of these women found inexpensive housing at YWCAs. Because most of them were untrained and had no marketable skills, the YWCA provided a natural site for a school.

Other early practical nursing programs included the Thompson School, founded in Brattleboro, Vermont, in 1907; the American Red Cross Program, begun in 1908; and the Household Nursing Association School of Attendant Nursing, begun in Boston in 1918.

During World War I and World War II the need for people who had some skills, but, more important, who could be prepared quickly, became crucial. As this need became more and more critical, the practical nurse, who until this time was primarily found in the home, moved out into the world.

In 1941 the Association of Practical Nurse Schools was founded; in 1942 membership was opened to practical nurses and the name was changed to the National Association of Practical Nurse Education (NAPNE). The first planned curriculum for practical nursing was developed in 1942, and in 1945 NAPNE established an accrediting service for schools of practical nursing. The National Federation of Licensed Practical Nurses was organized in 1949. This group, working in 1957 with the American Nurses' Association (ANA), attempted to clarify the role and function of the practical nurse, just as various groups throughout the nation have worked at delineating the roles of other nursing program graduates. The Council on Practical Nursing was established by the National League for Nursing (NLN) in 1957. In 1966 the Chicago Public School Program became the first practical nurse program to be accredited by the NLN.

The general curriculum, which is usually 1 year long, varies considerably from state to state and even from school to school. In many instances the education is weighed in clock hours instead of credit hours as used in the professional programs. Most of today's practical nurse educational programs stress clinical experiences, primarily in structured care settings such as hospitals and nursing homes. Basic therapeutic knowledge and introductory content from biological and behavioral sciences correlate with clinical practice. Usually about one third of the time is spent in the classroom and two thirds in the clinical areas.

The schools that provide practical nurse preparation vary tremendously. A program may be offered by a high school, trade or technical school, hospital, junior or community college, university, or independent agency. There has been a movement to incorporate practical nurse education and associate degree programs in the community college. All students are grouped together for "core" courses during the first academic year. At the end of this time, the student has the option of stopping the educational program and seeking licensure as a licensed practical nurse, or continuing for an additional year and seeking licensure as a registered nurse. Some students opt to do both. Graduates of these core programs in practical nursing usually possess a broader and more in-depth understanding of the biological sciences and, in some instances, the social sciences also because these are part of the core curriculum and may be college-level courses that are transferable to a 4-year institution.

Graduates of practical nurse programs take the NCLEX for practical nursing. The scope of their practice focuses on meeting the health needs of patients/clients in hospitals, long-term care facilities, and the home. LPNs or LVNs work with patients/clients whose conditions are considered stable and who are supervised by a registered nurse or a licensed physician.

Figures published by the NLN in 1986 indicate that there were just over 1,200 schools of practical and vocational nursing in the United States with 44 percent of the programs located in the South. Although the majority of programs exist in trade or technical schools (approximately 600), many are located in junior or community colleges (approximately 400), with decreasing numbers found in hospitals, high schools, military establishments, universities, and independent agencies.

DIPLOMA EDUCATION

Most registered nurses practicing today gained their basic, if not their only, nursing education in a diploma program administered by a hospital. Linda Richards generally is recognized as the first nurse graduated in the United States. In 1873 she received a diploma from the New England Hospital for Women and Children. Diploma, or hospital, schools of nursing flourished during the late 1800s and early 1900s. These training schools provided free or inexpensive staffing for the hospitals offering the educational program. Initially the education was largely apprenticeship in nature. Although some formal theory classes were conducted, learning was primarily achieved by "doing." There was no standardization of curriculum and no accreditation. Programs were developed to meet the service needs of the hospital rather than the educational needs of the students, and programs varied considerably from hospital to hospital.

The responsibility for administration of the educational program frequently was vested in the director of nursing service, who also had the role and title of director of nursing education. Many of the instructors were graduates of the program who undoubtedly possessed nursing skills but knew little of teaching-learning theories, teaching skills and techniques, curriculum design and development, or evaluation processes. In some instances the teacher was also a head nurse on one of the units in the hospital. Formal lectures often were delivered by members of the medical staff.

The curriculum generally was laid out in blocks of study that included medical nursing, surgical nursing, psychiatric nursing, obstetrics, pediatrics, operating and emergency room experience, as well as support courses in anatomy, physiology, nutrition, pharmacology, history of nursing, and often a course titled "professional adjustments." If a hospital was unable to provide certain learning opportunities, for example, psychiatric experience, students were sent on "affiliation" to a hospital where they could receive that education. Although the hospital dietitian may have been involved in teaching the nutrition course, nurses usually carried the responsibility for the remainder of the instruction, including the courses in biological sciences. The students usually were assigned to the hospital units during the early and late hours of the day (when the staffing needs were the greatest), working what were known as "split shifts." Lectures were given between 1 and 3 o'clock in the afternoon. Most days were at least 12 hours long.

Almost all the students were single young females who started the program after completing high school. They entered the school as "probies" (short for probationer) for a 6-week to 6-month probationary period. This was a testing time for both the student and the school, a time for the student to seriously look at nursing as a career and a time for the school to examine the student's aptitude for nursing. Although not exactly comparable to the experience of freshmen entering some private or Ivy League colleges, this situation had a few similarities. The probie often could be identified by dress; for example, the apron might be worn without a bib during this period. Although there was no real hazing at this time, the probie might be sent on errands that capitalized on her lack of knowledge and that might result in embarrassment later. (A typical assignment would be to send the probie to the central service area of the hospital for a supply of fallopian tubes.)

If the students survived the probationary period, they finished the remainder of the year as freshmen. They then became juniors for 1

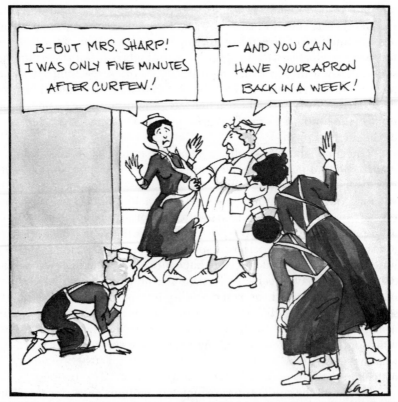

Figure 2–1. A student who had committed a minor infraction of the rules might have forfeited an article of apparel.

year, and completed the final year of the 3-year program as seniors. During the senior year the student often had the responsibility of supervising the units of the hospital, with perhaps a month spent on days, a month spent on evenings, and a month spent on the night shift. At the completion of the 3 years the students were awarded a diploma, but this was not recognized as an academic degree. Nor was academic credit given for the 3 years because legally, hospitals were not considered educational institutions.

The students were housed in dormitories that were attached to the hospital. The dorms generally had a housemother, and codes of behavior were strict and well enforced. For example, students who failed to adhere to 9:30 P.M. curfews, who were caught smoking in their rooms, or who committed other acts of indiscretion were at risk of expulsion from the school. Usually marriage was not permitted during the time the students were in training. Dress codes were rigid, and students who committed minor infractions of social behavior might lose an article of apparel (a cap or a bib) as evidence of misdemeanors.

By the late 1940s and early 1950s, many diploma schools had affiliated with nearby colleges and universities, and general education requirements such as anatomy, physiology, sociology, and psychology were offered. At this time also the National League of Nursing Education (later to become the NLN), was assuming an active role in curriculum guidance and accreditation. Programs became more educationally sound and were required to align themselves more closely with other types of postsecondary education.

Although the education described above may sound archaic by today's standards, a word must be said in defense of such programs. As a result of the many hours spent in hospital service, the students usually emerged from such programs skilled in "nursing arts" and were able to assume a position as staff or charge nurses without orientation. Although they may have shown weaknesses in knowing *why* something was done, they were certainly able to "do it." The graduate usually had a fairly good idea of her role as a nurse and was capable of functioning competently in that role, although some nurses today might not agree with that role. One often hears older nurses, hospital administrators, and physicians extol the virtues of the "good ol' days" when schools produced graduates "who could *do* something." Certainly, for more than a century, the diploma schools carried the major responsibility for producing graduates who could meet the health care needs of the nation.

Since the mid-1960s there has been a decline in enrollments in diploma schools and a decrease of about 3 percent in the number of programs each year. Graduations have decreased 26.4 percent since the early 1980s. In the fall of 1985 enrollments in diploma programs fell 19 percent—the greatest decrease ever.[2] There are several reasons for this. First and foremost is the expense. Hospitals derive funds from revenues collected from patient services, that is, the patient's hospital bill. Because hospitals are not chartered as institutions of higher education, they cannot formally charge tuition for educational programs they may offer. Therefore, the expense of operating programs of learning must be absorbed from funds collected through patient's bills. Second, the standards of education had to be met if schools were to be accredited. It became more difficult to find faculty members who were educationally qualified to be instructors. The last significant reason for the decline in diploma schools is the result of nursing education studies conducted throughout the nation that emphasized the need to provide nursing education in institutions of higher education; encouraged recruitment of large numbers of men, women, and minorities; and identified the need for nurses prepared with both 4-year and 2-year degrees (see Chapter 1). Gaining impetus from these studies, the ANA Committee on Education developed *The American Nurses' Association's First Position on Education for Nursing.* One of the stands the ANA took stated that the education for all who are licensed to practice nursing should occur in institutions of higher education (see Chapter 3). Given these explanations, it can be anticipated that the decline in the number of diploma schools and graduations will continue.

Most diploma schools in operation today have sound educational programs that meet the criteria necessary for accreditation, qualified faculty, and clinical learning experiences that meet the student's learning needs rather than hospital's service needs. Many have phased into associate degree or baccalaureate programs through affiliation with local colleges and universities, and a degree is awarded by the cooperating college or university at the completion of the studies.

Graduates of today's diploma programs have been provided a foundation of study in the biological and social sciences and may have some courses in the humanities. There is a strong emphasis in diploma programs on patient/client experiences, and the course of study also includes experience in nursing management (*i.e.*, being in charge of a nursing unit). Graduates work in acute, long-term, and ambulatory health care facilities.

ASSOCIATE DEGREE EDUCATION

The movement for associate degree education began in 1952. It has the distinction of being the first and, to date, the only type of nursing education established on the basis of planned research and experimentation. Three events undoubtedly influenced its beginning. First, it followed in the wake of the community college movement across the United States, which saw the organization and growth of 2-year community colleges that offered not only the first 2 years of a traditional 4-year college program, but also brought to the community many vocational and adult education programs. The goal of the community college was to make some form of college education available to all who would desire it. Second, the cadet nurse program was created during World War II and demonstrated that qualified students could be adequately educated in less than the traditional 3 years. Lastly, the development of associate degree education was influenced by the studies conducted about nursing education in the United States, as discussed earlier in this chapter.

Associate degree education, which had its birth in the Cooperative Research Project in Junior and Community College Education for Nursing, began at Teachers College, Columbia University and was directed by Mildred Montag. The original project included seven junior and community colleges and one hospital school, located in six regions of the United States. This type of nursing education has expanded from only 2 schools in 1952 to 778 programs in 1987, which produced more than 45,000 graduates.[3]

The basic characteristics of associate degree education include the following:

1. The unit in nursing is an integral part of the parent institution and is structured, controlled, and financed as is any other unit of the institution.
2. Faculty members in the unit in nursing have the same privileges and responsibilities as other faculty of the institution. They are responsible for development, implementation, and evaluation of the program of learning.
3. The program of learning usually is organized for completion within a 2-year period. It is based on a clearly stated rationale and a conceptual framework that are derived from its philosophy and objectives. The program of learning meets the requirements of the parent institution for granting an associate degree and of the state licensing agency for eligibility to write the examination for registered nursing.
4. Students meet the requirements of the institution and its nursing program for admission, continuation of study, and graduation. They share in the responsibilities and privileges of the total student body.[4]

Associate degree education was founded on the premise that the health care delivery system could incorporate a nursing technician whose function would be less autonomous than that of the baccalaureate-prepared nurse but greater than that of the practical nurse. The graduate would be prepared to work "at the bedside" under supervision, performing the routine nursing skills for patients. This would be a new type of worker, the nursing technician, to help meet nursing needs, and a new type of technical education program in nursing would exist in 2 years' time in junior and community colleges. One half of the curriculum comprised general education courses and the other half, nursing courses. Learning experiences were carefully selected to meet specific objectives. Dr. Montag considered the program to be terminal; that is, most students would conclude their education at this point and would not continue on to earn a baccalaureate degree. Graduates would be awarded an associate degree from the junior or community college sponsoring the program and would be eligible to write the examination for registered nurse licensure.

Over the years associate degree education has changed somewhat. There is a growing tendency to place more emphasis and time on nursing courses than on general education courses. Many programs, in an attempt to prepare graduates who can meet the demands of employers, have added courses in team leadership and physical assessment. More and more graduates are seeking additional education beyond the associate degree, and the "ladder" concept in nursing education is growing. Registered nurse baccalaureate and "two-on-two" programs are increasing as these graduates demand easier matriculation into 4-year institutions of learning. These programs are discussed later in the chapter.

The advent of associate degree education in nursing brought with it a change in the kind of students who enrolled. Nursing students were traditionally a homogeneous group mainly comprised of single white females ranging in age from 18 to 35 who were usually scholastically in the upper third of their high school class. Associate degree programs (although sometimes adding selective admission policies to the "open door" philosophy of the community colleges) attract older people, married women, minorities, men, and students with a wider range of intellectual abilities. Recent years have also seen persons who already possess baccalaureate or higher degrees in other fields seeking admission to associate degree programs.

Perhaps more has been written about associate degree education than about all the other nursing programs combined. In 1978 the NLN published *Competencies of the Associate Degree Nurse on Entry into Practice*, a document whose drafts were mailed to all associate degree programs and to individual members of the Council of Associate Degree Programs for input. This document began with assumptions basic to the scope of practice of the associate degree nurse on entry into practice.

The practice for graduates of associate degree nursing programs:

- Is directed toward clients who need information or support to maintain health.
- Is directed toward clients who are in need of medical diagnostic evaluation and/or are experiencing acute or chronic illness.
- Is directed toward clients' responses to common, well-defined health problems.
- Includes the formulation of a nursing diagnosis.
- Consists of nursing interventions selected from established nursing protocols where probable outcomes are predictable.
- Is concerned with individual clients and is given with consideration of the person's relationship within a family, group, and community.
- Includes the safe performance of nursing skills that require cognitive, psychomotor, and affective capabilities.
- May be in any structured care setting but primarily occurs within acute- and extended-care facilities.
- Is guided directly or indirectly by a more experienced registered nurse.
- Includes the direction of peers and other workers in nursing in selected aspects of care within the scope of practice of associate degree nursing.
- Involves an understanding of the roles and responsibilities of self and other workers within the employment setting.[5]

The document goes on to outline specific competencies of the associate degree nurse on entry into practice. The competencies are focused around five interrelated roles: the role as provider of care, the role as communicator, the role as a client teacher, the role as a manager of client care, and the role as a member within the profession of nursing.

Despite the planning and experimentation that preceded the instigation of associate degree nursing programs, hospital nursing service personnel often were not prepared for this new type of graduate. Sometimes referred to as "a 2-year wonder," the new graduate was criticized by nursing service for being prepared to function only as beginning practitioners and to *become* competent nurses instead of already being well-indoctrinated with the operations of the hospital and ready to slip into staff leadership roles. Although it levels similar complaints at today's baccalaureate graduate, nursing service appears to have the poorest understanding of associate degree education. This is not surprising when one realizes that a major issue in nursing as a whole is the delineation of roles of the various practitioners. What is technical education? How does it vary from baccalaureate programs? What constitutes a professional role? Whereas some accuse associate degree educators of offering "mini-baccalaureate" programs "watered down to encompass 2 years," others challenge baccalaureate programs to define a truly professional component of nursing and to develop a curriculum that will educate a graduate to function in that capacity.

Another problem involved with associate degree education stems from what might be called titling. Although technical education for nursing was well delineated by Montag, Matheney, and other leaders in associate degree education, and although it is honored in other fields of study, there has been little acceptance of graduates who are "technicians" in nursing. This resistance has come from the graduates of associate degree programs as much as from the general nursing public. In 1976 the Council of Associate Degree Programs, meeting in Washington, D.C., moved to change the name of the graduate of associate degree programs from "technical" to "associate degree" nurse.

Whereas questions regarding titling, licensure, entry level, and role delineation are yet to be answered, most nursing educators agree that associate degree education in nursing has a permanent place within the educational establishment and within the nursing profession itself.

BACCALAUREATE EDUCATION

The first school of nursing to be established in a university setting was started at the University of Minnesota in 1909. The program existed as a quasi-autonomous branch of the university's school of medicine. Close inspection of the curriculum would reveal a program little different from the 3-year hospital program; nothing was required in the way of higher general education, and graduates were prepared for the RN certificate only. Education was predominantly apprenticeship in nature, and students provided service to hospitals in exchange for education. It was not until 1919 that an undergraduate baccalaureate program in nursing was created at Minnesota. In the interim, baccalaureate programs had been initiated at a number of other schools.

Most of the baccalaureate programs were 5 years long. This provided for the 3 years of nursing school curriculum not vastly different from that of the hospital programs, and for the additional 2 years of liberal arts.

Although the development of baccalaureate education for nurses may not seem like a major step to young people of today, remember that in 1909 women had yet to be granted the right to vote; nursing was considered by many a less than desirable occupation, vocational in its orientation, overshadowed by militaristic and technical aspects, and confined to women. A liberal education, scholarship, and knowledge were thought to be incompatible with the female personality, and possibly posed problems for marriage later. The nursing curriculum, with its emphasis on performance of skills rather than the philosophical and theoretical approaches used in the humanities, was not well accepted by universities. The growth of these schools was not rapid. In 1919 there were eight baccalaureate programs; in 1985 there were 455 programs.[6]

Baccalaureate education has been advocated by nursing leaders as the minimum educational preparation for supervisory and administrative nursing roles. Baccalaureate education further provides the background needed for public health positions, including school nursing. In 1965 the ANA specified baccalaureate preparation in nursing as the minimum educational preparation for entry into professional nursing practice (see Chapter 3). This position has gained acceptance among nursing groups.

Baccalaureate nursing programs are located in 4-year colleges and universities. When the program of studies includes an upper division (junior and senior years), baccalaureate nursing major that is built on a basis of liberal arts and science courses taken during the freshman and sophomore years, it is known as a *generic* baccalaureate program.

Applicants to such programs must meet the entrance (and graduation) requirements established by the university and those of the nursing school. The admission requirements usually specify academic preparation at the high school (or preadmission) level, which includes courses in foreign language, higher-level study of mathematics and science, and a high cumulative gradepoint average. Relatively high scores on college admission tests may also be necessary.

During the freshman and sophomore years of study, students who pursue a nursing education take liberal arts, biological, and physical science courses with college students who are preparing for other majors. In some schools these courses may be completed on a part-time basis, but if this occurs, the entire course of study covers more than a 4-year span. The number of required liberal arts and science courses may vary from program to program but usually constitutes about one half of the total number of credits specified for graduation from the college or university. Students study specifically nursing content in their junior and senior years, thus the term *upper-division major in nurs-*

ing. Nursing theory can be taught that builds on an understanding of the physical and biological sciences and liberal arts studied the previous two years.

In recent years there has been some tendency for schools offering baccalaureate nursing education to introduce nursing content at some point in the sophomore year of study. These courses, if offered at this point, often include an overview of the nursing profession and some of the fundamental nursing skills.

Students in baccalaureate nursing programs learn basic nursing skills. They also learn concepts of health maintenance and promotion, disease prevention, and supervisory and leadership techniques and practices, and are provided with an introduction to research. Clinical course work includes experience in community health settings, and practice as leaders on a nursing team within the acute care hospital as well as basic care procedures. Emphasis is placed on developing skills in critical decision making, on exercising independent nursing judgments that call for broad background knowledge, and on working in complex nursing situations in which the outcomes are often not predictable. Acting as a patient-client advocate, the graduate of a baccalaureate nursing program collaborates with other members of the health care team in structured and unstructured settings and supervises those with lesser preparation. The baccalaureate graduates often work with groups as well as with individuals.

Recent years have seen changes in the nature of baccalaureate education. Some schools, seeking to add a serious professional component, have added courses that permit a degree of specialization at the baccalaureate level, for example, additional courses in coronary or intensive care nursing. Other schools are providing more grounding in research, either as preparation for graduate school or for a more varied role in nursing. One of the most interesting changes has occurred in California. In that state the rules and regulations for schools of nursing stipulate that all courses required by the Board of Nursing for licensure as a registered nurse be offered within the first 36 months of full-time training, the first 6 academic semesters, or the first 9 academic quarters, whichever is shortest.[7] In essence this means that all educational preparation required for application for licensure of students enrolled in baccalaureate programs in that state must be completed by the end of the junior year. This leaves the senior year to be filled with specialty experience, preceptorships, or whatever the school might deem appropriate education. This change in the licensure law has also caused some problems. Some students complete their junior year and successfully pass the licensing examination. They then elect to drop out of school and work as a registered nurse. Although they are licensed in the state of California, these students have no degree from any school, which creates problems if they seek licensure in another state.

In 1979 the NLN Council of Baccalaureate and Higher Degree Programs developed a statement on the "Characteristics of Baccalaureate Education in Nursing." This statement, as revised in 1986, concludes with the following list of activities that the graduate of the baccalaureate programs in nursing is able to do.

- Provide professional nursing care, which includes health promotion and maintenance, illness care, restoration, rehabilitation, health counseling, and education based on knowledge derived from theory and research.
- Synthesize theoretical and empirical knowledge from nursing, scientific, and humanistic disciplines with practice.
- Use the nursing process to provide nursing care for individuals, families, groups, and communities.
- Accept responsibility and accountability for the evaluation of the effectiveness of their own nursing practice.
- Enhance the quality of nursing and health practices within practice settings through the use of leadership skills and a knowledge of the political system.
- Evaluate research for the applicability of its findings to nursing practice.
- Participate with other health care providers and members of the general public in promoting the health and well-being of people.
- Incorporate professional values as well as ethical, moral, and legal aspects of nursing into nursing practice.
- Participate in the implementation of nursing roles designed to meet emerging health needs of the general public in a changing society.[8]

MASTER'S AND DOCTORAL PROGRAMS THAT PREPARE FOR LICENSURE

In concluding our discussion of the various educational programs that prepare the graduate to write the state licensing examination for registered nursing, we need to mention the generic master's programs. In addition, there is one program, located at Case-Western Reserve, in which the student earns a doctorate in nursing before being eligible to write the licensing examination.

The history of such programs goes back a number of years, to programs at Yale and several other schools of nursing where students were admitted with a baccalaureate degree in another area. They were granted a master's degree in nursing after completing an established program of study of approximately 2 years that prepared the graduate for registered nurse licensure. Interest in this type of educational preparation for nursing is increasing. It reflects, in part, the thinking of some nurse leaders that the minimum preparation for professional nursing should be the master's degree. It also provides a higher degree to those persons who possess basic baccalaureate preparation in another area of study and are making career changes. Many of these students have chosen to pursue a 2-year associate degree in nursing because of time and expense. With increasing emphasis being placed on the need for a baccalaureate degree for professional practice, making this type of program an option is certainly credible.

SIMILARITIES AMONG PROGRAMS

Currently there appear to be as many similarities in the various avenues to nursing education as there are variances. These similarities may be grouped into several broad classifications that include academic standards, administrative concerns, and areas relating to students.

In the academic realm three similarities stand out:

1. All graduates write the NCLEX for registered nursing in their state. All writers must meet the same minimum cutoff score to pass the test and become licensed.
2. All schools must meet the criteria established for state board approval and (in many instances on a voluntary basis) the criteria developed for national accreditation.
3. Members of the faculty are pushed to meet the increasing demands of education, clinical excellence, tenure, and possibly vocational certification. Work loads and the time invested in the performance of professional responsibilities often are disparate with that of instructors from other areas of the campus, even though they are considered colleagues in the educational setting.

From an administrative perspective, two similarities are noted:

1. All programs are relatively expensive to operate in comparison to other forms of education provided in colleges and universities. Federal and state agencies are tightening the reins on funding and are demanding greater accountability. Less finan-

cial assistance is available to students in the form of scholarships and loans than in the past. Tuition costs are rising.

2. Most programs find themselves searching and competing with other schools for learning experiences in clinical agencies. To some extent this competition is related to changes in societal values and the health care delivery system. Families are electing to have fewer children and, more recently in some societies, to deliver these children at home. The result has been fewer patients in the obstetrical units of hospitals. Pediatric patients are managed on an outpatient basis as much as possible, and hospitalization, when required, is kept to a minimum. The management of the client with psychiatric disturbances is moving from institutions to community mental health centers whenever feasible. Finally, the increase in the number and size of schools in urban areas creates high demand for clinical facilities in those areas.

When the area relating to students is considered, three similarities are mentioned:

1. All schools must develop sound educational programs while balancing student enrollments against faculty recruitment and retention factors. A serious drop in applicants to all programs in 1979–80 was followed by more applicants than could reasonably be accommodated in 1982–83. This resulted in the development of selective admission policies that were carefully scrutinized by school officials and then reviewed by the school's attorney for correct legal form and for legal ramifications before being accepted by the school's policymaking group. At the present time enrollments in nursing are plummeting, and in some instances schools are closing. The impact of these yo-yoing enrollments on nursing service and placement of new graduates is apparent.

2. Programs are caught up in more legal challenges than in the past, since applicants and students seek their "rights as individuals" and challenge admission and dismissal policies. The *N.S.N.A. Student Bill of Rights and Responsibilities*, which was designed by nursing students, is widely accepted by schools of nursing throughout the country. This bill sets forth the students' basic rights and establishes grievance procedures if a student believes that these rights have been violated (see Chapter 12, Figure 12–4). Another legal concern relates to mal-

practice coverage for students. Collegiate programs, now removed from the umbrella coverage of the hospital, ask that students purchase malpractice insurance to protect the students against financial losses that could occur as the result of suits that could be based on errors committed in the learning process.

3. All programs are seeing a wider diversity in the characteristics of applicants seeking admission to the programs. That is to say, programs are receiving more applications from males, minorities, older adults, and persons who possess degrees in other fields of study.

One usually finds nursing educators more or less united in their efforts to create quality programs that will graduate students who can function satisfactorily in a changing and challenging health care delivery system (see Table 2–1).

OTHER FORMS OF NURSING EDUCATION

Educational offerings in nursing have grown tremendously since the 1960s. This is due in part to the changing role of the nurse in health delivery and to the need for more adequate education to meet the preparation requirements of that role. Another contributing factor is the continuing push to make nursing truly professional in nature. The result is the need for practitioners, with master's and doctoral degrees, who are interested and competent in research techniques and skills. A third significant reason for advancing nursing education relates to requirements placed on the profession for leadership in nursing administration and education. Nurse educators, joining the ranks of other professionals in the academic environment, are required to possess equivalent educational background. Nurses who assume roles in nursing administration have found the need for a solid understanding of management and finance principles that is acquired by study at the master's and doctoral level.

Registered Nurse Baccalaureate Programs

Recent years have seen an increase in the number of RNB (registered nurse baccalaureate) programs. These programs are designed for nurses who have completed nursing in either diploma or associate degree programs that prepared for registered nurse licensure, and who are returning to school to complete baccalaureate degrees in nursing.

These programs carry various names in different parts of the country, including BRN (baccalaureate registered nurse) programs, two-on-two, and, in the Midwest capstone programs. There are several reasons for the increase in this form of nursing education. Employers are requiring greater preparation for supervisory roles. Highly qualified young men and women are entering associate degree programs because of cost and time factors and are then planning more education several years after completion of the original program. Nursing as a profession is pushing toward baccalaureate preparation as the minimum entry level for professional practice.

RNB programs vary greatly throughout the United States. In some instances they exist in universities that already offer the generic baccalaureate. The students may be integrated with generic baccalaureate students, partially separated, or totally separated. Another form of RNB preparation is the two-on-two approach, in which students transfer into the college or university with junior standing and complete an additional 2 years of upper-division nursing classes to achieve the baccalaureate in nursing. Some schools offer nurse practitioner preparation in conjunction with the baccalaureate degree, although the growing tendency is to place this at the master's level.

The general trend is to allow the transfer of credits from junior and community colleges in basic education courses such as psychology and sociology and sometimes in the biological sciences. Often some transfer credit is given for nursing, for example, 45 quarter credits, or the courses may be challenged. Distribution requirements of the particular college or university must be satisfied, and upper-division nursing courses must be completed in such areas as physiological nursing, community health, and supervision. A minimum of 2 years usually is required for completion of the program, although the time may be longer, depending on the number of requirements satisfied at the time of entry.

When the two-on-two programs were first launched, they were criticized by nurse educators. The criticism seemed to revolve around three central themes. The first involved the fact that the ladder concept in nursing education has been slow to develop. As we discussed earlier, many nurse educators perceived associate degree education as terminal and did not accept it as a stepping-stone to baccalaureate education.

The second concern related to the problems associated with evaluating previous learning and granting credit for that learning. How should one equate nursing process that one taught at the 100 level in the community college with nursing process that one taught at the 300 level in the senior university?

The third area that presented difficulties was that of determining
(Text continues on p. 63)

Table 2–1 *Educational Avenues to Registered Nursing: A Comparison*

Question	Diploma	Associate Degree	Baccalaureate
Where?	Is usually conducted by and based in a hospital	Most often conducted in junior or community colleges, occasionally in senior colleges and universities	Located in senior colleges and universities
How long?	Requires generally 24–30 months but may require 3 academic years	Requires usually 2 academic or sometimes 2 calendar years	Requires 4 academic years
Entrance?	Requires graduation from high school or its equivalent, satisfactory general academic achievement, and successful completion of certain prerequisite courses	Requires that applicants meet entrance requirements of college as well as of program	Requires that applicants meet entrance requirements of the college or university as well as those of program
Curriculum?	Includes courses in theory and practice of nursing and in biological, physical, and behavioral sciences	Combines a balance of nursing courses and college courses in the basic natural and social sciences with courses in general education and the humanities	Frequently concentrates on courses in the theory and practice of nursing in the junior and senior years

	May require that certain courses in the physical and social sciences be taken at a local college or university		Provides education in the theory and practice of nursing and courses in the liberal arts as well as the behavioral and physical sciences
Clinical?	Provides early and substantial clinical learning experiences in the hospital and a variety of community agencies; these focus on an understanding of the hospital environment and the inter-relationship of other health disciplines	Requires as a significant part of the program supervised clinical instruction in hospitals and other community health agencies	Provides clinical laboratory courses in a variety of settings where health and nursing care are given
Educational advancement?	Little or no transferability of courses unless affiliated with a community college or university	Is structured so that some credits may be applied to baccalaureate degree	Provides the basic academic preparation for advancement to higher positions in nursing and to master's degree
Cost[28]	From $250 – $4,250 if private $1,440 median	From $277 – $3,750 if private; $2,944 median	From as little as $386 tuition per year to nearly $4,375 per year, if private; $3,935 median

(Continued)

61

Table 2–1 Educational Avenues to Registered Nursing: A Comparison (continued)

Question	Diploma	Associate Degree	Baccalaureate
Terminal ability?	Graduate is prepared to plan for the care of patients with other members of the health team, to develop and carry out plans for the care of individuals or groups of patients, and to direct selected members of the nursing team. Has an understanding of the hospital climate and the community health resources necessary for the extended care of patients	Graduate is prepared to plan and give direct patient care in hospitals, nursing homes, or similar health care agencies and to participate with other members of the health team, such as licensed practical nurses, nurses aides, physicians, and other registered nurses in rendering care to patients	Graduate is prepared to plan and give direct care to individuals and families, whether sick or well, to assume responsibility for directing other members of the health team, and to take on beginning leadership positions. Practices in a variety of settings and emphasizes comprehensive health care, including preventive and rehabilitative services, health counseling and education, and care in acute and long-term illnesses Have necessary education for graduate study toward a master's degree and may move more rapidly to specialized leadership positions in nursing as teachers, administrators, clinical specialists, nurse practitioners, and nurse researchers
Licensing?	Must successfully complete state licensing examination	Must successfully complete state licensing examination	Must successfully complete state licensing examination

(Adapted from Your Career in Nursing, Publication No. 41-1562. New York, National League for Nursing, 1976) what additional courses in nursing should be offered and how they should be offered. A serious question existed as to whether the standards, program objectives, and educational structures that had been developed for the generic student were appropriate for the registered nurse group. What learning experience could be included that would help to "socialize" the student for the role of a baccalaureate graduate? What additional nursing courses were needed to form the upper-division major in nursing that would provide a basis for graduate education? Because the skills of the various graduates were not clearly delineated, it was difficult to develop a curriculum that would enable the RNB graduate to demonstrate specific terminal behaviors. When attempts were made to develop such programs, baccalaureate educators found themselves confronted with another concern: they were working mostly with adult students. This required them to rethink teaching-learning principles in order to educate these students effectively. Students were seeking a learning program that required different packaging, one that allowed for part-time study and more evening and weekend classes that would allow part- or full-time employment while pursuing more education. They wanted the education brought to them rather than going to the educational setting.

RNB education and two-on-two educational programs have recently gained more acceptance as a result of the push from the ANA Commission on Nursing Education to increase the availability of baccalaureate programs for registered nurses. As more and more states endorse the ANA position on entry into practice, nurse educators, steeped in the traditional approaches to baccalaureate education, are challenged to create and accept more innovative educational strategies.

Some of the programs now being developed provide for part-time study or for studies completed through evening courses. The desirability of such an approach for nurses who must work to support their education is obvious.

In some instances schools with both generic and RNB programs report graduating more RNB students than generic students. Figures obtained from the NLN indicate that the enrollment of registered nurses in baccalaureate programs increased from 452 in 1973–74 to 3,239 in 1982–83. Dramatic increases are anticipated after 1986.[9]

The External Degree

The concept of an external degree is not new. Universities in Australia, the Soviet Union, and England have long recognized independent study validated by examination. The University of London has awarded college degrees earned in this fashion since 1836. The major difference between the external degree and the traditional educational experience is that students awarded an external degree attend no classes and follow no prescribed methods of learning. Learning is *assessed* through highly standardized and validated examinations. This approach to education had not been developed in the United States until recently. Schools in the United States that were first to recognize the value of this self-directed learning were New York's Empire State College and the University Without Walls consortium.[10]

The New York Regents External Degree (REX) Program of the University of the State of New York has become part of this movement. The Board of Regents established the College Proficiency Examination Program in 1961. Similar to the College-Level Examination Program tests developed by the Educational Testing Service, the examination allows students to gain credit and meet the regents' external degree requirements without attending classes.

In 1971 the New York Board of Regents authorized an external associate degree program in nursing; the external baccalaureate degree in nursing was to follow in April 1976. In 1973 the W. K. Kellogg Foundation awarded a grant of $528,000 to ensure financial support for the first 2 years of the program. Since that time the Foundation has provided continuous support for the program in the amount of $3.5 million. By the end of 1983 approximately 2,200 candidates had earned associate degrees, with the first students completing the program in 1975. Another 600 candidates had earned baccalaureate degrees, with the first degrees awarded in 1979. An estimated 9,000 persons were actively enrolled in these nursing programs.[11] The programs are accredited by the NLN.

The nursing program, like other external degree programs in arts, science, and business, uses an assessment approach and is primarily — although not exclusively — designed for those with some experience in nursing. It is philosophically based on principles of the adult learner that advocate education that is flexible and learner-oriented. Specifically, the responsibility for demonstrating that learning has occurred is placed on the student, and the responsibility for identifying the content to be learned and objectively assessing that this has occurred rests with the faculty. The nursing major is divided into cognitive and performance components. The cognitive learning is documented through five nationally standardized and psychometrically valid written examinations. These examinations are available nationally through the American College Testing Program and are administered six times a year at nearly 200 sites. Clinical skills are evaluated through four criteria-referenced performance examinations. Five regional performance assessment centers have been established throughout the United States to make the performance examinations more accessible to candidates. Because performance examinations are quite different from typical evaluation procedures, the people who administer the examinations must complete a 100-hour training program. The major thrust of the training sessions is to exchange teaching-helping behaviors with those of the neutral observer whose role is to determine that criteria have been met. Testing centers are located at Long Beach Memorial Hospital and Stanford University Hospital in California, and in hospitals in Atlanta, Denver, and Milwaukee. In addition there are 12 testing centers located throughout New York State.

Collaborative relationships have been established with academic institutions that want to assist REX candidates who live in their area. The local colleges advertise the program to area nurses and offer

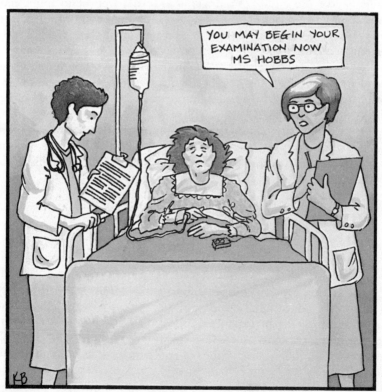

Figure 2–2. Clinical skills are evaluated through performance examinations.

courses designed to assist the student who is preparing for examination. Close collaboration occurs between the REX faculty and the local college faculty.

Dr. Carrie Lenburg has provided the major thrust for the concept of the external degree in nursing and the development of the programs at the University of the State of New York. Students who want to learn more about this program are encouraged to write to her at the University of the State of New York, Regents External Degree Program, Cultural Education Center, Albany, New York 12230.

In 1981 the California State University Consortium inaugurated the West Coast's first statewide external degree baccalaureate program in nursing for working RNs who have current California licenses. Fashioned after the New York model, the program received a Kellogg grant for $2,276,097 in 1982 to develop self-paced instruction modules and other nontraditional learning options. A number of hospitals also subsidized employee enrollment. Three degree routes are possible: some students take the New York Regents External Degree examinations; some complete a series of 53 one-unit courses that combine class work and group projects at learning centers located throughout the state; and some plan a combination of course work and challenge examinations. The program has emphasized flexibility in learning methods, pace, and site at which the learning occurs. Critics of the new program express concern about its ability to maintain prevailing standards of education. Cost is another factor.

Despite objections, alternative and nontraditional avenues to nursing education continue to grow and appeal to the learner. Nursing education, like nursing care, should be tailored to the consumer's needs.

NURSING EDUCATION AT THE GRADUATE LEVEL

Master's Preparation

The critical need for nurses who have had additional preparation, to function in educational settings, in supervisory roles, as clinical specialists, and to fulfill the expanded role of the nurse, has resulted in the increase of master's programs. In 1983, 154 master's degree programs were reported. The total number of students enrolled was 18,112 — the highest to date.[12]

A variety of models of master's preparation in nursing exist. Most could be classified as traditional in approach, but in a recent study 36 percent stated that they used nontraditional options, including outreach programs, summers-only programs, RN-to-MSN tracks that provide a direct route to master's degrees for RNs who have graduated from diploma or associate degree programs, programs for groups with special needs, such as registered nurses with non-nursing baccalaureate degrees or those seeking preparation as technical nurse educators, and programs that admit non-nurses and foreign graduates. Some schools offer off-campus classes, perhaps rotating sites, and some use telecommunication systems to deliver core content by way of television. In at least one school all classes are on Fridays. Several unique programs (*e.g.*, those at Yale University, Pace University, and the University of Tennessee at Knoxville) offer a master's degree in nursing after completion of a baccalaureate degree in another field.[13] Such programs, called generic master's degree programs, were discussed earlier in the chapter.

Most master's degree students in nursing have chosen the area of advanced clinical practice as their main interest, as opposed to supervision, administration, or teaching. Students are highly concentrated in the medical-surgical nursing specialty, with maternal-child the second highest area of concentration, psychiatric-mental health third, and public health the least often chosen specialty area.[14] Most programs require at least 1 full year for completion; many have been expanded to 2 years.

Master's programs in nursing are often found in senior colleges and universities that have baccalaureate programs in nursing. They have the option of seeking voluntary accreditation from the NLN.

Persons seeking information about master's degree programs in nursing should be aware of the NLN publication *Master's Education: Route to Opportunities in Contemporary Nursing.*

Doctoral Studies

The number of requests for admission to doctoral study in nursing has greatly increased since the early 1980s. In 1984, 30 doctoral programs in nursing were in operation. However, in response to the growing demand for nurses with doctoral degrees — the number is expected to reach 13,490 by 1990[15] — another 43 schools are planning to begin doctoral programs by 1988. The impetus for this movement stems from the need for advanced study for academic advancement or tenure in the educational setting and reflects the need in nursing research for the advancement of the profession as a whole.

Doctoral programs in nursing offer a variety of degrees such as the doctor of nursing science (DNSc.), the doctor of science in nursing

(DSN), the doctor of nursing education (DNEd.), or the doctor of philosophy (PhD.) in nursing. Other types of doctorates are also available to nurses, such as the doctor of education (Ed.D.) or the doctor of public health (DPH).

A doctorate outside the area of nursing was often the only doctorate available to the person seeking further education; doctorates in nursing are relatively new to the educational milieu, as opposed to such degrees in psychology, sociology, anthropology, or physiology. Certainly nursing can and has benefited from other disciplines. Before doctorates in nursing were offered, doctoral study in other fields allowed nursing into the mainstream of education in the United States.

The difference in preparation and function of graduates possessing these various degrees is confusing, but for the most part nurses with doctorates play leadership roles in education, often serving as dean or director of nursing programs, or they are involved in the research and development of a body of nursing knowledge.

Although assuming no role in the accreditation of doctoral programs, the NLN has published a pamphlet titled *Doctoral Programs in Nursing* that provides information about various programs of doctoral study in nursing.

DIRECTLY ARTICULATED PROGRAMS

Another recent innovation in nursing education is a program that provides direct articulation between lower-level and higher-level programs. The purpose of such a program is to facilitate opportunities for nurses to start and stop at some point, or keep moving up the educational ladder.

The plan, which is especially attractive to associate degree and practical nurse graduates, allows students to move up the *career* ladder in steps, usually of 2 years' academic and clinical work. Students in an articulated licensed practical nurse/associate degree program would spend 1 year preparing to be an LPN and another year completing the associate degree. If they want to continue after this 2-year period, they can earn a baccalaureate degree at another institution after 2 more years of study. From that point a student could continue work toward a master's degree.

Such programs usually involve planning between two or more institutions, but, depending on start-and-stop points, they may occur within a single institution. A program that involves several institutions is the Orange County – Long Beach consortium in southern California, which

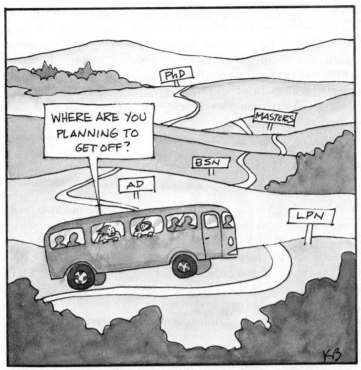

Figure 2–3. Among innovations occurring in nursing education over the last decade are programs that provide direct articulation between lower-level and higher-level programs.

includes five community colleges and two universities. In combination, these seven schools prepare licensed vocational nurses, registered nurses at the associate degree and baccalaureate levels, and specialization at the master's degree level.[16]

Another articulated program exists in the Agassiz region of northwest Minnesota, where a consortium was developed to provide a ladder program encompassing four levels: nursing assistant, practical nurse, associate degree nurse, and baccalaureate degree nurse. A fifth level, that of pursuing graduate study after completion of the baccalaureate, was assumed.[17]

These multiple-entry, multiple-exit programs are not without problems. Initially they are difficult to develop because of the tremendous amount of joint planning needed. For example, the development of a common philosophy to encompass all levels of education is imperative. Common terminal objectives must be developed at each level.

Leveling of content in supporting areas of natural and behavioral sciences is also important. Educators need to speak the same language and develop mutual respect. It is also difficult to keep the programs in operation once begun. As might be anticipated, a tremendous amount of faculty and administrative time is required to work out equivalent courses and to keep the programs "in sync" with one another; however, those involved in articulated programs agree that the effort is rewarding.

NONDEGREE PROGRAMS

Specialized programs have been developed to help to prepare the nurse as her role grows in breadth and scope. Some of these programs are incorporated into the preparation leading to a particular degree; others exist as part of a school's continuing education program.

The registered nurse anesthesia preparation and the midwifery program both award a certificate after completion of a standardized and rigorous course of study lasting from 18 months to 2 years. Each program stipulates its own admission requirements, some requiring licensure only, others requiring baccalaureate preparation.

Programs that have been introduced more recently include the nurse practitioner and nursing specialist preparation in areas of nursing practice such as pediatrics, gerontology, family health, genetics, and women's health care. Designed to meet the increasing demand of the medical and lay community, these courses provide concentrated study in specific areas over a period of time lasting from several weeks to several months. Requirements for admission vary tremendously. Some require licensure for admission, others stipulate the baccalaureate degree, while still other programs require that the education occur at the post-master's level.

The proliferation of such programs has been so great that a complete listing is impossible. A student interested in pursuing such preparation is encouraged to write to the college or university of choice for information about available programs.

INTERNSHIPS FOR THE NEW GRADUATE

When nursing education moved from hospital-based diploma programs into higher education, a new problem was created. Employers of the new graduates, who expected these graduates to function as experienced and qualified professionals on the day after graduation, complained that these new graduates were not prepared to assume staff nurse positions within their institutions. The changes that had occurred in nursing education, including changes in diploma education, had resulted in shortened clinical experience. Many graduates of diploma schools of the 1950s would have as much as 4,000 clock hours of clinical experience, albeit more as an apprenticeship and a service to the hospital than as a learning experience. Graduates of associate degree programs, with integrated curricula and objective-based learning experiences, emerged into the work world with clinical learning time of 800 or fewer clock hours. Baccalaureate and hospital-based programs also had decreased their clinical hours as curricula were reorganized. Critics in nursing service were distressed by a new type of graduate who could think, analyze, and synthesize, but who was inexperienced in "doing." Most graduates needed an orientation to the work facility, to their new role in that organization, and time to become efficient in the administration of their newly learned skills. Although few would question the need for internships and residencies for the new *physician*, the need for a similar experience for new *nursing* graduates was viewed as appalling. The new graduates, unable to live up to the expectations placed on them, became frustrated and discouraged, and often left the work market for a less stressful situation, sometimes even outside of nursing. Nursing educators, in defending the education provided, cited other professions, such as law and engineering, in which graduates needed a period of time to adapt to the world of work.

By the 1970s it was apparent that something must be done. Although the cost was a problem, internships and orientation programs for new graduates were instituted by hospitals. The programs were intended to ease the transition from the role of student to that of staff by providing the opportunity to increase clinical skills and knowledge as well as self-confidence. Programs can last from several weeks to a year and are designed for graduates of all nursing programs: associate degree, diploma, and baccalaureate. They often include rotations to various units within the hospital, including specialty areas, and they accommodate different shifts. Usually some formal class work is associated with the experience, but the majority of the time is spent in direct patient care, often under the supervision of a preceptor.

Some direct benefits to institutions, other than a better prepared new employee who remains in employment, have resulted from such programs. Inadequacies in policy and procedure books have been uncovered and, as a result, these books have been rewritten. Performance evaluation tools that are more objective in format have emerged. Nursing practice throughout an agency may have become more standardized. Job satisfaction has increased.[18]

Today more and more agencies are developing internship programs for new nursing graduates. In May 1986 the NLN listed 118 nurse-intern programs in 31 states and the District of Columbia. They acknowledged that their data were provided in response to numerous requests but that no definitive, single source for such a listing is available.[19] It is no longer unusual for hospitals to advertise planned orientation and internships as benefits offered to the new graduate who would seek employment at their institution.

CONTINUING EDUCATION

One of the most widely publicized issues in today's nursing literature and most frequently discussed at meetings and conventions is continuing education. Continuing education in nursing is defined as

> planned learning experiences beyond a basic nursing educational program. These experiences are designed to promote the development of knowledge, skills, and attitudes for the enhancement of nursing practice, thus improving health care to the public.[20]

Like so many other areas of nursing, this is not new. In an article titled "Nursing the Sick," written around 1882, Florence Nightingale wrote:

> Nursing is, above all, a progressive calling. Year by year nurses have to learn new and improved methods, as medicine and surgery and hygiene improve. Year by year nurses are called upon to do more and better than they have done. It is felt to be impossible to have a public register of nurses that is not a delusion.[21]

The first continuing education courses for nurses probably would be considered postgraduate instruction today. In 1899 Teachers College at Columbia University instituted a course for qualified graduate nurses in hospital economics. Nursing institutes and conferences were first offered to nurses in the 1920s. Often these were given to make up for deficiencies in basic nursing curriculums of the time. Hospital in-service or staff development programs were also beginning to be discussed in nursing literature around this time. Today most hospitals employ someone who is responsible for an in-service education program.

By 1959 federal funds became available for short-term courses, giving much thrust to continuing education. In 1967 the ANA published *Avenues for Continued Learning*, its first definitive statement on continuing education, and in 1973 the ANA Council on Continuing Education was established. The Council, which is responsible to the ANA Commission on Education, is concerned about standards of continuing education, accreditation of the programs, transferability of credit from state to state, and development of guidelines for recognition systems within states. In 1974 *Standards for Continuing Education in Nursing* was published by the ANA, and the federal government altered the Nurse Traineeship Act of 1972 to include an option that would provide continuing education as an alternative to taking increasing numbers of students into programs receiving federal capitation dollars.

By the 1970s almost all nursing publications had something to say about continuing education for nurses. Practically all states were organizing or planning to organize some method by which the nurse could receive recognition for continued education. These systems were called Continuing Education Approval and Recognition Program, or Continuing Education Recognition Program, and most state systems followed the guidelines and criteria prepared by the ANA.

The continuing education unit (CEU) became a rather uniform system of measuring, recording, reporting, accumulating, transferring, and recognizing participation in nonacademic credit offerings. The definition of a CEU was developed by the National Task Force on the Continuing Education Unit, which represents 34 educational groups. Although nursing was not one of the groups, the definition has been accepted by the profession. Ten hours of participation in an organized continuing education experience under responsible sponsorship, capable direction, and qualified instruction is equal to one CEU.[23]

Today colleges, universities, hospitals, voluntary agencies, and private proprietary groups are all offering continuing education courses to registered nurses. Cost of that education varies tremendously. Nurses attending meetings and conferences may earn a CEU, or part of one, for merely being in the meeting. No attempt is made to assess whether learning has occurred. Professional journals are including sections on programmed instruction that can be completed in the comfort of one's living room. These have an evaluation mechanism. Telecourses are offered by television. Workshops, institutes, conferences, short courses, and evening courses abound. Yet some nurses do not feel the need to keep up with these current offerings.

A system for accreditation and approval of continuing education in nursing was developed and implemented by the ANA in 1975. Accreditation is awarded for a period of 4 years and assures the public that the continuing education offerings provide consistent quality. A new system, put into operation August 1, 1987, allows organizations that offer

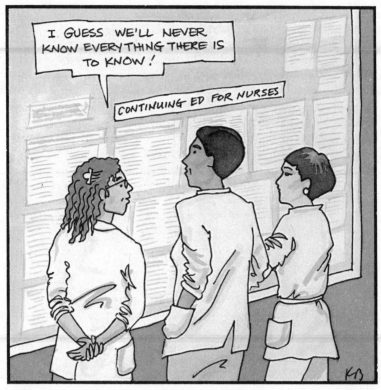

Figure 2–4. Today colleges, universities, hospitals, voluntary agencies, and
private proprietary groups are all offering continuing education
courses to registered nurses.

continuing education to seek accreditation as either a *provider* or an
approver. A provider was any organization that was responsible for the
development, implementation, and evaluation of courses. An approver
could be the state nurses' associations, the specialty organizations, or
the federal nursing services that have been designated to approve the
continuing education process. State nurses' associations, the specialty
organizations, and the federal nursing services could be both a provider
and an approver. The advantage of this program is that it made the
system more accessible to groups seeking accreditation.

An issue today is whether continuing education should be mandatory or voluntary. Mandatory continuing education affects licensure,
that is, any nurse renewing a license in a state requiring (mandating)
continuing education will have to meet that state's regulations for com-

pleting CEUs. Voluntary continuing education is not related to relicensure. Most states are moving toward mandatory continuing education. Government agencies and state legislatures are exerting pressure on nurses, as they have on physicians, attorneys, dietitians, dentists, pharmacists, and other professionals, to provide evidence of updated knowledge before renewal of license.

A position supporting mandatory continuing education raises some other issues. How shall the learning be measured? Who should accredit the programs? How can quality be ensured? By whom and where shall records be retained? Who should bear the cost? What should be the time frame for continuing education? How many hours, courses, and credits should be required?

In 1985 the ANA reported that 19 states required continuing education for continued licensure. Since that time in at least one state that requirement has dropped as a result of *sunset* policies, which require government programs and agencies to undergo a periodic review to determine the need for their continuation. Eleven of the states require continuing education for renewal of registered nurses' licensure and eight require continuing education of nurse practitioners, with some states requiring it of both. Two states require it only of nurse anesthetists. The hours required range from 15 to 30, with the number of hours required of nurse practitioners greater than that required of registered nurses. One state requires 100 clock hours of continuing education of the nurse practitioner.[22] (See Appendix A for specific requirements.)

CONCLUSION

The development of nursing education in the United States has resulted in three major avenues to preparation for licensure as a registered nurse. In addition, various other nontraditional approaches to nursing education have evolved. Much controversy currently exists over which of these routes best prepares the graduate to function in the beginning role of a registered nurse and which degrees should be required for the various expanded roles.

The answers are yet to be determined, but one thing is certain. As nursing grows as a profession and as technology expands and influences health care delivery, changes must and will occur in the education of persons prepared to deliver that care.

In addition, continuing education, whether it is represented by further education that results in a higher degree or whether it takes the form of classes, seminars, or workshops that update and increase expertise, is being mandated by more and more states for continued licensure as a registered nurse.

Nursing education has had a dynamic history. And it will have a dynamic future. It might be well for nurses to stop apologizing for the many and varied approaches to licensure, certification, and continuing education. It is time to applaud the innovations that exist and to perfect the quality of the education available. Only then will the public reap the benefits of this creativity.

REFERENCES

1. Nursing Data Review:1985, Publication No. 19-1994, p 150. New York, National League for Nursing, 1986
2. Gothler A, Rosenfeld P: Nursing education update: Enrollments and admission trends. Nurs Health Care 7 (10):555, Dec 1986
3. Gothler A, Rosenfeld P: Nursing education update: Enrollments and admission trends. Nurs Health Care 7 (10):555, Dec 1986
4. Characteristics of Associate Degree Education in Nursing, Publication No. 23-1500, p 2. Council of Associate Degree Programs. New York, National League for Nursing, 1973
5. Competencies of the Associate Degree Nurse on Entry into Practice, Publication No. 23-1731, p 3. Council of Associate Degree Programs. New York, National League for Nursing, 1978
6. Gothler A, Rosenfeld P: Nursing education update: Enrollments and admission trends. Nurs Health Care 7 (10):555, Dec 1986
7. Laws Relating to Nursing Education Licensure: Practice with Rules and Regulations, p 18. Sacramento, California Board of Registered Nursing, 1976
8. Characteristics of Baccalaureate Education in Nursing, Publication No. 15-1758, pp 2–3. Council of Baccalaureate and Higher Degrees. New York, National League for Nursing, 1987
9. Nursing Data Review:1985, Publication No. 19-1994, p 42. New York, National League for Nursing, 1986
10. Wozniak D: External degrees in nursing. Am J Nurs 73:1014, Jun 1973
11. Lenburg CB: Preparation for professionalism through Regents External Degrees. Nurs Health Care 5 (6):319–325, Jun 1984
12. Nursing Data Review:1985, Publication No. 19-1994, p 50. New York, National League for Nursing, 1986
13. Forni PR: Nursing's diverse master's programs: The state of the art. Nurs Health Care 8 (2):71–75, Feb 1987
14. NLN Nursing Data Book:1981. Publication No. 19-1882, pp 85–92. New York, National League for Nursing, 1982
15. Andreoli KG: Specialization and graduate curricula: Finding the fit. Nurs Health Care 8 (2):65–69, Feb 1987

16. Haase PT: Types of RN programs. In Pathways to Practice, No. 2 in a Series of Final Reports on the Nursing Curriculum Project, p 6. Atlanta, Southern Regional Education Board, 1982
17. Kintgen–Andrews J: The development and demonstration of an articulation model. Nurs Health Care 3 (4):181–188, Apr 1982
18. Haase PT: Acclimating the novice nurse: Whose responsibility? In Pathways to Practice, No. 4 in a Series of Final Reports on the Nursing Curriculum Project, p 1. Atlanta, Southern Regional Education Board, 1982
19. Nurse intern programs. Nurs Health Care 7 (5):270–271, May 1986
20. American Nurses' Association: Standards for Continuing Education for Nursing, p 11. Kansas City, American Nurses' Association, 1974
21. Nightingale F: Nursing the sick. In Seymer LR: Selected Writings of Florence Nightingale, p 349. New York, Macmillan, 1954
22. Facts About Nursing 84-85, p 109. Kansas City, American Nurses' Association, 1985

FURTHER READINGS

Allen VO, Sutton C: Associate degree nursing education: Past, present, and future. Nurs Health Care 2:496–497, Nov 1981

American Nurses' Association: A Case for Baccalaureate Preparation in Nursing. A.N.A. Publication No. NE-6 15M, Dec 1979

American Nurses' Association's First Position on Education for Nursing. Am J Nurs 65:106–111, Dec 1965

Bell F, Rix P: Attitudes of nurses toward lifelong learning: One hospital examines the issues. J Contin Educ Nurs 10:15–20, Jan/Feb 1979

Boyle R: Articulation: From associate degree through master's. Nurs Outlook 20:670–672, Oct 1972

Cal State launches off-campus program for the working R.N. Am J Nurs 82:893, 904–905, Jun 1982

Coleman E: On redefining the baccalaureate degree. Nurs Health Care 7 (4):193–196, 1986

Cooper S: This I believe about continuing education in nursing. Nurs Outlook 20:579–583, Sep 1972

Corona D: College education tailormade for registered nurses. Am J Nurs 73:294–297, Feb 1973

Craver DM, Sullivan PP: Investigation of an internship program. J Contin Educ Nurs 16 (4):114–118, Jul/Aug 1985

Dake MA: C.E.U.: A means to an end? Am J Nurs 74:103–104, Jan 1975

Fahy ET: Keying in on the business of graduate education in nursing. Nurs Health Care 7 (4):203–205, Apr 1986

Felton G: Harnessing today's trends to guide nursing's future. Nurs Health Care 7 (4):211–213, Apr 1986

Gibbs GE: Will continued education be required for license renewal? Am J Nurs 71:2175–2179, Nov 1971

Guidelines for Baccalaureate Education in Nursing for Registered Nurse Students in Colleges and Universities, Publication Series 79, No. 3. Washington, D.C., American Association of Colleges of Nursing, 1980

Hogstel MO: Associate degree and baccalaureate graduates: Do they function differently? Am J Nurs 77:1598–1600, Oct 1977

Hornback MS: Measuring continuing education. Am J Nurs 73:1576–1577, Sep 1973

Johnston SC: The use of the Rines model in differentiating professional and technical nursing practice. Nurs Health Care 3 (7):374–379, Sep 1982

Juneau PS: Dimensions of Practical/Vocational Nursing. New York, Macmillan, 1979

Kasprisin CA, Young WB: Nurse internship program reduces turnover, raises commitment. Nurs Health Care 6 (3):137–140, Mar 1985

Lee A: No, seven out of ten nurses oppose the professional/technical split, Part I. RN 42:82–93, Jan 1979

Lee A: No, there has to be a better way, Part II. RN 42:39–46, Feb 1979

Lee A: Why feelings run high on the professional/technical split, Part III. RN 42:52–58, Mar 1979

Lenburg C, Johnson W: Career mobility through nursing education. Nurs Outlook 22:265–269, Apr 1974

McGriff EP: A case for mandatory continuing education in nursing. Nurs Outlook 20:712–713, Nov 1972

McQuaid EA: How do graduates of different types of programs perform on state boards? Am J Nurs 79:305–308, Feb 1979

Mead ME, Berger S, Nicksic E: Contracts for continuing education. J Contin Educ Nurs 16 (4):121–126, Jul/Aug 1985

Montag ML: Community College Education for Nursing. New York, McGraw-Hill, 1959

Montag ML: Looking back: Associate degree education in perspective. Nurs Outlook 28:248–250, Apr 1980

O'Leary J: What employers will expect from tomorrow's nurses. Nurs Health Care 7 (4):207–209, Apr 1986

Popiel ES: Continuing education: Provider and consumer. Am J Nurs 71:1586–1587, Aug 1971

Ramphal M: This I believe about excellence in technical nursing. Nurs Outlook 16:36–38, Mar 1968

Rogers ME: Reveille in Nursing. Philadelphia, FA Davis, 1964

Rogers ME: Educational Revolution in Nursing. New York, Macmillan, 1961

Ross CF: Personal and Vocational Relationships in Practical Nursing. Philadelphia, JB Lippincott, 1981

Seymer LR: The Nightingale training school: One hundred years ago. Am J Nurs 60:658–661, May 1960

Shetland M: This I believe about career ladder, new careers, and nursing education. Nurs Outlook 18:32–35, Sep 1970

Skoblar SM, Amster LA: Doctors write an unsolicited Rx for nursing education. RN 40:39–42, Sep 1977

Wajdowicz EK: The Americanization of Florence: A look at associate degree nurses. Nurs Health Care 7 (2):97–99, Feb 1986

Wood LA: A.N.A. sets standards for continuing education. Am J Nurs 74:31, Jan 1974

Woolley AS: Defining the product of baccalaureate education. Nurs Health Care 7 (4):199–201, Apr 1986

3 | *The Future of Nursing Education*

Objectives

After completing this chapter, you should be able to

1. *Discuss the development of the **ANA Position Paper on Nursing Education.***
2. *Identify the major points outlined in the **ANA Position Paper.***
3. *Discuss the positions of other nursing organizations in regard to entry into practice.*
4. *Discuss the problems that will be encountered in the implementation of the ANA position on entry into practice.*
5. *Explain what is meant by a **grandfather clause** and why it is necessary when licensing laws are changed.*
6. *List some changes that may occur in the methods of nursing instruction in the future.*
7. *Discuss the impact of reduced federal funding on nursing education.*
8. *State the reason nursing theories are important to the profession.*
9. *Identify three nursing theories.*

In our discussion of nursing and nursing education thus far, we have provided a background for understanding the development of nursing as a profession and a discussion of the various educational paths that will prepare you for the practice of that profession. It seems fairly certain that there will be changes in nursing education. Social, technical, political, and financial factors will affect the way that nursing is practiced and the manner in which students will be educated for the profession.

THE AMERICAN NURSES' ASSOCIATION POSITION PAPER

In 1948 Esther Lucille Brown, in her report *Nursing for the Future* (see Chapter One), recommended

> that the term "professional," when applied to nursing education, be restricted to schools, whether operated by universities or colleges, hospitals affiliated with institutions of higher learning, medical colleges, or independently, that are able to furnish professional education as that term has come to be understood by educators.[1]

By the late 1950s and early 1960s the American Nurses' Association (ANA) began to look with concern at nursing education and the delivery of nursing care. The ANA believed that improvement of nursing practice depended on the advancement of nursing education. When the ANA House of Delegates met in 1960, they accepted as a basis for continued discussion a recommendation from the Committee on Current and Long-term Goals that would "promote the baccalaureate program so that in due course it becomes the basic educational foundation for professional nursing."[2] In 1962 a Committee on Education was appointed by the ANA Board of Directors to pursue this goal.

The recommendation was addressed again in June 1964, when the ANA House of Delegates voted to "continue to work towards baccalaureate education as the educational foundation for professional nursing practice." The Committee on Education was directed to "enunciate a precise definition of preparation for nursing at all levels."[3]

This activity was to result in the development and publication in 1965 of *A Position Paper on Educational Preparation for Nurse Practitioners and Assistants to Nurses.* This paper was the culmination of the work of the Committee, which for 2 years studied the major changes and trends in and around nursing, especially as these trends affected patient care. The position was developed in accordance with basic premises or assumptions, which are as follows:

1. Nursing is a helping profession and, as such, provides services which contribute to the health and well-being of people.
2. Nursing is of vital consequence to the individual receiving services; it fills needs which cannot be met by the person, by the family, or by other persons in the community.
3. The demand for services of nurses will continue to increase.
4. The professional practitioner is responsible for the nature and quality of all nursing care patients receive.
5. The services of professional practitioners of nursing will continue to be supplemented and complemented by the services of nurse practitioners who will be licensed.
6. Education for those in the health professions must increase in depth and breadth as scientific knowledge expands.
7. In addition to those licensed as nurses, the health care of the public, in the amount and to the extent needed and demanded, requires the services of large numbers of health occupation workers to function as assistants to nurses. These workers are presently designated: nurses' aides, orderlies, assistants, attendants, etc.
8. The professional association must concern itself with the nature of nursing practice, the means for improving nursing practice, and the standards for membership in the professional association.[4]

The paper took four major positions:

1. The education for all those who are licensed to practice nursing should take place in institutions of higher education.
2. Minimum preparation for beginning professional nursing practice at the present time should be *baccalaureate degree education* in nursing.
3. Minimum preparation for beginning technical nursing practice at the present time should be *associate degree education* in nursing.
4. Education for assistants in the health service occupations would be short, intensive preservice programs, in vocational education institutions rather than in on-the-job training programs.[5]

In general, the position paper was received in the nursing community with something less than overwhelming enthusiasm. The existence of three educational routes (baccalaureate, associate degree, and di-

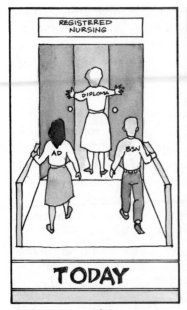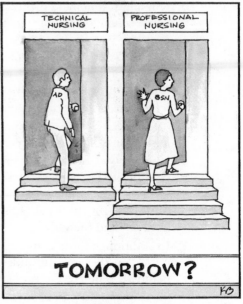

Figure 3–1. The proposed change in entry level would require a baccalaureate degree for professional nursing and an associate degree for technical nursing.

ploma) preparing graduates for registered nurse licensure created problems and confusion. The largest group of practicing nurses was composed of diploma graduates, who had no preparation beyond the original diploma and who saw themselves functioning as professional nurses. Advocates of associate degree programs were concerned that their graduates might have to assume the title "licensed practical nurse." The position paper also did not differentiate the educational preparation of the "assistants in the health service occupations" and virtually eliminated the 1-year practical nurse program as it was currently known.

Among the more perplexing of the problems was the lack of definitive statements on the competencies of the graduates of each of the programs, and the roles, functions, and responsibilities that each would fulfill in the health care delivery system. Although the position paper was fairly specific in describing the educational expectations of "professional" and "technical" nursing practice, most graduates of programs preparing for registered nurse licensure were employed by acute care hospitals. The role for the registered nurse in these institutions was primarily socialized around the diploma graduate of the 1950s. In addition, approximately 85 percent of the 1966 nursing work force was composed of diploma graduates for whom the diploma was the only educational credential. In the face of overwhelming objection to the position paper, ANA's newly appointed Commission on Nursing Education focused its energies on continuing education.

In 1978 the ANA House of Delegates decided to step up activity that would clarify and strengthen the system of nursing education. They adopted the following three significant resolutions:

1. That by 1985 the minimum preparation for entry into professional nursing practice be the baccalaureate in nursing, that the ANA would work closely with the state nurses' associations to identify and define two categories of nursing practice, and that national guidelines for implementation be identified and reported back to the ANA membership by 1980

2. That ANA establish a mechanism devising a comprehensive statement of competencies for the two categories of nursing practice by 1980

3. That ANA actively support increased accessibility to high-quality career mobility programs that use flexible approaches for those seeking academic degrees in nursing.[6]

Again in 1982 the ANA House of Delegates accepted a recommendation from the Commission on Nursing Education, which was amended to read that the ANA "move forward in the coming biennium to expedite implementation of the baccalaureate in nursing as the minimum educational qualification for entry into professional nursing practice."[7]

As you carefully look at these resolutions and recommendations you will notice that they become more and more directive and concrete. In 1960 the recommendations were accepted as a basis for continued discussion. In 1964 the ANA voted to work toward the baccalaureate as the foundation for professional nursing. In 1978 the 1985 date was established as a time when the *minimum* preparation for entry into professional nursing practice would be the *baccalaureate* in nursing and that they would identify and define two categories of nursing practice. In 1982 the charge was to *implement* in the coming biennium the baccalaureate as the *minimum educational preparation* for professional practice.

In June 1984, with issues relating to organizational structure settled 2 years earlier, the ANA again took an aggressive step toward implementation of the position statement. The Cabinet on Nursing Education introduced an initiative and won an unconditional endorsement of its plan to establish the baccalaureate for professional practice in 5 percent of the states by 1986, in 15 percent of the states by 1988, in 50 percent of them by 1992, and in 100 percent of the United States by 1995. At this time ANA's Board of Directors agreed to commit $100,000 a year over 5 years to assist the state associations to bring this plan into effect. Later an additional $500,000 was allocated for a nationwide public relations campaign to seek support for the changes in the states. The first states to receive these moneys were Maine, Montana, Oregon, and North Dakota. Illinois later received a $50,000 grant for a project that would establish two levels of nursing with legislative action slated for 1987.[8]

In 1985, 20 years after the publication of the original position paper, the ANA again pushed to make the statement a reality. The 680-member house of delegates decided that the title "registered nurse" be reserved for the professional nurse prepared with a baccalaureate degree. The title "associate nurse" was adopted as the title to be used for the technical nurse, a graduate of a state-chartered institution that would award an associate degree. The second title was not determined with any ease. Seventeen titles in all were considered by the delegates for the 2-year nurse.[9]

Activities of the State Associations

In 1974 the New York Nurses' Association became the first state to adopt a resolution regarding entry into professional practice that would make it mandatory by 1985 for all applicants for registered nurse licensure in New York State to have the minimum of a baccalaureate degree in nursing, with an upper-division major in nursing. The proposed legislation was also designed to change the educational requirement for the licensed practical nurse to an associate degree. As proposed, the law allowed for "grandfathering" the license of all current RNs and LPNs, and it specified 1985 as the date when new RNs would be required to have a baccalaureate degree and new LPNs to earn an associate degree. This would have eliminated the 1-year practical nursing program. Although the resolution did not move far in terms of legislation, it started movements in other states and became the springboard for vigorous debate in the entire health care field regarding the appropriate educational preparation required of a professional nurse.

Other states were soon to follow with position statements. By April of 1980, 34 state nurses' associations had voted to support the ANA stand. Of the 34 states supporting the ANA resolutions, 30 states endorsed the concept of two categories of practice; 10 had settled on titles, and 4 had developed competency statements for the categories.[10]

As of August 1986, at least 48 state nurses' associations had taken positions to change the educational requirements for entry into nursing practice. The change most commonly recommended was to stipulate the baccalaureate degree in nursing as the requirement for licensure at the professional level and the associate degree in nursing as the requirement for licensure at the technical level. This would mean that there would be one entry point for each level of licensure. Boards of nursing would need to redefine the legal scope of practice for each level.[11]

In January 1986 North Dakota promulgated administrative rules that would require nursing programs to develop specific curricula leading to the associate degree for practical nurse programs and the baccalaureate degree for registered nurse programs in order to be approved by the North Dakota Board of Nursing. This requirement would become effective January 1, 1987. The North Dakota legislature was not involved in changing the rules and regulations, although legislative action would have been necessary to change the act itself. Therefore, the rules were submitted to the attorney general for his review, as required by the Administrative Practices Act, and were subsequently approved "as to their legality." They were adopted by the Board on January 16, 1986.[12]

Action regarding this change actually started in May 1984, when a decision was made by members of the state board of nursing to revise the nursing education rules to more closely implement the two definitions of nursing (registered nurse and licensed practical nurse) contained in the North Dakota Nurse Practices Act. North Dakota had five baccalaureate nursing programs; three were located in state-supported institutions and two were in private schools. One of the five schools also offered an associate degree and two of the institutions offered a master's degree. The state also had three hospital-based diploma programs and two state-supported associate degree programs. There were seven programs in North Dakota that prepared licensed practical nurses. In accomplishing this change, numerous hearings were scheduled throughout the state. At one point a bill was introduced into the legislature that would have limited the authority of the Board, but the bill failed and the work proceeded. The final assault to these changes was an injunction filed by two of the hospitals with diploma programs, alleging that the law authorizing the Board to establish standards for all nursing education programs was an unconstitutional delegation of legislative power to the Board. On January 8, 1987, the North Dakota Supreme Court issued its opinion on the case, which affirmed the delegation of standard setting by the legislature to the North Dakota Board of Nursing and allowed the Board to enforce the nursing education rules. All of the state's nursing programs, with the exception of the two programs involved in the lawsuit, had voluntarily begun working toward compliance with the new administrative code. Because the Nurse Practice Act was not changed, only the rules, it was not necessary to add a grandfather clause. Nurses already licensed are protected because the revised rules set an effective date of January 1, 1987.

Other states that had nurse practice acts that would allow for the changing of educational requirements for licensure through the rules process carefully watched the activities that were taking place in North Dakota. Some states had organized groups dedicated to protecting the role of the associate degree graduate. One such state was Oregon, which became the first to have a bill passed in the state legislature that would bar the state board of nursing from making any change in entry-level requirements without legislative approval. Utah and Pennsylvania were to follow.[13,14]

Other Nurses' Associations and the Entry Issue

Gradually, other nursing specialty groups and associations have endorsed the baccalaureate degree as minimum preparation for entry into professional nursing practice. Among the first organizations to support the position was the National Student Nurses' Association, who voted in favor of this at their convention in 1976.

The Association of Operating Room Nurses (AORN) endorsed the baccalaureate degree as the minimum educational level for future entry into professional practice at the AORN Congress in March 1979; however, members did not support the ANA concept of two catagories of nursing practice. It was their belief that *one* level of entry, the baccalaureate degree, would promote a clear, unified, coordinated educational thrust for the future. They also believed that one level of entry would eliminate confusion about the nurse's role.

At an annual meeting of the Emergency Department Nurses' Association, held in October 1979, this group announced their formal support of the ANA resolution. The Association of Rehabilitation Nurses also supported the statement, as did the American Association of Occupational Health Nurses.

In December of 1979 the executive board of the Nurses' Association of the American College of Obstetricians and Gynecologists voted to support the move toward the baccalaureate degree in nursing being the minimum preparation for entry into professional nursing practice, provided that nursing address certain specific issues collectively. Included among these issues were concerns that currently licensed RNs and LPNs not be penalized by the move, that concepts of levels of nursing practice be clarified, that regional planning ensure availability and accessibility to baccalaureate degree programs, and that the heads of career mobility programs for diploma and associate degree graduates seeking the baccalaureate degree consider previous education and experience when awarding credit.

As time passed, more and more groups considered, debated, and supported the ANA position on entry into professional practice. In addition to the organizations mentioned earlier, the following nursing groups have taken positions supporting the baccalaureate degree as the educational requirement for professional practice:

American Association of Colleges of Nursing

American Association of Critical-Care Nurses

American Association of Nephrology Nurses and Technicians

American Association of Occupational Health Nurses

American Public Health Association/Public Health Nurse Division

Association of Rehabilitation Nurses

American Association of Nurse Anesthetists: Council on Accreditation of Nurse Anesthesia Educational Programs/Schools

National Association of Pediatric Nurse Associates and Practitioners

Oncology Nursing Society[15]

Two other significant nursing organizations, the American Organization of Nurse Executives (AONE) and the National League for Nursing (NLN), have taken positions supporting the baccalaureate. At its October 1986 annual meeting the AONE, a personal membership group of the American Hospital Association (AHA) composed of the chief nursing executives in hospitals, approved a "Position Statement on Educational Preparation for Nursing Practice." This statement recognized baccalaureate education in nursing as the basic preparation for professional practice as well as two levels of preparation, baccalaureate and associate degree. They also supported separate licensure processes; standardization among states of titles; and, to ensure adequate provision of nursing care during the transitional period, the establishment of a grandfather clause. The position taken by this group departs from that taken by their parent organization, the AHA, which continues its support for all three types of programs of nursing education: associate, diploma, and baccalaureate, while believing that a baccalaureate degree should be an attainable goal for each student and practicing nurse in or from an associate or diploma program.[16]

Of particular significance is the change in position of the second major nursing organization mentioned above. Historically, because the composition of the membership of the NLN includes educational councils representing practical, diploma, associate degree, and baccalaureate and higher-degree nursing preparation, the organization has voiced its support for all types of programs. A 1981 Position Statement on Preparation for Practice in Nursing affirmed its support for all programs, citing the "social reality" of different types of people seeking careers in nursing as its rationale. However, beginning in 1982, that position has changed. First, the Board of Directors approved a *Position Statement on Nursing Roles: Scope and Preparation.* Although supporting three levels of nursing (professional, technical, and vocational), it stated that "professional nursing practice requires a minimum of a baccalaureate degree with a major in nursing."[17] Many of the members of NLN, especially those from the Diploma Council, strongly objected to this position. However, it was supported by a vote of the membership at the 1983 convention. In response to concerns expressed by the Council of Associate Degree Programs in 1984, the NLN Board of Directors reaffirmed its support for the current system of licensure.

In October of 1985 the Board of Directors again moved the NLN toward a position change. They approved a motion that stated "NLN supports two levels of nursing practice, professional and associate. Further, NLN supports the councils working closely with ANA cabinets to help define the scope and practice of nurses within these levels."[18] After publication of this motion many members of NLN were up in arms, particularly those in the Council of Associate Degree Programs. They perceived the statement as paralleling that of ANA. Perhaps this one action gave more impetus to the development of the National Organization of the Advancement of Associate Degree Nursing than any other (see Chapter 12). In October of 1986, pressured by community colleges and from members of its four councils, the NLN Board sought a compromise position on entry. The proposal, a "trial balloon" as opposed to a position statement, would be sent to membership for discussion and feedback. It recommended that the titled "registered associate nurse" be used for graduates of associate degree and diploma programs and that baccalaureate and post-baccalaureate graduates be titled "registered professional nurse." It further called for "separate" examinations for the two levels of graduates. At the 1987 biennial convention, the membership "postponed indefinitely" resolutions addressing this issue.[19]

Discussion of the entry issue would not be complete without including decisions made by two other organizations. One of those organizations is the National Council of State Boards of Nursing. At an August 1986 meeting, representatives of the state boards voted without debate and opposition to take a "formal position of neutrality on changes in nursing education requirements for entry."[20]

The final group we will consider is the National Federation of Licensed Practical Nurses (NFLPN). This organization, faced with hospital layoffs of large numbers of practical nurses in favor of hiring more highly educated registered nurses, voted in August of 1984 to increase the length of study of the practical nurse program to 18 months and to award an associate degree at the completion of the program of study. It was the intent of the motion that much of the increased time would be spent in increasing clinical expertise and the written rationale for the resolutions was openly one of job security. The title of licensed practical nurse would be retained for graduates of such programs who had passed the National Council Licensure Examination for practical nursing (NCLEX-PN).[21] Three years later only one state had moved toward implementation, but the NFLPN continues to support this position. Because a large number of practical nurse programs exist in vocational-technical schools, the recommendation of ANA to place all nursing education in institutions of higher education remains unacceptable to the practical nurse group. They emphasize the critical need for the practical nurse in long-term care facilities.

PROBLEMS ASSOCIATED WITH IMPLEMENTATION OF THE ANA POSITION STATEMENT

A number of problems need to be resolved before the ANA position statement can become a reality.

Titling

One of the most controversial problems is that of titles. Although the position statement calls for two levels of nursing practice, the titles to be used by persons working at each level have not been identified by many states. Some state associations have incorporated titles into their position statements, generally using the title "RN" for the baccalaureate graduate and "LPN" for the 2-year associate degree graduate. This has caused widespread dissatisfaction among the ranks of associate degree graduates, students, and educators who believe that this denigrates the associate degree graduate, who currently may use the RN title if successful on state licensing examinations. The use of these titles is also upsetting to graduates of current diploma schools, from which no degree is granted. It would seem that neither title could be used by those graduates.

Following the decision of the ANA to title the associate degree graduate "associate nurse" and the NLN's suggestion to designate the title "registered associate nurse" to the 2-year graduate, there has been activity in some states to use those titles. Staunch supporters of associate degree education are not willing to make this compromise, arguing that since the beginning of the associate degree movement in the 1950s, the graduates have held the title "registered nurse." In supporting their stand on titling they point to the past success of the associate degree graduates on the NCLEX-RN.

Scope of Practice

Of equal concern to the issue of titling is that which relates to the description and delineation of the scope of practice for the two levels of caregivers. The scope of practice, as discussed in Chapter 4, is that section of the nurse practice act that outlines the activities a person with that license legally may do. As states have moved toward plans for implementing two levels of practice, the process of making nursing diagnoses and developing nursing care plans has been included in the scope of practice of the professional nurse only. Associate degree educators have been adamant in their contention that unless the scope of practice for the 2-year graduate also includes these behaviors, that graduate will be unemployable and able to do less than the LPN of today.[22]

The Grandfather Clause

Historically, the licensing of professions and occupations has been within the realm of the police power of each individual state. This power to license is used to safeguard the health and welfare of citizens. When a state licensure law is enacted, or if a current law is repealed and a new law enacted, the *grandfather clause* has been a standard feature that allows persons to continue to practice their profession or occupation after new qualifications that they might not meet have been enacted into law. The legal basis for the process is found in the Fourteenth Amendment to the U.S. Constitution, which says that no state may deprive any person of life, liberty, or property without due process of law. The Supreme Court has ruled that the license to practice is a property right.

The use of the grandfather clause in nursing is by no means a new process. For example, it was not until the mid-1950s that theoretical and practical experience in psychiatric nursing was required in all nursing curricula and that psychiatric content was included in state licensing examinations. When laws changed to make this a requirement, hundreds of practicing nurses had never had a formal course in psychiatric nursing and had not been required to write a psychiatric examination to qualify for licensure. The right of these nurses to continue to be licensed, and thus to practice their profession, was protected by a grandfather clause. (Some of these nurses are still practicing today without the psychiatric experience.)

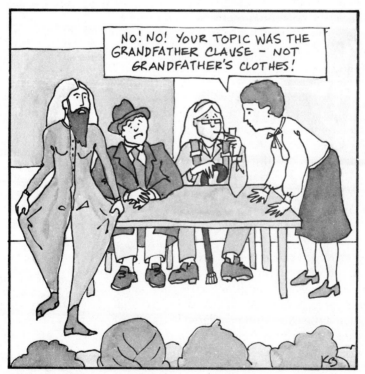

Figure 3–2. When a state licensure law is enacted or if a current law is repealed, the grandfather clause has been a standard feature that allows persons to continue to practice their profession.

When applied to the entry-into-practice issue, the grandfather clause would guarantee registered nurses who had been educated in associate degree or diploma programs before the date of any changes that would require a baccalaureate degree for registered nurse licensure the right to continue to be licensed and practice as registered nurses as long as their practice was safe. As an example of the application of the process, let us assume that changes in a state's licensure laws to require a baccalaureate degree as the minimum educational preparation for registered nurse licensure became effective June 1, 1990. After June 1, 1990, diploma and associate degree graduates would be licensed as *technical nurses.* All associate degree and diploma graduates licensed before June 1, 1990 would be considered *registered nurses,* as protected by the grandfather clause. Some people believe that the entry-into-practice resolutions would not have passed in state conventions without the assurance of a grandfather clause. Some voting delegates seemed more concerned "how will this affect me, personally" than about the impact of the resolution on nursing as a whole.

The grandfather clause is limited to the protection of a nurse's license. Additional qualifications can be established for certain jobs for RNs, and these are not included in nurse practice acts. For example, many head nurses, supervisors, and directors of nursing service are currently working in these positions with associate degree and diploma preparation only. Qualifications could be written that would require the minimum of a baccalaureate degree to work in the capacity of a head nurse, supervisor, or director of nursing service. Similar actions have already occurred with regard to qualifications for teachers in nursing schools, in which requirements have changed from a baccalaureate degree to a master's degree and, in some instances, to doctoral preparation. Similarly, changes have occurred in the educational preparation required of persons working in community health and school nurse positions.

Some nurses believe that the grandfather clause should be conditional. If it were conditional, persons licensed before the changes in the licensure law would continue to use their current title for a stipulated period, for example, 10 years. At the end of that period, if they had not completed the education mandated in the changes (or any other conditions that might have been added), they would have to use the title proscribed in the new law for persons with their educational preparation. Because of the complexity and the questionable legal status of the issue, there is little likelihood that conditional grandfathering will occur.

Interstate Endorsement

Another concern expressed over licensure changes is related to interstate endorsement or reciprocity for licensure among states. Nursing is one of the few professions to have developed a process by which national examinations with standardized scores are administered in each state or jurisdiction. This allows a nurse who has passed the licensing examination in one state to move to another state and seek licensure in that state, without the need to retake and pass the examination in the state to which the nurse is moving. Because nurses have been highly mobile, this has been a great advantage to many. As states move toward making changes in their practice acts, it is hoped that the movement will be similar across the nation so that interstate endorsement can be maintained without requiring re-examination.

Competency Expectations

A final and significant concern is the task of describing and differentiating the competencies and the scope of practice of the two levels of nursing specified in the ANA's position paper. Once these two levels of nursing are identified and described, different licensing mechanisms could be put into place. Graduates of baccalaureate nursing programs and graduates of 2-year associate degree programs currently write the same licensing examination for practice as a registered nurse. To suggest that the educational background provided in 4-year programs and that provided in 2-year programs is so similar in outcome as not to require separate expectations of the graduates seems faulty. It fails to recognize the broad range of functions in nursing and the potential for improving the quality of care that can be given to those needing that care. Because 2-year graduates are currently demonstrating success on the licensing examinations, it might also be suggested that the current licensing examinations are not testing those skills that the ANA would categorize as professional. Little differentiation of skill is required in beginning staff nurse positions.

Some work has been done toward describing the competencies of graduates of the different programs in nursing. In 1978 the NLN published *Competencies of the Associate Degree Graduate on Entry into Practice.* In 1979 an NLN Task Force presented a working paper on competencies of graduates of nursing programs that included descriptions of practical, associate degree, diploma, and baccalaureate graduates. This paper has now been published as *Competencies of Graduates of Nursing Programs;* however, these statements are largely theoretical. Many of the statements, especially those of the baccalaureate graduate, call for intellectual processes of critical decision making. These processes may be difficult to measure because they may be evidenced only when used inappropriately or not used at all. The need for realistic statements regarding competencies of each level or category of nursing are necessary so that appropriate testing can be developed, and so that each category can be used effectively and efficiently within the health care delivery system. Validated competencies will also provide a basis for the development of curriculum patterns that will ensure adequate preparation of each category of caregiver without running the risk of overeducation or undereducation at any one level. It can also serve as a foundation for the development of educational mobility patterns within the profession.

In 1982 two projects sponsored by the Midwest Alliance in Nursing were started. One, titled "Defining and Differentiating ADN and BSN Competencies, and Facilitating ADN Competency Development" was funded by the W. K. Kellogg Foundation. The second, titled "Continuing Education for Consensus on Entry Skills," was funded by a grant from the Division of Nursing of the Department of Health and Human Services. The goal of these studies was to achieve a regional consensus among nursing service persons and educators from both types of programs on differentiated statements of scope of practice for each level of graduate.

In 1986 the National Council of State Boards of Nursing published a study conducted for that organization by the American College Testing Program. The purpose of this study, titled "A Study of Nursing Practice and Role Delineation and Job Analysis of Entry-Level Performance of Registered Nurses," was to validate the NCLEX-RN. Five major areas were examined: role delineation, the influence of the setting, the transition from entry level practice to practice beyond entry level for registered nurses, the differences in RN practice as a function of education, and evaluation of the NCLEX-RN test plan. In looking at the role delineation, 17 categories of activities were identified. The study found that there was a high degree of consensus in nursing about the criticality of nursing activities (*i.e.*, which activities may sometimes be omitted and which can never be omitted). It further indicated that the specific setting strongly influenced the activities that occurred, that first-line managers were consistent in indicating that the transition time for a new graduate is about 6 months, and that the influence of educational background on the practice patterns of newly licensed registered nurses was not as great as one might expect. New baccalaureate graduates showed a greater tendency to be involved in some type of research activities than did new diploma and associate degree graduates, but on all other types of activities that were studied, no substantial differences were found.[23]

CHANGES IN NURSES' EDUCATION

Although we hold no claim to a crystal ball that would help foresee the changes needed in the education of the nurse of the future, enough evidence of change, or the need for it, is already present to alert us to the need for different approaches and perhaps different directions. Some modifications in traditional nurse education have already occurred. Outreach programs, which take the educational program to the student rather than requiring the student to come to the college, have been started in many parts of the country. These have been particularly useful in helping to meet the needs of the registered nurse seeking baccalaureate preparation.

Cable television and video instruction have extended the perimeter of the classroom. The use of television in the classroom and in the practice laboratory has already proved to be an effective and efficient method to extend the ability of one instructor to assist many students. Videotaped demonstrations eliminate the need for tedious repetitions of basic procedures for small groups. Students can view videotapes at their own convenience and can use videotaped playbacks to assess their own skills, freeing the instructor for other instructional activities.

Studies have been conducted that look at the characteristics of the person who wants to pursue a career in nursing. As a result of some of the information gained in these studies, programs have been designed that address the needs of the adult learner, rather than fashion all educational patterns toward the recent high school graduate. Programs that permit part-time study, and thereby allow the student to work while attending school, have also been developed. Classes that traditionally were conducted during peak morning hours are being moved to late afternoon hours or to weekends to appeal to and meet the needs of the working student. Remedial classes in basic mathematics, grammar, study skills, or English as a second language have been made available to students who may not have had the same educational opportunity as others.

Self-instructional modules have, in some instances, replaced the traditional lecture, and the whole area of computerized instruction is being developed in nursing education. Instruction in the use of the computer itself has been included in the curriculum pattern for many nursing programs. A questionnaire was distributed to all nursing education programs by NLN in 1984. Ninety-one percent of the nursing programs reported that at least a few faculty had attended or participated in computer-oriented classes or workshops during 1983–84. However, at that time few programs felt that either their recent graduates or their current students would be able to apply computer technology in practice.[24] Today we are beginning to see students who come to nursing education well equipped to address the concept of computer literacy. Many hospitals have completely computerized charting systems. The development of computer software in nursing education exceeds one's ability to know all the alternatives to instruction. Computer science is no longer a foreign language.

As nurses recognize the need to become more political to bring about the changes they see as necessary in the health care delivery system, courses will need to be developed that will provide the necessary

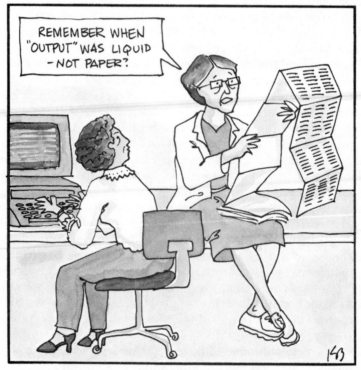

Figure 3–3. As hospitals, like other industries, put the computer to work in their agencies, the new graduate will be forced to have a beginning understanding of computer language and the operation of the machines.

information to allow the nurse to function in this new political role. Politics requires learning about power, a term some nurses want to reject as being incompatible with the aims of the profession. Kalisch and Kalisch have defined power as "the ability to affect something or to be affected by something. Power means the capacity to alter behavior."[25] Nurses, because they offer critically needed services, possess much potential power but need a basic understanding of how to make use of that potential to bring about desired change. As the nurse assumes a stronger patient advocacy role, she or he must possess better understanding of the social system, policy formation and implementation, the legislative process, lobbying, and political mobilization. Many programs have made a step in this direction by including courses in assertive behavior in their nursing curricula, but this is only a beginning.

Some nurses see themselves functioning as independent practitioners or in joint practices. This role requires additional understanding of business management and economics and a knowledge of advanced clinical skills. Alternative health care providers will find themselves in a competitive system. Escalating medical costs may mean that as a nation, we need to modify our concepts of health care delivery so that it responds to the needs of persons in all economic strata.

REDUCED FEDERAL FUNDING

One of the gravest problems facing nursing education today is that of funding. In 1964, through the Nurse Training Act (NTA), $238 million was authorized for the advancement of nursing education, and $4.6 million was authorized to administer the programs. The programs, five in all, included construction of nursing facilities, improvement of teaching, continuation of traineeship programs that reimbursed students for advancing their nursing education, provision of loans to nursing students, and monies specifically set aside to improve instruction in hospital-based schools. This act was responsive to the recognized shortage of trained health personnel. In 1963 the Consultant Group on Nursing in their final report, *Toward Quality in Nursing*, estimated that we would need 130,000 more nurses in 1970 than were available in 1960. This would mean that nursing schools would need to increase their graduates by 75 percent. The consultants also urged an increase in the number of nurses with graduate degrees and baccalaureate degrees, and an increase in the number of LPNs.

In the years immediately following the passage of the NTA, many schools and students were to benefit from these funds. When the NTA reached expiration in 1969, the Health Manpower Act continued most of NTA's programs. The 1971 NTA, which followed, authorized the largest expenditure of funds for nursing in the history of the country — $855 million. After that period the federal funding for nursing saw a constant decrease. The $160 million appropriated in 1973 dropped to $145 million in 1974. Congress enacted the 1975 NTA but authorized only $553 million for the entire 3-year period the act would be in effect. This bill was vetoed by the president but was saved when Congress overrode the veto.

Each of the last four Presidents of the United States, both Republican and Democrat, believed that the nurse shortage had ended. They also contended that nursing students could apply for the federal aid made available to students in general (*e.g.*, basic educational grants). All four thought that the amount of money allocated to nursing education was "excessive."

In 1979 Congress again was able to extend the NTA for 1 more year, with funding at $103 million. By 1983 the appropriations were cut to $48.9 million.

As funding was reduced, the purposes for which the funds were made available also changed. Fewer dollars were made available for the basic education of nursing students. Emphasis was placed on funding advanced training for nurses and the preparation of nurse practitioners. Funds were also available for nursing research. Student loans were continued, but the total amount was reduced and "forgiveness clauses," which required the student to repay only part of the loan if he or she became actively involved in nursing on graduation, were eliminated. At the same time tuition costs sharply increased. Capitation funding, which provided money to schools based on student enrollment, was eliminated.

We are only beginning to feel the impact of the loss of these dollars and will be unable to judge their effect on the profession of nursing until a few more years have passed. Capitation funds were often used by schools to provide time and reimbursement for curriculum work. These funds also were used to provide equipment for skills laboratories. They were used to send faculty to workshops in which they could learn more about curriculum and improve their skills as instructors. The funds might also have been used to pay for consultants who could help a faculty in the development of a sound program of study for the students. In some cases capitation monies were used to fund the cost of accreditation of the nursing program by the NLN. Such NLN accreditation attests to the quality of a particular program. Capitation funds might have been used to maintain agency membership in the NLN or in regional groups (*e.g.*, the Western Institute of Nursing).

We will not know how seriously these cuts will affect nursing programs for another 5 years. It is reasonable to assume that some of the time and money put into curriculum development will stop, which is regrettable in light of the changes being absorbed by nursing today. Some schools may decide that they cannot afford to be nationally accredited. Professional development of faculty may decrease because each faculty member will have to assume the cost of that development personally. All of these items have far-reaching effects on the quality of a program.

Nursing education is notorious for its costs. Equipment required to educate nursing students is expensive. Because student learning also requires hands-on experience within hospital settings, student-teacher ratios must be low. Although 100 or more students may be assigned to a psychology class taught by one instructor, it is impossible for a nursing instructor to guide more than 8 to 12 students safely in an acute care facility in which students are giving total patient care.

Nursing schools often used federal dollars to help offset the high cost of nursing education to a particular institution. Without those dollars many schools are cutting back on their programs by taking fewer students and hiring fewer faculty members. In some instances entire programs have been closed. It will be a challenge to nurses to continue working for the funding of nursing education and research in the future while at the same time being responsive to the economic situation of the nation.

Many people in nursing today are concerned that we will experience a serious nursing shortage in the 1990s. Historically, serious nurse shortages have spurred the investment of federal dollars into nursing education. The need for more nurses during World War II resulted in the nurse cadet program. Shortages of the 1950s resulted in the Nurse Training Act. If the shortage that is being predicted materializes, federal dollars may become available once again.

NURSING THEORIES

One of the innovations in nursing that has been receiving increasing emphasis, and will undoubtedly continue to do so, is nursing theory. The curriculum design of the nursing program in which you are enrolled may be based on concepts outlined by a particular nursing theorist. Perhaps one of the hospitals to which you are assigned for clinical experience also uses the principles of a nursing theory to structure the delivery of care.

A theory is a "scientifically acceptable general principle which governs practice or is proposed to explain observed facts."[26] Because nursing as a developing profession is seriously involved in research on which to build a sound body of nursing knowledge, theories are valuable to us. They provide the bases for hypotheses about nursing practice. They make it possible for us to derive a sound rationale for the actions we take. If the theories are testable, they will then allow us to build our knowledge base and to guide and improve nursing practice. Explained in the words of Barbara Stevens:

> A nursing theory . . . attempts to describe or explain the phenomenon called nursing. A theory is always a shorthand way to understand or characterize a phenomenon. It points out those components or characteristics that give the phenomenon its identity. It pulls out the salient parts of a phenomenon so that one can separate the critical and necessary factors (or relationships) from the accidental and unessential factors (or relationships).[27]

She goes on to describe a theory as a map whose purpose is "to give one a handle on the phenomenon with which it deals." Most nursing theories are developed around a combination of concepts. Among those concepts, four subject areas usually are included; an approach to the total person, an approach to health-illness, an approach to the environment (or society), and an approach to nursing.

Today there are many published nursing theories. In an attempt to structure and organize those theories, various authors have categorized or classified theories. Not all are classified similarly. Included are general classifications such as the art and science of humanistic nursing, interpersonal relationships, systems, and energy fields.[28] Others include groupings that include growth and development theories, systems theories, stress adaptation theories, and rhythm theories.[29]

Some examples of growth and development theories that are mentioned and with which you are probably familiar are those of Maslow, Erikson, Kohlberg, Piaget, and Freud. Most basic nursing texts incorporate a discussion of the concepts developed by these theorists. The theories are so named because they focus on the developing person. They have the common characteristic of arranging this development in terms of stages through which a person must pass to reach a particular level of development. From a nursing standpoint they allow us to monitor the progress through the various stages and evaluate the appropriateness of that progress. You will recognize Maslow for his approach to self-actualization, Erikson for his psychosocial development, Kohlberg for his theories of moral reasoning, Piaget for his approach to cognitive

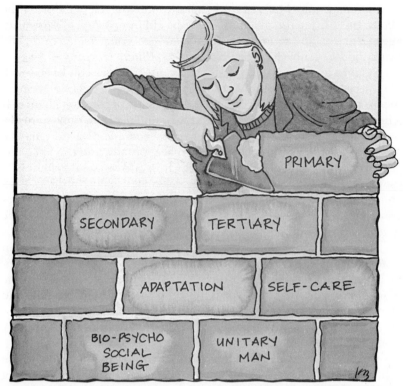

Figure 3–4. Nursing is in the process of building a body of scientific knowledge.

development, and Freud for psychosexual theories on which medicine would later base the school of psychoanalysis. These theories are not truly theories of nursing, however, because they were not developed for the purpose of explaining, testing, and changing the practice of nursing. They represent some of the "borrowed" knowledge around which we build our profession.

Theories that speak to the art and science of humanistic nursing were the earliest purely nursing theories developed. Some authors have looked back at the contributions of Florence Nightingale and have included her in that grouping. Among the others are Virginia Henderson and her *Definition of Nursing,* Faye Abdellah and the *Twenty-one Nursing Problems,* Lydia Hall and her *Core Care and Cure Model,* and Madeleine Leininger's *Transcultural Care Theory.*

Interpersonal relationships theories deal with interactions between and among people. Many of these theories were developed during the 1960s. Included in this grouping could be Hildegard Peplau's *Psychodynamic Nursing*, Joyce Travelbee's *Human-to-Human Relationship*, and Ernestine Wiedenbach's *The Helping Art of Clinical Nursing*.

Systems theories are so classified because they are concerned with the interactions between and among all the factors in a situation. A system is usually viewed as complex and in a state of constant change. It is defined as a whole with interrelated parts and may be a subsystem of a larger system as well as a suprasystem. For example, a person may be viewed as a system composed of cells, tissue, organs, and the like. The person is a subsystem of a family, which in turn is a subsystem of a community. In a systems approach the person is usually considered as a "total" being, or from a "whole" being point of view. Systems theories also provide for "input" into the system and "feedback" within the system. The systems approach was popular during the 1970s.

Stress adaptation models are based on concepts that view the person as adjusting or changing (adapting) in order to avoid situations (stressors) that would result in the disturbance of balance or equilibrium. The adaptation theory helps to explain how the balance is maintained, and therefore points the direction for nursing actions. Included in this group one often finds Sister Callista Roy's *Adaptation Model* and Betty Neuman's work, but both may also be considered systems models.

One of the latest classifications of theories is by energy fields. These theories, although they may have been started earlier, have been a product of the 1980s. Included in this group are the works of such persons as Myra Levine, Joyce Fitzpatrick, Margaret Newman, and Martha Rogers.

It is not our purpose to discuss and critique all the many approaches to nursing theory. The student who wants to pursue nursing theorists further is encouraged to consult the section on further reading at the end of the chapter. A brief discussion of four of the major nursing theorists today follows.

Sister Callista Roy. This model is organized around concepts that describe how a person can adapt behavior to allow him or her to deal (cope) with stimuli from the environment that are stressors. Stressors disrupt the dynamic state of equilibrium and result in illness. Four adaptive modes, or ways in which a person adapts, are identified: through physiological needs, self-concept, role function, and interdependence relations. Nursing's role is to assess a patient's adaptive behaviors and the stimuli that may be affecting him or her and manipulate the stimuli in such a way as to allow the patient to cope.

Dorothea Orem. This model has a goal of "constancy" for the person and speaks to the concept of self-care. Self-care is the person's own action that has pattern and sequence and, when effectively performed, contributes to the way he or she develops and functions. Nursing's role is to help the person meet the self-care requisites thereby limiting self-care deficits.

Betty Neuman. Identified as a health care systems model, this approach to nursing is organized around stress reduction. It is primarily concerned with the effects of stress and the reactions to stress and the development and maintenance of health, and therefore also speaks to maintaining equilibrium. The person deals with stressors through "lines of defense" and is protected from stressors through "lines of resistance." Nursing's role is focused on reduction of stress factors and through prevention that is "primary, secondary, or tertiary."

Martha Rogers. Known as the science of unitary man, the essence of this model is the assumption that the person is a unified energy field that is continually interacting and exchanging matter and energy with the environment. These exchanges result in increasing complexity and innovativeness of the person. Health and illness are not viewed as separate states. Nursing's role is to repattern human beings and environment in order to achieve maximum health potential. This model has been used by the North American Nursing Diagnosis Association [NANDA] in developing the nursing diagnosis taxonomy and the language used within that taxonomy. However, the group substituted the term "human response patterns" for the more unfamiliar "patterns of unitary man."

CONCLUSION

Changes occur in our society almost faster than we can adjust to them. Technical advances have fueled an information explosion. The economy hits peaks and suffers setbacks. Life expectancy increases. Innovations occur in the delivery of health care, but the cost of that care continues to increase. Medical advances make it possible to save many lives that would have been lost a decade ago. Nursing education must be responsive to all of these. Curriculum patterns need to be scrutinized to assure that nursing programs prepare their graduates appropriately for roles in the health care delivery system. Those roles themselves need to be more clearly defined and delineated. Nursing educators will also need to be responsive to new innovations in our society and incorporate these into the teaching methods. Perhaps the biggest challenge to nursing education will be accomplishing all of the above while at the same time adjusting to severe cuts in federal funding to nursing programs.

REFERENCES

1. Brown EL: Nursing for the Future. New York, Russell Sage Foundation, 1948
2. Hanson HC: Supplemental Report. In Proceedings of the Forty-Second Convention (May 2–6, 1960) of the American Nurses' Association, p 54. New York, The Association, 1960
3. Reiter F: Supplemental Report. In Proceedings of the Forty-Fourth Convention (June 15–19, 1964) of the American Nurses' Association, p 49. New York, The Association, 1964
4. American Nurses' Association's First Position on Nursing Education. Am J Nurs 65:106, Dec 1965
5. American Nurses' Association's First Position on Nursing Education. Am J Nurs 65:107, Dec 1965
6. A Case for Baccalaureate Preparation in Nursing. American Nurses' Association Commission on Nursing Education Pub. No. NE–6 ANS, pp 5–7. Kansas City, American Nurses' Association, 1979
7. ANA votes federation. Am J Nurs 82:1251, Aug 1982
8. ANA gears up new drive for entry level change: Despite opposition, some SNAs see success soon. Am J Nurs 85:194, Feb 1985
9. ANA delegates vote to limit RN title to BSN grad; "associate nurse" wins vote for technical level. Am J Nurs 85:1016, 1017, 1020, 1022, 1024, 1025, Sep 1985
10. Stand on BSN taken by 34 state associations. Am J Nurs 80:582, 624, 628, Apr 1980
11. Edge S: State positions on titling and licensure. In Looking Beyond the Entry Issue: Implications for Education and Service, Publication No 41-2173, p 129. New York, National League for Nursing, 1986
12. North Dakota rule changes require associate, baccalaureate education. Issues 7 (2):1–3, 1986
13. ADNs, community college bar entry-level change in Oregon. Am J Nurs 85:921, 923, Aug 1985
14. Pennsylvania legislature bars change in entry rules. Am J Nurs 87:113, 126, Jan 1987
15. Hartung D: Organizational positions on titling and entry into practice: A chronology. In Looking Beyond the Entry Issue: Implications for Education and Service, Publication No 41-2173, p 122. New York, National League for Nursing, 1986
16. Hartung D: Organizational positions on titling and entry into practice: A chronology. In Looking Beyond the Entry Issue: Implications for Educa-

tion and Service, Publication No 41-2173, p 123. New York, National League for Nursing, 1986

17. NLN calls for baccalaureate preparation for professional nursing practice. Nurs Health Care 3 (3):154, Mar 1982

18. Board supports move to two levels of nursing practice. Nurs Health Care 6 (10):521, Dec 1985

19. Directors focus on entry related issues; titling and licensure proposal to go to membership. Nurs Health Care 7 (10):560, Dec 1986

20. Hartung D: Organizational positions on titling and entry into practice: A chronology. In Looking Beyond the Entry Issue: Implications for Education and Service, Publication No 41-2173, p 124. New York, National League for Nursing, 1986

21. NFLPN oks "two nursing levels" 18 month curriculum for LPNs. Am J Nurs 84:1303, 1312, 1314, Oct 1984

22. Illinois RNs seek compromise on scope of practice. Am J Nurs 86:77, 84, 90, Jan 1986

23. A Study of Nursing Practice and Role Delineation and Job Analysis of Entry Level Performance of Registered Nurses. Chicago, National Council of State Boards of Nursing, 1986

24. Gothler AM: Nursing education update: Computer technology. Nurs Health Care 6 (9):509–510, Nov 1985

25. Kalisch BJ, Kalisch P: Politics of Nursing, pp 1,2. Philadelphia, JB Lippincott, 1982

26. Riehl JP, Roy SC: Conceptual Models for Nursing Practice, p 3. New York, Appleton-Century-Crofts, 1974

27. Stevens BJ: Nursing Theory: Analysis, Application, Evaluation, 2nd ed, p 1. Boston, Little, Brown, 1984

28. Marriner A: Nursing Theorists and Their Work. St. Louis, CV Mosby, 1986

29. Leddy S, Pepper JM: Conceptual Bases of Professional Nursing, p 117. Philadelphia, JB Lippincott, 1985

FURTHER READINGS

ADN "mavericks" found national group to fight title change. Am J Nurs 86:79, 82, Jan 1986

A first for the nation: North Dakota and entry into nursing practice. Nurs Health Care 7 (3):135–141, Mar 1986

AHA, RN Execs go separate way on entry. Am J Nurs 86:1421, Dec 1986

Brower HT: Potential advantages and hazards of non-traditional education for nurses. Nurs Health Care 3 (5):268–272, May 1982

Bullough VL, Bullough B: The Emergence of Modern Nursing. New York, Macmillan, 1969

Christ T: Entry into practice: A recurring issue in nursing history. Am J Nurs 80:485–488, Mar 1980

Dakota nurses aim to be first to act on entry. Am J Nurs 86:76, 83, Jan 1986

Felton G: Harnessing today's trends to guide nursing's future. Nurs Health Care 7 (4):211–213, Apr 1986

Fighting odds, NFLPN seeks 18-month curriculum. Am J Nurs 86:1420, 1428, Dec 1986

Fitzpatrick JJ, Whall AL: Conceptual Models of Nursing: Analysis and Application. Bowie, Md, Robert J Brady Co, 1983

George JB (ed): Nursing Theories: The Base for Professional Nursing Practice. The Nursing Theories Conference Group. 2nd ed. Englewood Cliffs, NJ, Prentice-Hall, 1985

Glick M: Educational entry level into nursing practice. J Contin Educ Nurs 16:185–188, Nov/Dec 1985

Illinois RNs brace for battle over entry-level bill. Am J Nurs 87:244, 247, Feb 1987

Johnston SC: The use of the Rines model in differentiating professional and technical nursing practice. Nurs Health Care 3 (8):374–379, Sep 1982

McCloskey JC: Nursing education and job effectiveness. Nurs Res 32:53–58, Jan/Feb 1983

Maine SNA: LPNs argue on entry: Now it's up to the legislature. Am J Nurs 86:326, 340, 342, 344, Mar 1986

Midwest schools pioneer "expanded" LPN program. Am J Nurs 86:1420, 1429, Dec 1986

NLN seeks compromise on entry: ADNs hold out for RN licensure. Am J Nurs 18:113, 124, 125, Jan 1987

NLN switches position, back two entry levels. Am J Nurs 86:78, 82, Jan 1986

Orem DE: Nursing: Concepts of Practice. 2nd ed. New York, McGraw-Hill, 1980

Primm PL: Entry into practice: Competency statements for BSNs and ADNs. Nurs Outlook 34:135–137, May/Jun 1986

Roy SC, Roberts SL: Theory Construction in Nursing: An Adaptation Model. Englewood Cliffs, NJ, Prentice-Hall, 1981

Schoen D: A study of nurses' attitudes toward the BSN requirement. Nurs Health Care 3 (8):382–387, Sep 1982

Smullen BB: Second-step education for R.N.s. Nurs Health Care 3 (8): 369–373, Sep 1982

State Boards declare "neutral stance" in entry-level debate. Am J Nurs 86:1180, Oct 1986

Stull MK: Entry skills for BSNs. Nurs Outlook 34:138–139, May/Jun 1986

Torres G: Theoretical Foundations of Nursing. E Norwalk, Conn., Appleton-Century-Crofts, 1986

Trachtenberg SJ: What universities will be like in the year 2000. Phi Delta Kappan 64:327–330, Jan 1983

WV legislators block board's move to boost entry standards. Am J Nurs 86:326, 344, Mar 1986

Unit II
Legal and Ethical Accountability for Practice

4

Credentials for Nursing Practice

Objectives

After completing this chapter, you should be able to

1. Outline the history of nursing licensure.
2. Differentiate between **permissive** and **mandatory licensure** for nursing.
3. State those factors that contributed to uniformity in nursing education across the country.
4. Outline the role of the state board of nursing.
5. Discuss the content of the various sections of the Model Nurse Practice Act.
6. Define **certification**.
7. State the problems associated with certification in nursing.
8. Discuss the recommendations of the "Study of Credentialing in Nursing."

Credentials are proof, in writing, of qualifications. They communicate to others the nature of one's competence and can be used as a tool for evaluating one's ability to perform. There are many types of credentials, for example, diplomas, degrees, licenses, and certificates.

ESTABLISHING LICENSURE

Credentials were not always available for nurses. Before the Nightingale schools became prevalent in England and nursing schools were established in the United States, anyone could claim to be a nurse. Formally educated nurses and noneducated persons worked side by side to deliver care. A rudimentary means of differentiating between them was the certificate of completion that was issued by nursing schools to those who had completed a program of study in nursing.

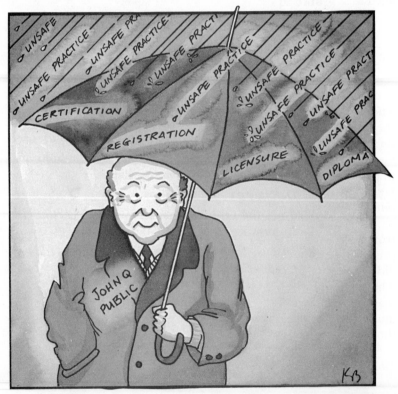

Figure 4–1. Various forms of credentialing assure the public of qualified care givers.

However, because the quality of education that was offered in the nursing schools differed widely — programs varied in length from 6 weeks to 3 years — it became apparent that a completion certificate was not an adequate guarantee of competence. Nursing leaders were concerned about the situation. They believed that the patient had no way to judge whether a given nurse's education was sound and often suffered from the quality of care administered by poorly prepared nurses.

In 1896 the Nurses' Associated Alumnae of the United States and Canada was created. (This organization later evolved into the American Nurses' Association [ANA].) One of the major concerns of the association was the establishment of a credentialing system that was firmly based in laws passed by a legislative body. This form of credential is called *licensure*. The route of legal licensing for credentialing was long and difficult. Nurses, legislators, and the public had to be educated about the value of legislation to govern the profession and to be encouraged to support it. Chart 4–1 is a chronology of nursing licensure.

Permissive Licensure

The ANA campaigned vigorously for the adoption of state licensure laws. These laws provided a voluntary process by which a nurse who met predetermined standards would be licensed to practice, and the license would be registered with the state. This is called *permissive licensure* because the person is "permitted" to be licensed if requirements are met. A nurse who was so licensed could legally call herself (there were virtually no male nurses at that time) a registered nurse. Under this system no one was required to have a license to practice nursing.

The standards for permissive licensure included (a) graduating from a school that satisfied certain requirements and (b) passing a comprehensive examination. A person who did not meet the legal standards did not receive a license and could not use the title registered nurse. The community benefited because there was an established credential that attested to a level of competence. The licensee profited in regard to job availability and salary if the community differentiated between those who were licensed and those who were not licensed.

The first laws providing for permissive licensure were passed in 1903 by North Carolina. By 1923 all the existing 48 states had permissive licensure laws. Alaska and Hawaii passed licensure laws while still territories and continued to recognize these laws when they became states.

Chart 4-1.   The History of Nursing Licensure

1867   Dr. Henry Wentworth Acland first suggested licensure for nurses in England.

1892   American Society of Superintendents of Training Schools for Nurses organized and supported licensure in the United States

1901   First nursing licensure in the world: New Zealand.

1903   First nursing licensure in the United States: North Carolina, New Jersey, New York, and Virginia (in that order).

1915   ANA drafted its first model nurse practice act.

1919   First nursing licensure in England.

1923   All 48 states had enacted nursing licensure laws.

1935   ANA endorsed mandatory licensure.

1938   First mandatory licensure act in the United States: New York (effective 1947).

1946   Ten states had definitions of nursing in the licensing act.

1950   First year the same examination used in all jurisdictions of the United States and its territories: State Board Test Pool Examination.

1965   Twenty-one states had definitions of nursing in the licensing act.

1971   First state to recognize expanded practice in the nursing practice act: Idaho.

1976   First mandatory continuing education for relicensure: California.

1983   Change to nursing process format examination: National Council Licensure Examination for Registered Nurses (NCLEX-RN).

1986   First state to require baccalaureate degree for registered nurse and associate degree for licensed practical nurse: North Dakota (effective 1987).

Mandatory Licensure

After permissive licensure laws came into being, nurses' activity regarding licensure became less intense. There was still concern, however, that some persons were practicing nursing without having demon-

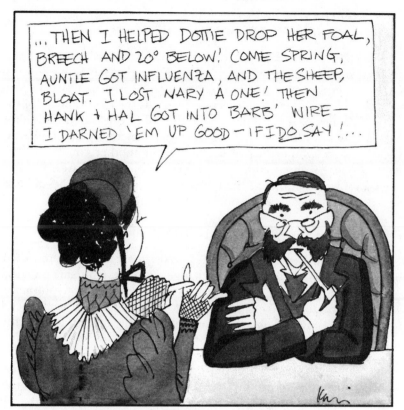

Figure 4-2. A standard credential makes hiring easier.

strated skill and knowledge. The majority of those functioning without licenses were nursing school graduates who had failed the licensing examinations. They were referred to as graduate nurses, as opposed to registered nurses. In addition, some nurses were employed who had been educated in foreign countries and did not meet the licensure requirements in the state in which they were residing.

To eliminate this situation and provide greater protection to the public, many nurses began to call for *mandatory licensure*, which requires that all those who wish to practice nursing meet the established standards and be licensed. The first mandatory licensure law took effect in New York State in 1947. Throughout the years additional states changed their laws relating to the practice of nursing and required licensure.

Concerns About Permissive and Mandatory Licensure

The continued existence of permissive licensure laws in Texas presents some problems to nurses practicing in that state. One concern is that patients are jeopardized by potentially lower-quality care. Another issue is that permissive licensure retards the development of the nursing profession as a whole because the public does not differentiate between those without an appropriate education and standard of practice and those who are more qualified. Still another concern is economic. Those without education and credentials often are willing to work for lower salaries, and this tends to hold down the salaries of those who do have formal preparation.

Enacting Licensure Legislation

During the late 1960s and the 1970s many states altered their nursing practice acts to reflect the changes in modern nursing practice. New legislation is usually initiated through the nurses' association at the instigation of the nursing community. The association may spend months preparing and planning the content of the bill and gaining the support of legislators.

The proposed law enters the legislative process through an elected member of the legislature. It must go through the entire committee, hearing, and voting procedure before it can become a law. During this process individuals and organizations may affect the content of the bill by influencing the legislators. The originators of the law may either support the proposed changes or favor the original content. For example, in 1974 in New York State a bill was introduced that would have changed the educational requirements for entry into practice to require a baccalaureate degree. During the legislative process changes were made in the bill that were acceptable to some original supporters but distressed others. The bill was defeated and the proposed changes in educational requirements did not become law.

Rules and Regulations

Each state has its own set of rules and regulations to carry out the provisions of the law regulating nursing. These rules and regulations are established by the administrative body, usually the board of nursing, which is given that responsibility by law. Most states require that public hearings be held in regard to the proposed rules and regulations, but the board has the authority to make the final decision. The rules and regulations must be within the scope outlined by the law. Those that are accepted by the appropriate board have the force of law unless they are challenged in court and are found to be not in accord with the law.

In some states the nursing practice act is detailed and specifies most of the critical provisions regarding licensure and practice. In other states the nursing practice act is broad, and the administrative body is given a great deal of power in making decisions through rules and regulations. One example of this difference is in the educational requirements for licensure. In some states the law specifies that a diploma, an associate degree, or a baccalaureate degree is an acceptable preparation for registered nursing. In those states, in order for the educational requirements to change, the law itself would have to be changed. In states where the educational requirement is established by the board of nursing through rules and regulations, as in North Dakota, changes can be made by the board without going through the legislative process. Thus it is important that you investigate both the actual nursing practice act and the rules and regulations governing nursing in your state.

Licensure Law Content

Early in the 1900s the ANA, as part of its leadership role in nursing licensure, formulated a model nurse practice act that could be used by state associations when planning legislation.[1] This model was revised in 1981 by the ANA Congress for Nursing Practice and a more up-to-date approach to nursing licensing legislation was published. A year later the National Council of State Boards of Nursing also developed a model nurse practice act.[2] Most state nurse practice acts have recently been rewritten to more accurately reflect modern-day nursing practice. Where this has not been done, revisions are being considered. We recommend that you carefully read the nurse practice act for the state in which you will be practicing. A copy of the act may be obtained from the state board of nursing (see Appendix A for addresses).

In some states one act covers both practical nursing and registered nursing, while other states have two separate, but similar, acts. The following general topics are usually covered in state licensure laws.

Purpose

The purpose of regulating the practice of nursing is twofold: to protect the public and to make the individual practitioner accountable for actions. Note that the protection of the status of the licensed individual is not the reason for licensure. With this in mind you can better understand the inclusion of some other topics in the act.

Definitions

All the significant terms in the act are defined for purposes of carrying out the law. This is where the legal definition of nursing is spelled out. The ANA model act suggests the following:

> The practice of nursing means: the performance for compensation of professional services requiring substantial specialized knowledge of the biological, physical, behavioral, psychological, and sociological sciences and of nursing theory as the basis for assessment, diagnosis, planning, intervention, and evaluation in the promotion and maintenance of health; the casefinding and management of illness, injury or infirmity; the restoration of optimum function; or the achievement of a dignified death. Nursing practice includes but is not limited to administration, teaching, counseling, supervision, delegation, and evaluation of practice and execution of the medial regimen, including the administration of medications and treatments prescribed by any person authorized by state law to prescribe. Each registered nurse is directly accountable and responsible to the consumer for the quality of nursing care rendered.[3]

Although no state uses this exact wording, among the concepts commonly included are the reference to performing services for compensation, the necessity for a specialized knowledge base, the use of the nursing process (although defined differently), and components of nursing practice. Ten states include some reference to treating human responses to actual or potential health problems. This definition first appeared in New York State's license law and was incorporated in ANA's Social Policy Statement. [4] All but 6 states refer to the execution of the medical regimen and 24 include a general statement about additional acts, which has been interpreted to recognize that nursing practice is evolving and that the nurse's area of responsibility can be expected to broaden.[5]

Definitions of practical nursing are more restrictive and usually designate that the individual must function under the supervision of professionals and in areas demanding less judgment and knowledge.

Board of Nursing

The board is the agency that is legally empowered to carry out the intention of the law. The membership of the board, the procedure for appointment and removal, and the qualifications are important aspects of the act because the board has the power to write the rules and regulations that will be used in daily operations.

The members of the state board of nursing usually are appointed by the governor. North Carolina is the only state in which the registered nurse members of the state board are elected by the registered nurses in the state. The law specifies the occupational background of the candidates, but nominations are made by nurses.

Boards of nursing range in size from 7 to 17 members. Prerequisites regarding the educational background of nurses who serve as board members vary from state to state, and some states require that the board include nurses from differing occupational areas, such as education and nursing service. All but nine states have at least one public member of the board. Three states have at least one physician on the nursing board. A government official is on the board in one state.[6]

In all but six states there is a combined board for registered nurses and licensed practical nurses. In these six states two separate boards exist. Each state board has a paid staff that usually is headed by a registered nurse who is employed as the executive director of the state board of nursing. The executive director is responsible for administering the work of the board and seeing that rules and regulations are followed.

The ANA recommends that the board of nursing have the authority to carry out the following:

- Govern its own operation and administration
- Approve or deny approval to schools of nursing
- Examine and license applicants
- Renew licenses, grant temporary licenses, and provide for inactive status for those already licensed
- Regulate specialty practice
- Discipline those who violate provisions of the licensure law through conducting hearings, issuing subpoenas to witnesses, revoking, suspending, or refusing to renew a license, or setting limitations or conditions on practice[7]

Some of these functions were performed by a centralized state licensure agency. In 1984, 33 states had such an agency.[8] These agencies range from those that have responsibility only for housekeeping matters, such as collecting fees, managing routine license renewals, and providing secretarial services, to those that have all decision-making authority, relegating the individual boards, such as the board of nursing, to advisory status.

Each state board must operate within the framework of its own state law regarding the practice of nursing, but all cooperate with one another and with the ANA and the National League for Nursing (NLN). For example, state boards acting together have contracted with CTB Testing Service (a subsidiary of McGraw – Hill Publishing Co.) to prepare the licensing examinations that are used throughout the United States.

Qualifications for Licensure Applicants

The qualifications may be described in detail, or only general guidelines may be given, leaving the details up to the board of nursing. The most common basic requirements are graduation from an approved educational program and proficiency in the English language. Some states make the educational requirements more specific, such as requiring high school graduation and either an associate or baccalaureate degree or a diploma in nursing. All states require a passing score on a comprehensive examination but do not name the examination in the law. The current licensing examination is discussed later in this chapter. Twenty-two states require that the applicant be of "good moral character" and 14 require "good physical and mental health."[9] Those who are licensed in other states must meet the same requirements. The process of obtaining an additional license is called "licensure by endorsement" (for further information, see "Obtaining a License").

Titling

The titles registered nurse, licensed practical nurse, and licensed vocational nurse, as well as sometimes additional titles for advanced practice, are reserved for those meeting the requirements of the law. This makes it illegal for an unlicensed person to call himself or herself a registered nurse.

Grandfathering

Whenever a new law is written, a statement is usually included specifying that anyone currently holding the license may continue to hold that license, even if some requirements are changed. Without this provision the enactment of a new law would require that every person who is currently licensed reapply and show that they meet the new standards.

Renewal

The length of time for which a license is valid is specified, as well as any requirements for renewal. In some states license renewal requires only payment of a fee. In 16 jurisdictions continuing education is required for renewal. One state (Washington) dropped its continuing education requirement after a brief period. Documenting continuing education may require submission of records or may be attested to by signing a form. In many states where the applicant is not required to submit records at the time of renewal, a procedure for random checking assures compliance with the law. Continuing education requirements vary greatly, for example, from as many as 24 hours every year to as few as 15 hours every 2 years. State requirements for continuing education are outlined in Appendix A.

Financial Concerns

Although the act itself does not usually specify the fees to be charged, general restrictions on the method of calculating fees and on how the fees may be used are often included in the act. The act may specify how the expenses of the board of nursing are to be met and who has legal authority to make decisions regarding the use of funds.

Nursing Education Programs

Some state laws describe the requirements of a nursing education program in only the most general terms, leaving the details up to the board of nursing. In other states the law is specific. It may specify the number of years of education, the courses or content that must be included, and the approval process for a program. If the law is general, then the board sets more specific standards. All nursing education programs in a state must fulfill the requirements of the state law.

Disciplinary Action

Disciplinary action may take the form of license withdrawal, or restrictions may be placed on the license, such as working only in a setting where narcotics are not administered. Such disciplinary action can only be taken based on criteria that are stated in the law. In the past most state acts contained general statements with regard to such matters as immoral and unprofessional conduct. Because of the vagueness, they proved to be unenforceable in court. In addition, most courts have only supported reasons for revocation of the license when the offense was in some way related to performance. Therefore, most modern laws contain specific concerns, such as the following, which are recommended by the ANA:

- Fraud in gaining a license
- Felony conviction
- Addiction to drugs

- Harming or defrauding the public
- Willfully violating the nurse practice act[10]

Violations and Penalties

Specific power is provided to prosecute those who violate the provisions of the law. The board may be authorized to ask a court to halt a specific practice that it believes is contrary to the law until a full hearing can take place. This is called "injunctive relief," referring to the court order called an injunction.

Exceptions

Certain provisions may allow those who are not licensed to act as nurses in specific situations. Performing as a student while in an educa-

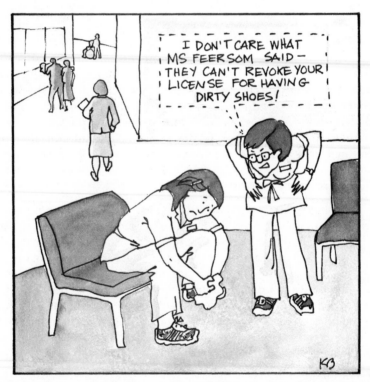

Figure 4-3. A nursing license may be revoked by the State Board of Nursing for reasons clearly spelled out in the law. These reasons may include fraud in obtaining a license, conviction of a felony, and conduct likely to harm the public.

tional program is usually the primary exception. In addition, those who are caring for family members or friends without pay are exempted, as are those who are acting in an emergency situation. Those licensed in another state who are practicing in a federal agency, such as a military hospital, are usually exempted from the law.

Miscellaneous Provisions

Each law requires "housekeeping" details that specify when it will become effective, that the previous act will no longer be in force, and other details pertaining to the individual state. Such provisions are usually of special interest when the law is first passed because nurses want to know when they will be affected by any changes.

Expanded Nursing Roles

Some nurse practice acts provide for the practice of nurses in expanded roles, including nurse midwives, nurse anesthetists, and nurse practitioners. Often the law requires that the person be certified for advanced practice by the ANA or a nursing specialty organization (section on certification later in the chapter). In some states no specific mention is made of expanded roles, but the board of nursing has approved specialty practice based on the provisions in the basic act. In still other states practice in special roles is not legally sanctioned. Appendix A provides information about specialty practice in each state.

The ANA opposes the inclusion of expanded practice in the licensure law. The association believes that the licensure law should regulate minimum safe practice and that the profession should regulate advanced practice. This is the case in medicine, where there is only basic licensure as a physician and specialty practice is regulated by specialty boards within the profession. An additional concern is that some of the laws regulating specialty practice have provided for physician review of nursing's scope of practice. This takes away from nursing autonomy and allows medicine to control some aspects of nursing. A third concern is the rigidity, which may not allow for evolving nursing roles.

OBTAINING A LICENSE

The Licensing Examination

The establishment of a licensing examination was an important part of early efforts to achieve a high standard for the registered nurse. When each state adopted a licensing law it also established a mechanism for the examination of license applicants. A major achievement in the history of licensure was the formation of the Bureau of State Boards of Nurse Examiners, which eventually led to the use of an identical examination in all states by 1950. The original examination, called the State Board Test Pool Examination, was prepared by the testing department of the NLN under a contract with the state boards. Each state set its own standards for a passing score.

Historically, content of the examinations was divided into subject categories of medical, surgical, obstetric, pediatric, and psychiatric nursing. Because nursing has changed in nature and these topics no longer reflect the totality of nursing practice, the current state board organization, the National Council of State Boards of Nursing, adopted a new plan for the examination, which was implemented in July of 1982.[11]

The Testing Division of the NLN prepared the first test under the

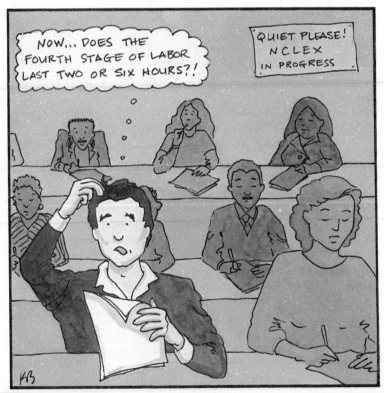

Figure 4–4. Licensing examinations are designed to measure the basic knowledge needed for safe practice.

direction of the National Council. Beginning with the examination in February 1983, the examination was prepared by CTB Testing Service. In addition to preparing the tests, the company scores the examinations and provides statistical information related to the examination to the National Council, the states, and individual schools.

The new examination, called the National Council Licensure Examination for Registered Nurses (NCLEX-RN), consists of a single examination for which a single score is given. The National Council had supported a research study to identify nursing behaviors that are significant in maintaining a safe and effective standard of care.[12] These critical behaviors were organized into ten major areas and further divided into 49 categories (see Chart 4–2). These categories were analyzed and test items were written to reflect the knowledge, abilities, and traits necessary to perform effectively within them. The behaviors occur in three kinds of health care situations:

1. those in which decision making is centered in the nurse;
2. those in which decision making is centered in the patient/client;
3. those in which decision making is shared.

Further organization of the behaviors reflects an emphasis on the nursing process, which is divided into the following five steps[13]:

(Text continues on p. 126)

Chart 4–2. Critical Requirements for Practice

I. Exercises Professional Prerogatives Based on Clinical Judgment

A. Adapts care to individual patient needs
B. Fulfills responsibility to patient and others despite difficulty
C. Challenges inappropriate orders and decisions by medical and other professional staff
D. Acts as patient advocate in obtaining appropriate medical, psychiatric, or other help
E. Recognizes own limitations and errors
F. Analyzes and adjusts own or staff reactions in order to maintain therapeutic relationship with patient

II. Promotes Patient's Ability to Cope with Immediate, Long-range, or Potential Health-related Change

A. Provides health care instruction or information to patient, family, or significant others

(continued)

Chart 4-2.   Critical Requirements for Practice (continued)

B. Encourages patient or family to make decision about accepting care or adhering to treatment regimen
C. Helps patient recognize and deal with psychological stress
D. Avoids creating or increasing anxiety or stress
E. Conveys and invites acceptance, respect, and trust
F. Facilitates relationship of family, staff, or significant others with patient
G. Stimulates, remotivates patient, or enables patient to achieve self-care and independence

III. Helps Maintain Patient Comfort and Normal Body Functions

A. Keeps patient clean and comfortable
B. Helps patient maintain or regain normal body functions

IV. Takes Precautionary and Preventive Measures in Giving Patient Care

A. Prevents infection
B. Protects skin and mucous membranes from injurious materials
C. Uses positioning or exercise to prevent injury or the complications of immobility
D. Avoids using injurious techniques in administering and managing intrusive or other potentially traumatic treatments
E. Protects patient from falls or other contact injuries
F. Maintains surveillance of patient's activities
G. Reduces or removes environmental hazards

V. Checks, Compares, Verifies, Monitors, and Follows up Medication and Treatment Processes

A. Checks correctness, condition, and safety of medication being prepared
B. Insures that correct medication is given to the right patient and that patient takes or receives it
C. Adheres to schedule in giving medication, treatment, or test
D. Administers medication by correct route, rate, or mode
E. Checks patient's readiness for medication, treatment, surgery, or other care
F. Checks to insure that tests or measurements are done correctly
G. Monitors ongoing infusions and inhalations
H. Checks for and interprets effect of medication, treatment, or care, and takes corrective action if necessary

(continued)

Chart 4-2.   Critical Requirements for Practice (continued)

VI. Interprets Symptom Complex and Intervenes Appropriately

A. Checks patient's condition or status
B. Remains objective, further investigates, or verifies patient's complaint or problem
C. Uses alarms and signals on automatic equipment as adjunct to personal assessment
D. Observes and correctly assesses signs of anxiety or behavioral stress
E. Observes and correctly assesses physical signs, symptoms, or findings, and intervenes appropriately
F. Correctly assesses severity or priority of patient's condition, and gives or obtains necessary care

VII. Responds to Emergency

A. Anticipates need for crisis care
B. Takes instant, correct action in emergency situations
C. Maintains calm and efficient approach under pressure
D. Assumes leadership role in crisis situation when necessary

VIII. Obtains, Records, and Exchanges Information on Behalf of the Patient

A. Checks data sources for orders and other information about patient
B. Obtains information from patient and family
C. Transcribes or records information on chart, Kardex, or other information system
D. Exchanges information with nursing staff and other departments
E. Exchanges information with medical staff

IX. Utilizes Patient Care Planning

A. Develops and modifies patient care plan
B. Implements patient care plan

X. Teaches and Supervises Other Staff

A. Teaches correct principles, procedures, and techniques of patient care
B. Supervises and checks the work of staff for whom she or he is responsible

(Jacobs A, Fivars G, Fitzpatrick R: What the new test will test. Am J Nurs 82:626, Apr 1982)

1. Assessing
2. Analyzing (or diagnosing)
3. Planning
4. Implementing
5. Evaluating

The examination is offered twice a year, for 2 days in July and for 2 days in February. It is given on the same date in all states. The score reported is not a raw score, but one derived from a complex process in which the test was examined for content necessary for minimum safe practice. The passing score is 1600 out of a possible 3200; the mean is 2000.

In order to prepare students to take the examination, the National Council has authorized the preparation of a study book that explains the examination, how it was written, and the scoring system, and provides sample questions to familiarize an applicant with the way the test is written.[14]

Licensure by Endorsement

Obtaining a nursing license in a state after first being licensed in another state is called licensure by endorsement. There are no reciprocal agreements between states that provide for moving licensure from one state to another. Each case is considered independently, based on the rules and regulations of the state. However, owing to the uniformity of licensing laws throughout most of the United States and its territories, nurses have enjoyed easy mobility between geographical areas.

Because the same licensure examination is used nationwide, no state requires that the examination be retaken. Some states, however, do require that a nurse moving into the state meet the current criteria for new licensure. In other states a nurse must fulfill the requirements that were in effect at the time of the original licensure. A state may require a nurse to meet other criteria, such as those for continuing education, before granting licensure by endorsement.

A temporary license that allows the applicant to be employed while credentials are being verified and processed is available in some states. This is not permitted in other states; a license must be obtained before any employment is legal. All states charge a fee for processing an application for licensure. For information on licensure fees, temporary permits, and continuing education requirements, see Appendix A. For more detailed information, write to the board of nursing of the state in which you are interested.

At the time of this writing, North Dakota is the only state that differentiates between an associate degree and a baccalaureate degree in the matter of licensure. In North Dakota an associate degree is required for licensure as a licensed practical nurse and a baccalaureate degree is required for licensure as a registered nurse. This change was made by the North Dakota Board of Nursing without the need for legislative action, and it was challenged in court. Although all currently registered nurses and licensed practical nurses were grandfathered into their licenses, this does not apply to nurses who were licensed in other states. The action of the board was sustained by the court; therefore North Dakota represents an exception to the general pattern of easy mobility for all registered nurses.

Licensure of Graduates of Foreign Nursing Schools

Nurses who have graduated from a nursing school in a foreign country and want to practice nursing in the United States must satisfy the board of nursing in their state that their education meets the requirements of the state and take the NCLEX-RN examination. To prevent the exploitation of foreign graduates who come to the United States to practice nursing and fail to pass the licensing examination, and to help assure safety in health care for the U.S. public, the ANA and the NLN have sponsored an independent organization called CGFNS (Committee on Graduates of Foreign Nursing Schools), which administers an examination to foreign-educated nurses. The examination covers proficiency in both nursing and English and helps the foreign-educated nurse to determine the possibility of passing the actual licensing examination. Nurses may take the CGFNS examination while still in their own country, although it is also given in the United States.

To obtain a nonimmigrant preference visa from the U.S. Immigration and Naturalization Service or a work permit from the U.S. Labor Department, the foreign-educated nurse must first pass the CGFNS examination. The majority of states also require the CGFNS examination as a preliminary step for foreign educated nurses applying for licensure.

REVOCATION OF A LICENSE

A license to practice any occupation becomes a property right of the individual after the state has awarded it. As long as the individual renews by paying the appropriate fees and meets any continuing requirements, such as continuing education, a license cannot be revoked without cause. The possible reasons for revoking a license are spelled out in the law. (The common reasons are listed earlier, in the discussion of disciplinary action.)

The procedure for revoking a license includes the right of the individual to have a hearing, which functions in many ways like a court proceeding. The state board or a specially designated hearing board is responsible for conducting the hearing and handing down a decision. The board's decision may be appealed to a court of law in most states. The individual being threatened with revocation of a license should have an attorney for legal counsel throughout the proceeding.

CERTIFICATION

Certification is a type of credentialing that has professional, but not legal, status. A certificate usually is awarded by a professional group and is based on the applicant's meeting certain standards. The definition of certification adopted by the Interdivisional Council on Certification of the ANA states: *"Certification is the documented validation of specific qualifications demonstrated by the individual registered nurse in the provision of professional nursing care in a defined area of practice."*[15] Certification is available from a variety of professional nursing organizations.

ANA Certification

When the ANA first began a certification program, it planned to certify for "excellence" rather than for "competence." This created confusion over terminology and resulted in some nursing certificates verifying excellence in practice while others verified basic competence in practice. All certificates previously awarded under this system remain in effect for the time specified, but a change has been made in the certification process to provide more uniformity.

Currently, ANA certification is a method of recognizing nurses who provide *direct* patient care. Applicants must demonstrate current practice, which is beyond that required for licensure as a registered nurse. The applicant must take a national examination and submit evidence of personal nursing practice in a specific clinical area. Certificates are valid for a period of 5 years, after which the nurse must submit further evidence related to clinical practice and continuing education for certification renewal. Chart 4–3 lists the various certification credentials available from the ANA.

Chart 4–3. *ANA Certification Areas Available*

Clinical Specialist Certifications (Require Master's Degree)

Clinical Specialist in Adult Psychiatric/Mental Health Nursing
Clinical Specialist in Child/Adolescent Psychiatric/Mental Health Nursing
Clinical Specialist in Medical-Surgical Nursing

Nurse Practitioner Certification (Require Specific Specialty Educational Program)

Adult Nurse Practitioner (BSN required)
Family Nurse Practitioner (BSN required)
Gerontological Nurse Practitioner
Pediatric Nurse Practitioner
School Nurse Practitioner (BSN required)

Other Nursing Specialty Certification (No Specific Specialty Educational Program Requirement)

Child and Adolescent Nurse
Community Health Nurse (BSN required)
Gerontological Nurse
High-risk Perinatal
Maternal Child Health
Medical Surgical Nurse
Nursing Administration (BSN required)
Nursing Administration, Advanced (master's degree required)
Psychiatric and Mental Health Nurse

For further information about any of these programs, write to Certification Unit, American Nurses' Association, 2420 Pershing Road, Kansas City, MO 64108.

Other Certification Programs

The Nurses Association of the American College of Obstetricians and Gynecologists (NAACOG) established a joint certification procedure with the ANA for the maternal–gynecological–neonatal nurse. The NAACOG withdrew from joint sponsorship of this program in 1979 and began providing independent certification in 1980. The National Association of Pediatric Nurse Associates Practitioners (NAP-NAP) offers certification for the pediatric nurse practitioner. Thus there are currently two certificates being awarded in the same area by two organizations. NAPNAP and the ANA have had joint conferences regarding certification, and it was hoped that one jointly sponsored certification might result. Fundamental differences still exist, however, between the two organizations on how authority for determining standards should be established.

The American College of Nurse Midwives provides a certification program for nurses specializing in nurse midwifery. Nurses graduating from approved midwifery programs apply for certification through this organization. Approved programs may be at a basic level or at a master's degree level. The license to practice as a midwife depends, however, on the state licensure laws. Some states do not allow the practice of nurse midwives; in other states the law recognizes the certification as an appropriate credential for practice; and in still other states no decision has been made.

Certification as a registered nurse anesthetist is provided by the American Association of Nurse Anesthetists (AANA). Since 1952 the AANA, with the approval of the American Hospital Association, has accredited programs for preparing nurse anesthetists and has administered an examination for certification of graduates of these programs. According to the AANA, certified registered nurse anesthetists today administer more than half of all anesthetics. Nurse anesthetists were the first nurses to be certified beyond the basic level.

Many other specialty organizations in nursing have certification programs (Chart 4–4). Most of these are administered by a separately titled and funded certification organization that is closely related to the specialty organization. This administrative structure is set up to protect the sponsoring organization from economic liability, to preserve tax-exempt status, and to provide a more objective approach to the credentialing process. Information on any of these specialty certification programs can be obtained by writing directly to the organization (see Appendix B).

Certification as a Basis for Licensure

Some states are using certification as a means of identifying competence in an expanded or specialized role, and thus are giving legal status to the certification. The requirements and methods for obtaining certification remain under the control of the organization granting the

---

Chart 4–4. Certification Available Through Other Organizations

Nurse Practitioner Certification

  Nurse Midwife (ACNM)
  Pediatric Nurse Practitioner (NAPNAP)
  Ob/Gyn Practitioner (NAACOG)

Nursing Specialty Certification

  Critical Care Nurse (CCNA)
  Emergency Room Nurse (EDNA)
  Enterostomal Therapy (ETA)
  Hemodialysis Nurse (AANNT)
  Infection Control Specialist (APIC) (not exclusively nurses)
  Inpatient Obstetric Nurse (NAACOG)
  Neonatal Intensive Care Nurse (NAACOG)
  Neonatal Nurse Clinician (NAACOG)
  Neurosurgical Nurse (AANN)
  Nurse Anesthetist (AANA)
  Nursing Home Administrator (ACHCA) (not exclusively nurses)
  Occupational Health Nurse (AOHN)
  Operating Room Nurse (AORN)
  Rehabilitation Nurse (ARN)
  Urological Nurse (AANNT)

  For further information on certification in any of these areas, contact the organization shown in parentheses. Addresses appear in Appendix B.

---

certification. The nurse receives a license from the state to practice in the expanded role.

Titles being used in these expanded roles vary from state to state. Some current titles are advanced registered nurse (ARN), specialized registered nurse (SRN), nurse practitioner (NP), independent nurse practitioner (INP), advanced registered nurse practitioner (ARNP), and certified registered nurse (CRN). In some states the specialized nurse uses the title of the specific certification, such as family nurse practitioner (FNP) and pediatric nurse practitioner (PNP).

Problems Related to Certification

The problems associated with certification have yet to be resolved. Programs that prepare nurses in these various specialties lack uniformity. The situation is reminiscent of the early years of nursing education. Some advanced programs accept any registered nurse and are completed in 6 to 9 months. Other programs that prepare nurses for the same specialty may be at the master's degree level. Thus the title awarded by the program is not a reliable indication of the degree of competence achieved by the nurse specialist. It is hoped that the certification program will improve the situation by defining the common standard of performance that must be demonstrated in order to attain the certificate.

Another concern is the disparity from state to state in credentialing nurses in specialty areas. This can hamper mobility and interfere with meeting the health care needs in areas of the United States where these nursing specialists are not recognized. Some believe that the certification program will be of help here also because it sets national standards that states may adopt. When different states adopt certification as an appropriate way of credentialing, reciprocity between those states is facilitated.

A third problem is related to the equivalency of certificates in different specialties. Not all specialists have the same educational, testing, or practice requirements. Some certify persons in independent areas of primary care, while others certify persons in what are essentially specialty areas of hospital nursing. To identify the exact meaning of a certificate in a nursing specialty, one would have to investigate the specific requirements of that certificate. Certification has not solved the problems related to credentialing in nursing specialties.

THE FUTURE OF CREDENTIALING

Both the public and nurses have been confused because credentialing in nursing involves so many aspects related to both licensure and certification. Because the ideal credential clearly communicates qualifications and competence, it is necessary to create a uniform credentialing system.

To clarify the matter, the ANA, in cooperation with 47 other interested groups, funded a major research study on credentialing in the field of nursing. Professional researchers at the University of Wisconsin, Milwaukee School of Nursing conducted the study under the guidance of a committee appointed by the ANA. The study assessed all current credentialing mechanisms, including licensure, certification, and granting of degrees. In addition, the researchers suggested means of increasing the effectiveness of credentialing and recommended plans for implementation of the proposed changes. The final report of the study was presented to the public and the members of the ANA in December 1978.[16]

The major recommendation of the study was that an independent, free-standing center for nursing credentialing be established. The study committee believed that this move toward an independent center would provide the checks and balances necessary to preserve equity for all in the system and would be an efficient, cost-effective service that would avoid duplication of efforts and provide for geographical mobility for nurses. The committee wrote that the profession of nursing must move its leadership and resources toward supporting this concept and reshaping the system.

Although the recommendations for a central credentialing center for nursing was made in 1978, and further study and discussion resulted, the organizations involved have not yet moved toward this goal. The threats to organizational autonomy and power involved in giving up an existing certification program are great and indeed may be insurmountable. The topic shall certainly continue to be hotly debated.

CONCLUSION

An awareness of the various credentials in use in the field of nursing will help you to plan more effectively for your own future in nursing. Whether the future holds a credential other than that of a registered nurse, understanding the extent of the issue and the significance of credentialing for the future of the nursing profession will help you to respond in a more knowledgeable way. Certainly the debate regarding credentials is not finished. Students of today will be responsible for shaping the nursing practice of tomorrow.

REFERENCES

1. Snyder ME, LaBar C: Issues in Professional Practice. Vol 1, Nursing: Legal Authority For Practice. Kansas City, MO, American Nurses' Association, 1984
2. National Council of State Boards of Nursing: Model Nursing Practice Act. Chicago, NCSBN, 1982

3. Congress for Nursing Practice. The Nursing Practice Act: Suggested State Legislation. Kansas City, MO, American Nurses' Association, 1981
4. Nursing: A Social Policy Statement. Kansas City, MO, American Nurses' Association, 1980
5. LaBar C: Statutory Definition of Nursing Practice and Their Conformity of Certain ANA Principles. Kansas City, MO, American Nurses' Association, 1984
6. Ibid.
7. Congress for Nursing Practice: The Nursing Practice Act, op. cit.
8. Boards of Nursing: Composition, Member Qualifications, and Statutory Authority. Kansas City, MO, American Nurses' Association, 1985
9. LaBar C: Statutory Requirements for Licensing of Nurses. Kansas City, MO, American Nurses' Association, 1984
10. Congress for Nursing Practice: The Nursing Practice Act, op. cit.
11. Test Plan of the RN Licensure Examination: Changes, Concerns, Issues, Process of Test Development, Pub. No. 23-1842. New York, National League for Nursing, 1981
12. Jacobs AM et al: ANA Council of State Boards of Nursings. Critical Requirements for Safe, Effective Nursing Practice, Pub. No. B-41. Kansas City, MO, American Nurses' Association, 1978
13. Test Plan for the National Council Licensure Examination For Registered Nurses. Chicago: National Council of State Boards of Nursing, 1982
14. Ibid.
15. American Nurses' Association: The Study of Credentialing in Nursing: A New Approach. Vol 1, The Report of the Committee. Kansas City, MO, American Nurses' Association, 1978
16. Ibid.

FURTHER READINGS

American Nurses Association: The Study of Credentialing in Nursing: A New Approach. Vol 1, The Report of the Committee. Kansas City, MO, American Nurses' Association, 1978
Bullough B: Nurse practice acts: How they affect your expanding role. Nursing 77:73–81, Feb 1977
Congress for Nursing Practice: The Nursing Practice Act: Suggested State Legislation. Kansas City, MO, American Nurses' Association, 1981
Credentialing in nursing: A new approach. Am J Nurs 79:614–683, Apr 1979
deTornyay R: The task ahead: Acceptance and implementation. AORN J 31:53, Jan 1980
Fickeissen JL: Getting certified. Am J Nurs 85:265–269, Mar 1985
Grinberg E: Why form a certification corporation? Oncol Nurs Forum 12:89, May/Jun 1985
Hipp RJ: Individual vs. institutional licensure: Part of the credentialing dilemma. Nurs Leadership 3:27–29, Jun 1980

Jacobs AM et al: ANA Council of State Boards of Nursing. Critical Requirements for Safe, Effective Nursing Practice. Pub. No. B–41. Kansas City, MO, American Nurses' Association, 1978

LaBar C: Boards of Nursing: Composition, Member Qualifications, and Statutory Authority. Kansas City, MO, American Nurses' Association, 1985

LaBar C: Statutory Definitions of Nursing Practice and Their Conformity of Certain ANA Principles. Kansas City, MO, American Nurses' Association, 1984

LaBar C: Statutory Requirements for Licensing of Nurses. Kansas City, MO, American Nurses' Association, 1984

Levine ME: Does continuing education improve nursing practice? Hospitals 52:138–140, Nov. 1, 1979

Licensure: State boards of nursing. Regan Rep Nurs Law 20:1, Jun 1979

Lipman M: Your rights before a state disciplinary court. RN 36:44–49, Dec 1973

McQuaid EA et al: How do graduates of different programs perform on state boards? Am J Nurs 79:674–683, Feb 1979

McQuaid EA, Sheridan P: A new licensing exam for nurses. Am J Nurs 80:723–725, Apr 1980

McCarty P: Certification allows nurses to show their competence. Am Nurse 17:6, May 1985

Nursing: A Social Policy Statement. Kansas City, MO, American Nurses' Association, 1980

Questions and Answers: Sunset Laws and Nursing. Kansas City, MO, American Nurses' Association, 1984

Snyder ME, LaBar C: Issues in Professional Practice. Vol 1, Nursing: Legal Authority for Practice. Kansas City, MO, American Nurses' Association, 1984

Task force proposed timetable: Five activities identified for credentialing center. Am Nurs 12:3, May 1980

Test Plan for the National Council Licensure Examination For Registered Nurses. Chicago, National Council of State Boards of Nursing, 1982

Test Plan of the RN Licensure Examination: Changes, Concerns, Issues, Process of Test Development, Pub. No. 23–1842. New York, National League for Nursing, 1981

The study of credentialing in nursing: A new approach. Nurs Outlook 27:263–271, Apr 1979

Trandel–Korenchuk DM et al: How state laws recognize advanced nursing practice. Nurs Outlook 26:713–719, Nov 1978

5 | Legal Responsibilities for Practice

Objectives

After completing this chapter, you should be able to

1. Differentiate between **common law** and **statutory law**.
2. Explain the role of institutional policy in legal decision making.
3. Differentiate between **civil law** and **criminal law**.
4. Define **negligence** and **malpractice**.
5. Explain the standard of the reasonably prudent nurse.
6. Define **liability**.
7. Identify situations in which liability is shared by employers or supervisors.
8. State points to be considered in the purchase of professional liability insurance.
9. Discuss the nurse's responsibility in the specific issues presented.
10. Identify factors that contribute to a suit being instituted against a health care professional.
11. Discuss a variety of actions by the nurse that might prevent the initiation of a suit.
12. Explain the various aspects of testifying for a legal proceeding.

Discussion about the individual nurse's responsibility for his or her own actions is appearing more frequently in nursing literature. Certainly as a nurse you will need to be very aware of your responsibilities.

Your professional responsibilities rest on a dual framework of legal and ethical constraints. Ethics are the principles of conduct governing one's relationships with others.

Ethics are at the basis of a decision to go to work in the morning, even if you do not want to. It is possible to pretend to be sick and stay home in bed for the day. There are no laws governing your action in such a situation. What is right is a personal decision. However, because the community as a whole would agree that to pretend illness to escape work was inappropriate behavior, the employer would be supported in a decision to dismiss you from your job if you should do this. Ethical decisions, therefore, have consequences both for oneself and for others. In this very simple case, you lost your job and the employer did not have anyone to do the necessary work.

Law includes those rules of conduct or action recognized as binding or enforced by a controlling authority. Ethics and the law may go hand in hand, with one supporting the other. Situations in which this occurs are the easiest to understand. For example, if you choose to steal money from your employer, that would be considered unethical behavior. It would also be a violation of the law. Many laws were written to provide a basis for the community to enforce those ethical principles of conduct that were felt to be essential to the well-being of the majority of people.

In some instances ethics may address entirely different questions than the law does. The first example of reporting to work as expected is an instance that would not be addressed by laws, although most people would have a similar view of right and wrong in that instance.

In still other situations some people will find that the law and their own ethics are divergent. These are the most difficult circumstances to face. An example of the law setting different standards than those set by ethics occurs in the case of a member of the armed forces killing an enemy soldier during a war. No country considers this to be an illegal act, but many people believe that such action is unethical and have therefore become conscientious objectors during times of war.

The purpose of this chapter is to show how the law affects nursing practice. Ethics are discussed more completely in Chapter 8. Examples are given throughout this chapter to help you understand the concepts

Jane Fantel, J.D., with the Seattle firm of Francis, Lopez, and Ackerman, served as a consultant regarding the legal material presented in this chapter.

discussed. The situations are not meant to be exhaustive. In an actual incident many more factors would be considered than can be presented in a brief paragraph. It is the interaction of these multiple factors that makes it impossible to make absolute predictions regarding legal outcomes in specific situations that occur in the real world of practice. Another point that you need to understand is the importance of the specific factual data in each case. Often cases appear to be similar on the surface, but some precise facts that differ may contribute to differing decisions in the apparently similar cases.

If you have a question about a specific situation, you would be well advised to consult an attorney who is experienced in medicolegal matters. The facility where you are employed may have a legal counsel who is available to you. Another source of legal aid is your nurses' association attorney. If you desire private counsel, suitable names may be recommended by your local bar association.

SOURCES OF LAW

Statutory Law

There are two general sources of law: statutory law and common law. *Statutory law* comprises two groupings. One contains those laws enacted by legislative bodies such as a county or city council, a state legislature, or the Congress of the United States. Nurse practice acts are in this category and are passed by state legislatures. Laws enacted by legislative bodies carry the greatest weight in a court. The other group includes the rules and regulations established by governmental agencies such as licensing boards and regulatory bodies. These agencies are authorized through enacted laws to establish regulations. These rules and regulations have the same force as enacted law unless found by a court to be outside the scope of or contrary to the intent of the enacted laws. Rules and regulations formulated by the state board of nursing are in this category.

Common Law

Common law derives from common usage, custom, and judicial decisions or court rulings. Previous judicial decisions or court cases are used to establish precedents for interpretations of statutory and common law. These decisions are binding within the jurisdiction of that particular court but are used in a more general way for guidelines in other jurisdictions. Common law is fluid and cannot be defined with precision. In general, statutory law carries more weight in the court than does common law.

The circumstance of abandoning a patient demonstrates how common law applies to nursing. There are no statutory laws dictating that nurses cannot leave a seriously ill patient unless they assure that someone else will provide care, but common practice and custom, which could be supported through testimony of nurses and other health care workers, require this of a nurse. Failure to meet this standard might be deemed a violation of common law.

Rulings

A ruling made by a state attorney general is an attempt to provide guidelines based on an interpretation of the statutory and common law relative to a specific situation and is not common law. Different attorneys general might vary in their opinions. The validity of an opinion only stands until a court rules on the situation. The final decision in any legal issue rests with a court.

The Role of Institutional Policy

Institutional policies are developed as guidelines to protect the institution itself and the employees of the institution from legal difficulties. Most often policies are developed by members of the hospital staff, who have expertise in a variety of practice areas, in consultation with an attorney.

Policies provide guidance as to the proper actions to be taken in given situations. These policies do not simply restate laws, but offer much more concrete direction. Established hospital policies may be considered by the court as indications of common usage (common law) and therefore may become important as a basis for legal decisions.

Institutional policies are changed in response to new situations and new expectations occurring in society. Usually there is an established institutional route for the change or expansion of hospital policy. Nurses may be in a position to recognize the need for such a change as they use policy from day to day.

CLASSIFICATION OF LAWS

Criminal Law

Law can be divided into civil and criminal components. Both statutory law and common law may be subdivided in this way. The term *criminal law* applies to law that affects the public welfare as a whole. A violation of criminal law is called a crime and is prosecuted by the government. On conviction, a crime may be punished by imprisonment, parole conditions, a loss of privilege (such as a license), a fine, or any combination of these. The punishment is intended to deter others from committing the crime as well as to punish the violator.

Civil Law

Civil Law applies to laws that regulate conduct between private individuals or businesses. A *tort* is a violation of a civil law in which another person is wronged. Private individuals or groups may bring a legal action to court for breach of civil law. Judgment of the court results in a plan to correct the wrong and may include a monetary payment to the wronged party. Because a private wrong has occurred, there is a private remedy.

Nurses may find themselves involved with both civil and criminal laws, either separately or within the same situation (see Fig. 5-1).

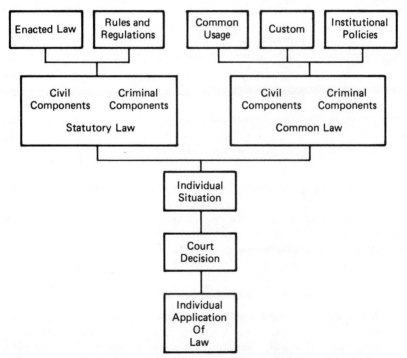

Figure 5-1. Civil law and criminal law both may affect a nursing situation.

CRIMINAL LAW AND NURSING

Because a violation of any law governing the practice of any licensed profession may be a crime, it is important to be aware of the extent of the nurse practice act. In instances in which the nurse practice act restricts functioning to acting under the direction of a physician or other licensed person, that explicit authorization must exist. Standing orders that refer to specific situations as well as the usual orders written for an individual patient may be adequate authorization. Custom or usual practice will not substitute for the specific authorization required by law. A violation of a professional practice act may be prosecuted as a crime even if no actual harm occurred to the patient.

Situation: Violation of a Practice Act

A nurse in a physician's office is contacted by a patient. The patient describes a problem that the physician commonly treats. The physician is unavailable, and there are no standing orders. The nurse proceeds to give the medication she believes the physician would have prescribed.

The nurse practice act does not give the nurse the authority to diagnose disease and prescribe the medication to treat. The medical practice act contains this authorization. This, then, is a violation of the law and is a crime, even though the patient was not harmed.

Violation of laws related to the care and distribution of controlled substances is also a crime.

Situation: Violation of Narcotic Laws

In making the routine check of the narcotic record before going off duty, the night nurse notes that the record does not match the actual count in relationship to the morphine in the supply. She is tired and does not wish to spend the time searching the record and correcting the mistake. Instead she makes a false entry for a patient who did not receive a narcotic so that the record appears correct.

Because the laws regulating the controlled substances are quite rigid, this would be a violation of the law.

It is costly to the state to undertake criminal prosecution; therefore, even when discovered, some violations of criminal law are not prosecuted in court. Knowing this, some nurses make the error of believing that "minor" violations are acceptable. Even when not prosecuted in court, criminal action could result in the loss of a job and in loss of a license to practice nursing.

CIVIL LAW AND NURSING

Torts

Torts (civil wrongs against a person) may be either intentional or unintentional. An *intentional tort* is one in which the outcome was planned. The wrong is not limited to physical harm.

Situation: Intentional Tort

An elderly, oriented, and competent patient decides to leave the hospital in the evening without medical consent, although additional treatment has been planned.

The evening nurse decides that this patient needs the planned treatment and should not be allowed to leave. She removes the patient's clothes from the room, disconnects the telephone so that the patient cannot call for a taxi, and tells the patient that he will not be allowed to leave.

The patient expresses anger and states that he will leave as soon as he finds a way. The next morning he makes a call to his son and leaves the hospital.

If legal action is taken, the nurse may be found to have committed an intentional tort. The nurse purposefully acted to keep the patient in the hospital against his will. The patient's loss of liberty was the wrong that occurred.

An *unintentional tort* is a wrong occurring to another person or property, although it was not intended to happen. *Negligence* is the failure to act as a reasonably prudent person would have acted in a specific situation. If harm is caused by negligence, it is termed an unintentional tort, and damages might be recovered. Negligence is a broad term that has many applications throughout society.

Situation: Negligence

A homeowner fails to pick up an object from the floor of his home, and a guest falls over the object in the dark and is injured. Negligence could be charged. The injury is the wrong; a reasonably prudent person would have picked up the object or provided light for the guest, and the injury can be shown to be a direct result of the failure to act prudently.

Malpractice

Malpractice is a term used for a specific type of negligence. It refers to the negligence of a specially trained or educated person in the performance of his or her job. Therefore, malpractice is the term used to describe negligence by nurses in the performance of their duties. The definition remains the same with one modification: the outcome was unintentional, but the wrong occurred to another person or to the property based on failure to act as a reasonably prudent *professional* would have acted in the situation. This is a higher standard than required of the general public. Thus all malpractice has the following three essential characteristics:

1. The person must be working in a professional capacity (either for pay or as a volunteer).
2. The wrong must be demonstrated.
3. The wrong must be shown to have been caused by the failure of the professional to act as a reasonably prudent member of that profession would have acted in that situation. This might include either doing what should not have been done or failing to do what should have been done.

Situation: Omission of Correct Action

An elderly, disoriented person is admitted to an acute care facility. At bedtime the nurse fails to put protective side rails on the bed. The patient falls out of bed, sustaining a fractured hip.

This could be found to be malpractice. The nurse was working in a professional capacity. The patient can be shown to have an injury. It may be demonstrated through testimony by nurses, and by reference to standard nursing texts, that a reasonably prudent registered nurse would have been expected to take action to protect this patient from falls. Failure to act could then constitute malpractice.

Situation: Commission of Inappropriate Action

A postoperative patient has an order to ambulate. The nurse assigned to this patient finds that the patient's condition has changed drastically since the order was written. The patient has a high temperature and a rapid pulse and is complaining of severe acute abdominal pain. The nurse proceeds to have the patient ambulate. The patient faints, sustaining a head injury in the fall. This necessitates additional hospitalization, x-ray films, and diagnostic procedures.

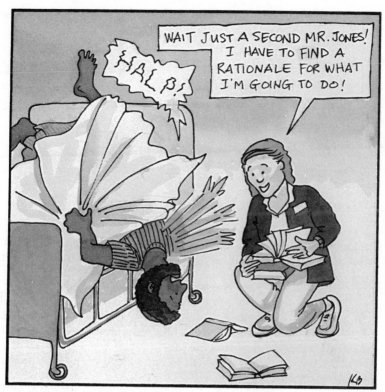

Figure 5–2. A reasonably prudent nurse uses common sense as well as nursing theory.

Again, this could be found to be malpractice. The nurse was working as a professional. The patient can be shown to have sustained injury. It may be demonstrated that a reasonably prudent nurse would have recognized that the change in the patient's condition called for consultation with the physician before proceeding with ambulation. Therefore malpractice could be found owing to inappropriate action on the part of the nurse.

LIABILITY

A person found guilty of any tort (whether intentional or negligent) is considered legally *liable,* or legally responsible, for the outcome. The person legally liable usually is required to pay for damages to the other person. This may include actual costs of care, legal services, loss of earnings (present and future), and compensation for emotional and physical stress suffered.

Personal Liability

As an educated professional, you are always responsible or liable for your actions. Thus, if a physician or supervisor instructs you to do something that is contrary to your best professional judgment and says, "I'll take responsibility," that person is poorly informed about the law. The physician or supervisor giving the directions may also be liable if harm results, but that would not lessen your personal liability.

Situation: Personal Liability

The registered nurse giving medications on a large medical unit notes that an order for digoxin (a heart medication) is considerably larger than the usual dose. She looks up the medication in a reference book and finds her view of the dose size confirmed. The ordered dose is several times the usual dose. The RN then calls the supervisor and explains the situation.

The supervisor double checks the order with the RN and then states: "Dr. Jones is an outstanding physician. I am sure he has a good reason for ordering this dose. Go ahead and give the medication as ordered." The RN then gives the medication, and the patient suffers a toxic reaction.

The RN would very likely be held liable for giving the incorrect amount of medication. She had the knowledge and judgment to recognize the dose as erroneous and failed to check with the physician. A statement by the supervisor does not remove the nurse's personal responsibility for her own actions. Because even a competent physician might make an error, the nurse had a responsibility to clarify that order.

The supervisor and the physician might also be held liable, but that would not necessarily lessen the RN's liability.

Although each person is legally responsibile for his or her own acts, the example above illustrates that there are also situations in which a person or organization may be held liable for actions taken by others.

Employer Liability

The most common situation in which others are held responsible is the employer-employee relationship. In many instances the employer can be held responsible for the torts committed by an employee. This is called the doctrine of *respondeat superior* (let the master respond). The law holds the employer responsible for having hired qualified persons, for establishing an appropriate environment for correct functioning, and for providing supervision or direction as needed to avoid errors or harm. Therefore, if the nurse, as an employee of the hospital, is guilty of malpractice, the hospital may also be guilty of malpractice. The employer's liability may exist even if the employer appears to have taken precautions to prevent error.

It is important to understand that this doctrine does not remove any responsibility from the individual nurse, but it extends responsibility to the employer in addition to the nurse. If, for example, a hospital has a procedure that does not conform to good nursing practice as you know it and you follow that procedure, you will still be liable for any resulting harm. You are expected to use your education and training to make sound judgments regarding your work.

Situation: Employer Responsibility

A nurse working in a long-term care facility is giving medications. This RN is not in the habit of checking identification bands, since he has worked at the facility for some time and feels that he knows the patients well. He mistakenly gives an elderly woman a medication that is intended for her roommate. The elderly woman is allergic to the medication she receives and has a severe reaction.

Both the RN in this situation and the long-term facility might be found liable for the harm that resulted. The RN had a personal, professional responsibility in giving medications. The facility also had a responsibility for making sure that employees carry out procedures safely and correctly.

Charitable Immunity

In some states nonprofit hospitals have "charitable immunity." This means that the nonprofit hospital cannot be held legally liable for harm done to a patient. The employees of that nonprofit hospital are still legally liable for their actions. The trend in legislation is toward the repeal of laws providing for charitable immunity. Those active in the consumer movement have argued that no institution should be relieved of responsibility in such a blanket fashion. If you are employed by a nonprofit institution, it is important that you know whether the law in your state provides for charitable immunity.

Supervisory Liability

When a nurse is in the role of charge nurse, head nurse, supervisor, or any other category in which the job involves supervision or direction of other persons, there is a potential for liability for the actions of others. The supervising nurse is responsible for exercising good judgment in a supervisory role. This includes making appropriate decisions about assignments and delegation of tasks. If an error occurs and the supervising nurse is shown to have exercised sound judgment in all decisions made in that capacity, the supervising nurse may not be held liable for the error of a subordinate. If poor judgment was used in assigning an inadequately prepared person to an important task, the supervisory nurse might be liable for resulting harm. The extent of the subordinate's responsibility would rest on his or her level of education and training. Persons without education or training might not be liable for error. The more education subordinates have, the more likely they will be liable also.

Situation: Supervisory Responsibility for Educated Person

Two sudden admissions to the coronary care unit create a situation in which additional help is needed to care for the patients in the unit.

The staff supervisor calls the person whose name appears first on the list of temporary-placement RNs. This nurse agrees to come in immediately. The nurse is not asked whether she has education or experience in coronary care, nor does she volunteer this information. She has no background or experience in coronary care.

While working in the coronary care unit, the temporary RN is assigned to complete care of two patients. Because of her lack of ability to read the monitors, a potentially life-threatening problem is not identified until the patient "arrests." Resuscitation efforts are successful, but the patient suffers some brain damage.

Both the staffing supervisor who placed the inadequately prepared RN in the unit and the temporary nurse herself could be found liable — the supervisor for incorrectly placing the nurse and the nurse for not recognizing her own limitations. The educational preparation of the temporary nurse gave her the background to understand that expertise was needed in this situation and that she herself did not possess it.

Situation: Supervisory Responsibility for Uneducated Person

The evening nursing supervisor is responsible for adjusting personnel assignments when employees are absent. He decides to send an extra aide to the emergency room to help out. This aide has never been assigned to the emergency room before and has no education or training other than the orientation to direct care given by the hospital. The supervisor instructs the aide to take care of the desk and answer the phone while others are busy.

While the aide is at the desk alone, a family enters the emergency room with an infant in acute distress. The aide instructs the family to sit down and wait until a nurse comes out of one of the rooms.

It is a long time before the nurse appears and care for the infant is instituted. The infant has a complicated recovery that later could be shown to be due to the delay in initial treatment.

The supervisor might be found negligent in this case for assigning the aide to the emergency room without proper direction or supervision. The aide might not be found negligent because she had no basis for recognizing the seriousness of the situation or for recognizing her own lack of ability to meet the responsibilities involved in being at the desk in an emergency room.

LIABILITY INSURANCE

Liability insurance transfers the risk of the costs of being sued and of any settlement from the individual to a large group. The expectation is that most individuals will not be able to afford such costs and that the pool of premiums will adequately cover the costs plus a profit for the insurance company that manages the financial plan.

There is currently a liability insurance crisis in the United States. The cost of liability insurance has escalated at an extraordinary rate. Some of the factors that have caused this to happen are the large judgments that have been made, the number of suits that have been brought, the large fees that attorneys receive, and the high profits of insurance companies. Regardless of the causes, the problem is a very real and serious one for all professionals.

Nurses in advanced practice have been especially affected by this change because their incomes have traditionally been quite moderate, and they cannot raise fees enough to cover insurance costs that may match those of physicians. Some hospitals may further limit the coverage that their policies provide for individual employees in an effort to hold down costs. Individual nurses have been named in an increased number of suits.

Some states have initiated legislation that allows for awards to cover actual losses and costs of care, but that limits awards for pain and suffering and other nontangible factors. Sometimes this has been accompanied by restrictions on insurance company rates. Some laws are also being amended to restrict the monetary liability of any party to the percentage of responsibility. For example, if damages were set at $10,000 and each of two defendants were determined to be responsible for 50 percent of the problem, one party could not be made to pay more than $5,000, even if the other party had no assets and could not pay. Liability laws continue to be a major concern for nurses.

Institutional and Individual Insurance

Many hospitals or other institutional employers carry liability insurance that covers both the institution and its employees. Liability insurance pays for the legal defense of a civil charge as well as for a settlement or judgment up to the limits of the policy.

Even if an employer carries liability insurance, it is often advisable for the individual professional to carry an independent policy. An independent policy may cover the person in voluntary activities as well as on the job. It also will follow the person who moves from one employer to another. If a legal action is instituted against the professional, the individual liability insurance policy may provide independent legal counsel.

Some nurses state that they do not carry insurance because it might encourage people to bring suit against them. They are under the mistaken assumption that persons will not sue if it means financial hardship for the person being sued. Judgments may be levied against tangible assets, such as a house, a car, or savings, as well as against future earnings. Married nurses who reside in community property states should realize that one half of the assets of the family may be vulnerable to a judgment reached. Community property states at this time include Arizona, California, Idaho, Louisiana, Nevada, New Mexico, Texas, and Washington. These factors combine to support the need for the individual professional to carry liability insurance that will provide legal counsel and protection in the case of any judgment.

Analyzing Insurance Coverage

Individual liability insurance for registered nurses is available from a variety of insurance companies directly through their agents and through professional organizations that offer coverage as a service to members. When investigating individual liability insurance, ask yourself the following questions:

- In what situations would I, as an individual, be covered?
- In what situations would I not be covered?
- How is my coverage affected by my actions? For example, if I failed to follow hospital policy, would I still be covered?
- What are the monetary limits of the policy?
- Does the policy provide me with legal counsel?

- Is the policy renewable at my option? What factors affect renewability?
- Does the insurance cover incidents that occurred while the policy was in force, regardless of when the claim is brought (claims occurred coverage), or does it cover incidents only if I am currently insured (claims brought coverage)?
- What is the cost compared with other policies?

Liability insurance coverage, which is carried by the hospital, should be carefully investigated by the nurse employee. "Full coverage" is not a very comprehensive statement. Questions 1 through 4 above apply to institutional policies as well as to individual policies. In addition, you should ask the following questions in regard to an institutional policy?

1. Does the policy provide me with individual legal counsel, or will the same attorney be working for the hospital?
2. At what point would the hospital no longer be responsible and I would be personally responsible?
3. How would my job be affected if action is instituted or a judgment is rendered against me? (Check institutional policy as well as the insurance company policy.)
4. Does the insurance company have the right to seek restitution from me if it pays a claim based on my actions?

It is important that you have accurate answers to these questions in order to make an informed decision regarding your need for an individual policy.

Insurance Cost and Coverage

The current American Nurses' Association (ANA) policy providing $1 million per claim and $1 million total in 1 year is adequate coverage for the registered nurse. This can be expected to increase with inflation. The cost for such coverage in 1987 was approximately $60 per year. Again, inflation can be expected to increase this cost. Since the 1970s the cost of the level of coverage recommended by the ANA rose from approximately $12 per year to its current amount. Coverage for specialty practice as a nurse practitioner, nurse anesthetist, or nurse midwife is a much greater problem. Some insurance companies have refused to cover these groups. Others have dramatically increased costs. Nursing organizations are working to resolve this problem.

LEGAL ISSUES IN NURSING

Some individual issues recur continuously in nursing practice. It is wise for the nurse to consider and try to understand these particular issues as they relate to individual practice.

Confidentiality and Right to Privacy

Confidentiality and the right to privacy with respect to one's personal life are very basic concerns in our society. With increased computerization of records, which can result in easier retrieval and cross-referencing of records from a variety of sources, the general public is becoming more concerned about potential invasions of privacy.

All information regarding a patient belongs to that patient. A nurse who gives out information without authorization from the patient or from the legally responsible guardian can be held liable. If you have any question about who the legally responsible guardian is, be sure to consult with your administrative authority. There may be a court-appointed legal guardian, or the situation may be governed by specific state laws regarding who becomes the responsible guardian when the person is unable to give personal consent. The hospital administration should be able to ascertain the correct action.

Only those professional persons involved in the patient's care who have a need to know about the patient can be allowed routine access to his record. A physician who is not involved in the patient's care or who does not have an administrative responsibility relative to that care is not allowed routine access. Persons not involved in care can be allowed access to the record by specific written authorization or by court order.

You should be cautious about what information you share verbally and with whom. In some instances, especially those involving treatment for alcoholism and drug abuse, even revealing the diagnosis or reasons for hospitalization would be considered a legal violation of confidentiality.

A *directory information policy* has been adopted by many acute care hospitals. This policy gives specific guidelines about what must be revealed according to freedom of information laws but will not violate confidentiality. Usually you are allowed to reveal the patient's name and sex and a general statement of condition (satisfactory, serious, and so on). If your hospital has no written policy, this is a wise standard to follow.

Situation: Breach of Confidentiality

A well-known political figure is hospitalized for a hysterectomy. The registered nurse in charge on the evening after the surgery answers the telephone. The call is from a man who identifies himself as a reporter from the community newspaper. He states that he has heard of the hospitalization and wonders how the patient is doing. The nurse responds that the patient is doing as well as could be expected for someone who has just had a hysterectomy for possible cancer. The column written in the paper suggests that because the political figure has cancer, she is an inappropriate candidate for office in the next election, and this becomes a major campaign issue.

The nurse could be held liable in a suit for revealing information to the press.

Privileged Information

Some information divulged to a nurse by a patient in the course of the professional relationship may be considered privileged. This means that if the nurse is called on to testify in court, that information need not be divulged. Not all communication between patients and nurses is considered privileged, and not all states recognize the nurse–patient relationship as one in which privileged communication exists. It is important that you understand that privilege is a very limited concept. Only a court can determine if privilege exists in any specific case. If the court does not determine information to be privileged, then you are legally obligated to testify about the communication.

Informed Consent

Legal Requirement

Everyone has the right to make decisions about oneself. Part of the right to make one's own decisions is the right to either consent to or refuse medical treatment. The law places the responsibility for obtaining consent for medical treatment on the physician. As a nurse you may be involved in this in some ways.

The law requires that the person give *voluntary* and *informed* consent. *Voluntary* means that no coercion existed; *informed* means that the person clearly understood the choices being offered. This consent may be either verbal or written. Written consent usually is preferred in health care in order to have a record and proof of consent.

A signature alone does not prove that the consent was informed. A blanket consent for "any procedures deemed necessary" is not sufficient. The form should describe the proposed medical treatment. The patient's medical condition is usually not accepted by the courts as a valid reason for not giving complete and accurate information. Currently there are no clear guidelines as to what constitutes complete information. Courts have generally supported the idea that usual risks need to be disclosed, but that rare or unexpected risks do not have to be discussed. It is the physician's responsibility to provide this information, and he or she is liable if the patient charges that the appropriate information was not given. The nurse may present a form for the patient to sign, and the nurse may sign the form as a witness to the signature. This does not transfer the legal liability to the nurse. If the patient does not seem well informed, it would be prudent for the nurse to notify the physician so that further information can be given.

Consent for Nursing Measures

Nurses must obtain consent for nursing measures undertaken. This does not mean that exhaustive explanations need to be given in each situation, since courts have held that patients can be expected to have some understanding of usual care; however, it is well for the nurse to remember that the patient is free to refuse any aspect of care that is offered. Consent for nursing measures may be implied. The nurse may state: "I have the injection the doctor ordered for you. Will you please turn over?" If the patient turns over, this is implied consent. Consent may also be verbal. The nurse may ask, "Are you ready for your bath now?" The patient answers, "Certainly."

Good nursing care requires that you use all of the means at your disposal to help the patient comprehend the value of the proposed care. For example, the postoperative patient needs to understand that getting into a chair is part of the plan of care, not a convenience for the nurse or simply a change to prevent boredom. Thus a patient's refusal of care is accepted after the patient has been given complete information so that an informed decision was made.

Withdrawing Consent

Consent may be withdrawn after it is given. People have the right to change their minds. Therefore, if after one intravenous infusion the patient decides not to have a second one started, that is his or her right. As a nurse you have an obligation to notify the physician if treatment is refused.

Consent and Minors

For a minor, consent usually is given by a parent or legal guardian. You should also obtain the minor's consent when he or she is able to give it. Courts are emphasizing increasingly that minors be allowed a voice in their own lives when it concerns matters that they are capable of understanding. This is especially true for the adolescent, but you need to consider it with any child who is 7 years of age or older. When the minor refuses care and the legal guardian has authorized that care, you should not proceed until legal clarification is given. Your nursing supervisor should be consulted.

Minors who live apart from their parents and are financially independent or who are married are termed *emancipated minors*. In most states an emancipated minor can give consent to his or her own treatment. Some states have additional specific laws allowing minors to give personal consent without also obtaining parental consent to treatment of venereal disease or for obtaining birth control information and supplies. You would need to be sure of the law in your own state if you practiced in an area where this would be a concern. An institution should develop policies to guide employees in making correct decisions in this and other areas dealing with consent.

Consent and the Mentally Incompetent

For a person who is legally determined to be mentally incompetent, consent is also obtained from the legal guardian. A difficult area involves those for whom no legal determination of competence has been made, but who do not seem able to make an informed decision. This might include the unconscious person, the very confused elderly person, or the inebriated person. The law in each state specifies who is allowed to give consent in such situations. There are also guidelines to follow in making the decision that the person cannot give his or her own consent. Your hospital policy may provide guidelines for the correct procedure. If it does not, you should consult an administrative person for a decision. Determining who is able to give legal consent is not a nursing responsibility.

Emergency Care

Care in emergencies has many legal repercussions. If a true emergency exists, consent for care is considered to be implied. The law holds that if a reasonable person were aware that the situation was life-threatening, he or she would give consent for care.

An exception to this is made if the person has explicitly rejected such care in advance, such as a Jehovah's Witness who is carrying a card stating his personal religion and that he did not wish to receive blood or blood products. This is one reason emergency room nurses should check a patient's wallet for identification and information related to care. If this is done with another person and a careful inventory of contents is made and signed by both, there should be little concern for liability for taking such an action.

Institutional Emergency Care

Most facilities that provide emergency care have policies designed to ensure that there is adequate support for claiming that an emergency exists. Thus the policy will often state that at least two physicians must examine the patient and concur that there is an emergency. This assures maximum legal protection for the physician and the institution.

In hospital emergencies the nurse sometimes may be in the position of identifying the needed action to be one that only a physician usually performs. If "life or limb" is truly in danger, the courts have held that the nurse can do those immediate things necessary even if they usually are considered a medical function, provided the nurse has the essential expertise to perform the action safely and correctly. The hospital would be expected to have a policy, which the nurse would follow, to verify and document the situation fully. This usually involves consultation with a supervisory nurse and verification of attempts to obtain medical assistance.

Situation: Nursing Action in An Emergency

In an orthopedic unit it is common to care for patients with new casts. A young man with a newly applied long-leg cast is admitted by way of the emergency room at 6 P.M. The nurse assigned to this patient's care carefully makes all the appropriate observations throughout the evening and documents his findings. He notes that the leg is beginning to swell and that the edges of the cast are beginning to cut into the skin. At that time the RN notifies the supervisor that a problem is developing and that he thinks the physician should be notified. The supervisor agrees and the nurse begins to try to contact the physician. Continuous observations are made, noting increasing swelling, color changes in the exposed toes, and loss of sensation. The physician cannot be reached and no other physician is immediately available. After consultation with the supervisor, the RN decides that an emergency exists and that the cast needs to be cut open to relieve the pressure. The RN has been taught to use a cast cutter and is familiar with the procedure. Cutting a cast open is considered a medical procedure in this hospital. The RN, with the concurrence of the supervisor, cuts open the cast and secures it in place with an elastic bandage. All observations made, consultations carried out, attempts to notify the physician, and the final action taken are carefully documented in the chart.

Hospital policy was followed throughout the situation to make sure that all necessary steps had been taken. Although this was going beyond the usual nursing practice, this would not be considered a violation of either the nursing or the medical practice acts because an emergency existed, and the results of inaction would have been serious.

Noninstitutional Emergency Care

Emergencies encountered outside the health care environment present other problems. Anyone rendering aid in an emergency is expected to behave as a reasonably prudent person would in such a situation. The nurse rendering aid in an emergency must behave as a reasonably prudent *nurse* in that setting. Thus the standard is higher than for the nonprofessional person, although the nurse is not expected to perform as if he or she were in an institutional setting. The physical situation and the psychological situation are both considered when determining what is reasonably prudent nursing action.

Many states have "good Samaritan" statutes that encourage health professionals to give aid in emergency situations. The first of these statutes was enacted in California in 1959. These statutes vary in content and comprehensiveness but relieve a professional of some liability when reasonable care is used. These laws often make people feel securer when rendering aid.

Different legal authorities give differing opinions in regard to rendering emergency aid outside of the health care setting. In their text, Rothman and Rothman advise caution and restraint in emergency situations, based on the potential for liability.[1] In contrast Bernzweig, in his text, encourages nurses to render aid and suggests that nurses should feel confident in the support of the community when carrying out emergency aid, as long as reasonable judgment is exercised.[2] Both sources agree that there is no documentation of any case in which a physician or nurse was held liable for malpractice in giving emergency care.

In 1968 the state of Vermont enacted a statute that *requires* all persons to provide assistance to others exposed to "grave physical harm." There are penalties for violation.[3]

Each nurse must make an individual decision about rendering emergency aid in a specific situation. This involves ethical as well as legal considerations.

Fraud

Fraud is a deliberate deception for the purpose of personal gain and is usually prosecuted as a crime. Situations of fraud in nursing are not common. One example would be trying to obtain a better position by giving incorrect information to a prospective employer. By deliberately stating that you had completed a nurse practitioner program to obtain a position for which you would otherwise be ineligible, you are defrauding the employer. This may be prosecuted as a crime because you also put members of the community in danger of receiving substandard care. You may also commit fraud by trying to cover up a nursing error to avoid legal action. Courts tend to be more harsh in decisions regarding fraud than in cases involving simple malpractice because fraud represents a lack of trustworthiness that could be damaging to other patients for whom you are responsible.

Situation: Fraud

A registered nurse is giving medications to the patients to whom she is assigned. In the course of the morning she presents a patient with his pills. He states that he was sure the doctor had discontinued the red pill because he had had a reaction to it the evening before. The nurse states that she is sure these are the correct medications. The patient takes the pill and the nurse charts the medication. The patient subsequently has a reaction. The nurse becomes frightened, goes back, and alters the medication record to make it appear that the medication was not given. This situation could be considered fraud. The deception was the changing of the record, and the personal gain was freedom from responsibility for the error.

Defamation of Character

Any time that shared information is detrimental to the patient's reputation, the person sharing the information may be liable for *defamation of character*. Written defamation is called *libel*. Oral defamation is called *slander*. Defamation of character involves communication that is malicious and false. Sometimes such comments are made in the heat of anger. Occasionally statements written in the chart are libelous. Severely critical opinions may be stated as fact. An example of such a statement might be "The patient is alcoholic," or "The patient is rude and domineering." The patient may charge that these comments in the chart adversely affected his care by prejudicing other staff against him. The prudent nurse will chart only objective information regarding a patient and give opinion in professional terms, well documented with fact. In conversations the prudent nurse avoids discussing patients.

Situation: Slander

Two registered nurses are leaving the floor for their coffee break. They are discussing the patients in their care as they wait for the elevator. They enter the elevator with a number of other people and continue their conversation. The first RN says: "That Mrs. Johnson in Room 201. I don't know whether I can take another day of her! She's impossible!" The other RN replies: "I know just what you mean. I had her last week and she was just on the bell all the time. If you ask me, there's nothing wrong with her that a good swift kick wouldn't cure!" First RN: "Do you really think she's faking?" Second RN: "I'm sure of it. Have you ever watched her when her husband comes to visit?"

A relative of the patient is in the elevator and overhears the conversation. She reports it to the patient. If the patient brings suit, the RNs involved might be found guilty of slander.

The nurses were discussing the patient in a place where others could hear the conversation. The comments clearly identified the patient, reflected opinions that were not supported with fact, and potentially would jeopardize the quality of the patient's care.

Assault and Battery

Assault is saying or doing something to make a person genuinely fear that he or she will be touched without consent. *Battery* is unconsented or unlawful touching of a person. Neither of these terms implies that harm was done. Harm may or may not have occurred.

For an assault to occur, the person must be afraid of what would happen even if the threatening person would not or could not carry out the threat. "If you don't take this medication, I will have to put you in restraints" is an example of an assault. The nurse who resorts to threats to achieve an end is in danger of being charged with assault.

For battery to occur, the touching must take place without consent. As you already have learned, implied consent is acceptable. Therefore, if the patient extends an arm for an injection, he cannot later charge battery, saying that he was not asked. But if the patient agreed because of a threat (assault), the touching would still be considered battery, since the consent was not freely given.

If you have an order to give a patient an iron injection and the patient says, "No. I had one of those before and they hurt!" and you persist and give the injection, a charge may be filed against you for battery. This is true even though the iron greatly benefited the patient and was a valid physician's order. The patient always has the right to refuse treatment.

False Imprisonment

Making a person stay in a place against his wishes is false imprisonment. The person can be forced to stay by using either physical means or verbal means. It is easy to understand why restraining a patient or confining a patient to a locked room could constitute false imprisonment if proper procedures were not first carried out.

Keeping a patient confined by nonphysical means is perhaps less clear. If you removed a patient's clothes for the express purpose of preventing his leaving, you could be liable for false imprisonment. Threats to keep a person confined, such as "If you don't stay in your bed, I'll sedate you," can also constitute false imprisonment. Any time a patient needs to be confined for his or her own safety or well-being, it is best to help the person understand and agree to that course of action. If

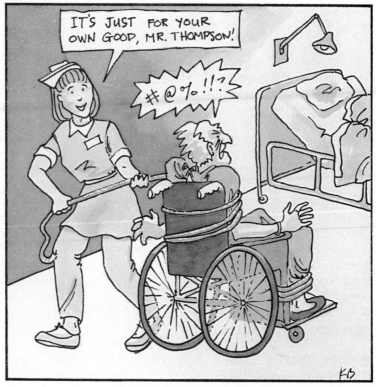

Figure 5-3. The improper use of restraints may constitute "false imprisonment."

the patient is not responsible, the guardian or legal representative may give permission. (This returns to the issue of who may give consent.) The third alternative is to objectively document the need in the patient's record and obtain a physician's order as soon as possible. Be sure to follow the policies of the facility.

In the conventional care setting you cannot restrain or confine responsible adults against their wishes. All persons have the right to make decisions for themselves, regardless of the consequences. The patient with a severe heart condition who defies orders and walks to the bathroom has that right. You protect yourself by recording your efforts to teach the patient the need for restrictions and by reporting the behavior to your supervisor and the physician.

In the same context the patient cannot be forced to remain in a hospital. If a patient wants to leave against medical advice, that is the patient's right. Again, you document your efforts in the record and follow applicable policies to protect the facility, the physician, and yourself from liability.

A hospital may not detain a patient for nonpayment of a bill. The hospital is free to take legal action against the person who does not pay, but refusing discharge would constitute false imprisonment.

False imprisonment suits are a special concern in the care of the psychiatric patient. Some particular laws relate to this situation. In the psychiatric setting you may have patients who have voluntarily sought admission. The same restrictions on restraint or confinement that apply to the patients in the general care setting apply to these patients. Other patients in the psychiatric setting may have been committed involuntarily through the applicable laws of the state. Specific measures may be used to confine the involuntarily committed patient. These are usually defined by law in terms of situations covered, type of restraint allowed, and length of time restraining may be used. If you work in a psychiatric setting, you should review the specific policies that have been developed about restraint to assist staff in functioning within the legal limits.

FACTORS THAT CONTRIBUTE TO MALPRACTICE CLAIMS

When poor results or harm do occur in the course of nursing practice, they usually are not followed by a suit. An understanding of some of the factors that enter into whether or not a suit is instituted may help you.

Social Factors

Much is currently being written about changes in the public's attitudes toward health care personnel. Health care is big business, and patients complain increasingly of not being known individually. This results in a patient being more willing to bring suit against someone who is part of the large, impersonal system.

Health costs are high, and some people see hospitals and physicians as having the ability to pay a large settlement, whether directly or through insurance. If the patient's own income is lessened or disrupted by the illness, he or she might bring suit as a solution to economic difficulties. Increased public awareness of the size of monetary judgments that are awarded in some instances may also be an economic incentive to instituting a suit.

In the past, nurses' salaries were low, and therefore there was little economic incentive to bring suit against a nurse. As nurses achieve better economic conditions, they, too, face the possibility of suit.

Suit-Prone Patients

Some people are more likely to bring suit for real or imagined errors. If these people are recognized as being suit-prone patients, it is possible for you to protect yourself through increased vigilance in regard to care and by special emphasis on thorough record keeping. Although we would warn you to guard against stereotyping, these general descriptions may help you to prevent problems. The suit-prone patient usually is identified by overt behavior in which he or she is a *persistent fault finder* and *critic* of personnel and of all aspects of care. He or she may be *uncooperative* in following the plan of care and very sensitive to any perceived slight.

The person who exhibits a *hostile attitude* may extend his or her hostile feelings to the nurses and other health care persons with whom he or she has contact. The nurse who becomes defensive in the face of hostility only widens the breach in the nurse-patient relationship. It is necessary to pay careful attention to those principles for care learned in psychosocial nursing that dealt with how to help the hostile patient. Assisting the patient to solve his or her own problems and supporting the patient are the best protection for the nurse.

Another type of patient who appears more suit-prone is the very *dependent* person who uses projection to deal with anxiety and fear. This person tends to ascribe fault or blame for all events to others and is unable to accept personal responsibility for his or her own welfare.

Again, meeting this patient's needs in a well-considered plan of care is the answer.

A common error when confronting a suit-prone patient is for staff to become defensive and withdraw. This is done partly because the situation is unpleasant and partly because staff members feel personally threatened by the patient's behavior. This increases the likelihood of a suit if a poor result occurs.

Another possible nursing response to the suit-prone patient is to become more directive and authoritarian. This tends to increase the patient's feeling of separation and distance from the staff and again increases the likelihood of suit.

If the staff is helped to view the patient as a very troubled person who manifests his or her problems in this manner, sometimes they find it easier to be objective. The patient is in need of all the nursing skill that the well-prepared nurse can bring to the emotional problems. The suit-prone patient does not always end up suing. Much depends on the response of health care personnel.

Suit-Prone Nurses

Nurses may also be suit-prone. A nurse who is insensitive to patients' complaints, who does not identify and meet patients' emotional needs, or who fails to identify the limits of his or her own practice may contribute to suits instituted not only against the nurse, but also against the employer and the physician. The nurse's self-awareness is critical in preventing suits.

PREVENTING MALPRACTICE CLAIMS

The most significant thing you can do to prevent malpractice claims is to work at improving your own nursing practice and the general climate for nursing practice where you work. You can do this in a variety of ways.

Self-awareness

Identify your own strengths and weaknesses in practice. When you have identified a weakness, seek a means of growth. This may include education, directed experience, or an opportunity for discussion with colleagues.

Be ready to acknowledge areas of weakness to supervisors, and do

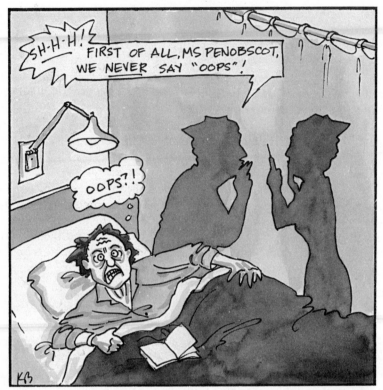

Figure 5-4. There are things that can be done to prevent malpractice suits.

not accept responsibilities for which you are not prepared. The nurse who has not worked in pediatrics for 10 years and accepts an assignment to a pediatric unit without orientation and education is setting the stage for an error to occur. Lack of current familiarity with the area is not a defense against liability. As a professional you should not accept the position if you cannot meet the criterion of being a reasonably prudent nurse *in that setting.* In instances of true emergency (disaster, flood, and so forth), courts may be more lenient, but "we need you there today" is not an emergency.

Adapt Proposed Assignments

It is reasonable to be assigned to assist an overworked nurse in a special area in which you can assume duties that are within your own competence and allow the specialized nurse to assume the specialized duties. It is not reasonable for you to be expected to assume the specialized duties. Thus, if you are not prepared for coronary care, you might go to that unit, monitor the IVs, take vital signs, and make observations to report to the experienced coronary care nurse. The experienced nurse would then be able to check the monitors, administer the specialized medications, and make decisions. Note that this does fragment the patient's care and would not be appropriate as a permanent solution, but could alleviate a temporary problem in a safe manner. It would be unsafe to assign you to *total* care of patients in that unit because you do not have the skills needed to plan and carry out care.

Following Policies and Procedures

It is your responsibility to be aware of policies and procedures of the employing institution. If they are sound, they can be an adequate defense against a claim, providing they were carefully followed.

For example, the medication procedure may involve checking all medication cards against a central Kardex that the charge nurse maintains. If you have done this and there was an error in the Kardex, you might not be liable for the resulting medication error. You had followed all appropriate procedures and acted responsibly. The liability would rest with the person who made the error. If, however, you had not followed procedure in checking, you might also be liable because you did not do your part in preventing error. As discussed previously, policies are often designed to provide legal direction.

Changing Policies and Procedures

As nursing evolves, changes are needed in procedures. Part of your responsibility as a professional is to work toward keeping all procedures up to date. These are part of nursing expertise. Are there written policies to deal with emergency situations? Statements such as "Oh, we've always done it this way" are not adequate substitutes for clearly written, officially accepted policies. Often facilities that are reluctant to make changes based on the suggestions of individual nurses are much more receptive to new ideas when the legal implications are noted.

Record Keeping

Nurses' records are unique in the health care setting. They cover the entire period of hospitalization, 24 hours a day, in a sequential pattern. Your record can be the crucial factor in avoiding litigation. Documentation in the record of observations made, decisions reached, and actions taken are considered much more solid evidence than verbal testimony, which depends on the vagaries of memory. For legal purposes observations and actions that are not recorded may be assumed not to have occurred. Properly kept records may also protect you from becoming liable for the error of another by demonstrating that you did all in your power to prevent harm, including consulting with others. Because each case is determined by the facts as well as by the applicable law, a clear documentation of all relevant data is important.

One concern over the problem-oriented records is that this format provides less detailed information and is less helpful in defense against litigation. This does not have to be the case. Any system of charting and record keeping can be used to provide the documentation of care needed. If you identify something that needs to be recorded and cannot find a provision within your system to make that recording, you can be sure that others have experienced the same difficulty. Rather than shrugging it off with the assumption that this means the record does not have to be kept, you might begin inquiries toward establishing a clear mechanism for the record keeping that concerns you. When nurses serve on committees to review and plan charting procedures, it is wise for them to seek consultation with the attorney for the facility. This would help ensure that the plan for record keeping is legally sound and professionally useful.

THE NURSE AS WITNESS

In the course of your practice as a registered nurse a time may arise when you will be asked to serve as a witness in a legal proceeding. Usually there are two kinds of cases that would involve the nurse as a witness. The first type is a personal injury action in which a person has been injured, for example, in an automobile accident, and you or your organization has been involved in the care of that person. Your testimony in that case might be on behalf of the person to help describe his or her injuries and care received for those injuries. The second type of lawsuit that involves the nurse as witness is one in which a patient brings a lawsuit against persons or organizations who have provided care for that patient, and in which the patient believes that the care was below the standard of the community. Medical malpractice is therefore alleged.

Purposes in Testifying

As a nurse you may be asked to testify in these legal actions for different reasons, perhaps as to the facts of the case in question in either of the situations above. For example, you may be asked to testify regarding the care given in a burn center to a victim of an electrical accident who received considerable nursing care during the recovery period, or you may have to give evidence regarding medical record notes or care given to a patient who has sued the facility for which you work.

As an expert witness, you may be asked to testify because of your expertise in a particular area of nursing. In this situation you would be giving a professional opinion of the facts of the case as they relate to your area of expertise. For example, if you are an operating room nurse, you may be given medical records from another hospital and asked to render an opinion, on the basis of your expertise, whether the standard of nursing care given at the first hospital was within the standards of the community. An expert witness, under Rule 702 of the Federal Rules of Evidence, accepted in the federal courts and many state courts, is defined as "a witness qualified as an expert by knowledge, skill, experience, training, or education" who may testify in the form of an opinion or otherwise.

Discovery

In a *civil lawsuit*, one between parties for the recovery of money damages, there is a lengthy discovery process that leads up to the trial itself. Often cases are settled before trial by the testimony developed in the discovery process. Discovery involves gathering information through document examination, interrogatories (written questions answered under oath), and depositions. Sometimes depositions are taken to preserve the testimony of a witness for trial under certain circumstances and act in lieu of live testimony at trial. Most depositions in which you would participate, however, would be depositions for discovery purposes. A *deposition* is a formal proceeding in which each attorney has an opportunity to question the witness, and a sworn verbatim record is made by a court reporter. Depositions are often held in attorneys' offices or in the health care facility for the convenience of the health care providers.

Testimony as a Witness in Deposition or at Trial

It is wise always to consult an attorney before talking to anyone about a matter in which you have been asked to testify, especially a malpractice action. It is possible for the person who is bringing suit to alter or amend the original complaint to include new defendants. Therefore, it is unwise for anyone who is asked to give a deposition or testify to do so without first consulting with an attorney. Many people believe that because they have done nothing wrong they do not need legal counsel. The law is complex, and you could jeopardize the position of an institution for which you work, or even jeopardize yourself and your professional future, with unwise statements. If you have liability insurance, you should advise your carrier and an attorney will be assigned to talk with you. If you are covered by an employer's policy, you should consult with the appropriate administration representative immediately to obtain counsel.

When you are being asked to consult as an expert witness, or to testify as a witness in a personal injury matter, the attorney who asks you to testify should be able to provide you with information you need about your testimony. Feel free to inquire of that attorney what your role is in the case and in which areas your testimony is expected. The attorney is

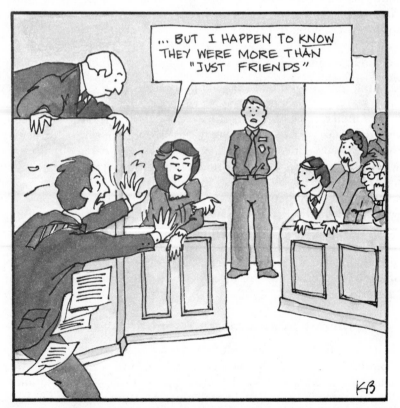

Figure 5–5. When testifying in court you should answer only the questions asked. Do not introduce other information.

likely to discuss at length what questions will be asked of you and ask you what your answer would be to those question.

As a witness, you will be required to swear or affirm to tell the entire truth. Failure to do this is *perjury.* You are expected to answer the questions asked of you to the best of your ability; however, you do not have to provide an answer that would incriminate yourself, nor do you have to answer a question for which you do not remember or know the answer.

If hypothetical situations or cases are presented for your response, be sure to note the differences between the hypothetical case and the one currently under consideration before you respond.

Be brief and direct when answering questions. Do not volunteer additional information that has not been asked for by the attorney. It is the attorney's job to ask the question so as to bring out the facts to which he or she wants you to testify. The opposing attorney will have an opportunity on cross-examination to ask you additional questions that that attorney believes are necessary for the facts of the case. It is helpful if you use words and terms that can be understood by those who are not familiar with medical terminology, or explain medical terminology where its use is essential. The purpose of your testimony is to provide facts that can be used by the court in making a decision. When you appear as an expert witness, your testimony provides an opinion that will assist the trier of fact to understand the complex areas in which expertise is necessary.

CONCLUSION

As a registered nurse, you will have a considerable legal responsibility for your own practice. It is important that you understand all the many ramifications of this responsibility. In addition, you are an important factor in preventing legal action against yourself, your employer, and other professionals with whom you work. Knowledge of the many factors involved in legal questions will be important to you in your career as a nurse.

REFERENCES

1. Rothman DA, Rothman L: The Professional Nurse and the Law, p 40. Boston, Little, Brown, 1977
2. Bernzweig EP: The Nurse's Liability for Malpractice, p 43. New York, McGraw-Hill, 1981
3. Vermont Statutes Ann, Title 12, Section 519. Supp 1971

FURTHER READINGS

Bandman E. Bandman D: There is nothing automatic about rights. Am J Nurs 77:867–872, May 1977

Bernzweig EP: The Nurse's Liability for Malpractice. 3rd ed. New York, McGraw-Hill, 1981

Bernzweig EP: Why you need your own malpractice policy. RN 48:59–60, Mar 1985

Bernzweig EP: How to spot the suit prone patient. RN 48:63–64, Jun 1985

Bullough B: The Law and the Expanding Nursing Role. 2nd ed. New York, Appleton-Century-Crofts, 1980

Carey KW: Refusing to follow orders: What's the cost of saying no? NursLife 5:53–56, Jul/Aug 1985

Creighton H: Law Every Nurse Should Know, 5th ed. Philadelphia, WB Saunders, 1986

Cushing M: The legal side: How a suit starts. Am J Nurs 85:655–656, Jun 1985

Fink JL: Legal implications of drug errors. Am Health Care Assoc J 10:37–40, Jul 1984

Guidelines for Boards of Inquiry. Publication No. L-05. Kansas City, MO, American Nurses' Association, 1979

Hemelt MD, Mackert ME: Dynamics of Law in Nursing and Health Care, 2nd ed. Reston, VA, Reston Publishing, 1982

Hemelt MD, Mackert ME: Your legal guide to nursing practice. Nurs79 9:57–64, Oct 1979

Horty JF: Healthcare law. Mod Health Care (regular column)

Isler C: Six mistakes that could land you in jail. RN 42:64–71, Feb 1979

The legal side. Am J Nurs (regular feature)

Mumme JL: Seven surefire ways to lose a malpractice case. RN 40:60–64, Nov 1977

Murchison I, Nichols TS, Hanson R: Legal Accountability in the Nursing Process. St Louis, CV Mosby, 1978

Northrop CE: The in's and out's of informed consent. Nurs 15:9, Jan 1985

Regan Reports on Hospital Law. Providence, Medica Press (quarterly publication)

Regan Reports on Medical Law. Providence, Medica Press (quarterly publication)

Regan Reports on Nursing Law. Providence, Medica Press (quarterly publication)

Regan WA: Legally Speaking. RN (regular column)

Regan WA: OR Nursing Law. AORN J (regular column)

Rothman DA, Rothman NL: The Professional Nurse and the Law. Boston, Little, Brown, 1977

Rozovsky LE: Answers to the 15 legal questions nurses usually ask. Nurs 78:73–77, Jul 1978

Rubbert TE: What to do if you are sued. Nurs 15:64D–E, 64G, 64I, Mar 1985

6 | *Ethical Concerns in Nursing Practice*

Objectives

After completing this chapter, you should be able to

1. Discuss reasons why ethical concerns are prominent in nursing.

2. List common bases used for ethical decision making and discuss their impact on the nurse.

3. Identify the basic concepts central to most ethical situations.

4. Discuss sociocultural factors that affect ethical decision making for nurses.

5. Identify how ethics relates to commitment to the patient/client, commitment to personal excellence, and commitment to nursing as a profession.

Concerns about right and wrong and good and evil are ethical issues that relate to fundamental beliefs in our society. These concerns have always been with us, and each generation has examined its own issues and the setting in which they occur, and has made its own decisions. Today we might find it difficult to understand the position of those people in the 1800s who believed that it was wrong to alleviate the pain of childbirth. These people held that pain was meant to be part of childbearing, according to their interpretation of biblical scriptures. Two hundred years from now people may have a similar difficulty understanding the positions that we take on ethical issues.

Because of a number of societal factors that have placed these problems squarely before us, ethical issues are currently being intensively discussed and debated. Many of the issues discussed in this chapter and the next are emotionally charged. If the various positions were not controversial, they would not be considered *issues*. Controversy means conflict. Conflicts can exist in values, in opinions, in solutions, and in judgments. As you read about these issues and discuss them in your classroom or with a classmate, we urge you to remember this. Only by considering all aspects of an issue can we seek understanding for ourselves. This allows us to deal more positively with the personal stress we may experience in our own lives as we attempt to find answers to ethical questions.

Throughout these chapters we emphasize personal decision making as the basic task when confronted with an ethical question. Ethical decision making cannot be escaped in nursing. The issues constantly confront us. Some nurses are tempted to back away and say, "That is not my concern," but the old saying "Not to decide is to decide" was never truer. Doing nothing is indeed a decision.

A BASIS FOR DECISION MAKING

Each person must determine his or her own basis for making ethical decisions. Some people rely on formal philosophical or religious beliefs that define matters in relation to truth or to good and evil. Others make a decision in each situation by attempting to weigh what is the greatest good for the greatest number. Still others reach a decision on the basis of personal life experience or on the basis of the experience of someone dear to them. By these and other mechanisms people come to different conclusions when confronted with ethical problems.

An additional dilemma may be created when different people come to different ethical conclusions. Many times it is possible and appropriate for you to accept another person's ethical decision as appropriate for them; however, there are other times when your own position will cause you to say, "I must oppose this action." This may bring you into direct conflict with others.

Personal Religious and Philosophical Viewpoints

Your personal viewpoint certainly will be a major factor in your ethical decision making. Achieving self-understanding in values is a lifelong learning task, and undoubtedly your position on various issues will change as you move through life. Values represent the concepts, ideals, behaviors, social principles, and major themes that give meaning to our personal life and make us unique. Values are the product of our life experiences and are influenced by family, friends, culture, environment, education, and many other conditions. Because of this our values may change. Recognizing your own value system is a goal of the classes, seminars, and books on the topic of values clarification. *Values clarification* is a growth-producing process of assessing, exploring, and determining what our personal values are and what priority they hold in our process of personal decision making. Often we do not fully explore our own values until we are confronted with a specific situation in which a decision is necessary. Although you should not feel pressured to alter your personal value system, it is important for you to seriously explore your own feelings and beliefs about various issues.

Religious beliefs form the basis for some of the decisions a person may make. However, a person who is a member of a religious group may or may not abide by the tenets of that faith. The individual makes his or her own decisions with regard to each situation, and that attitude may or may not parallel the doctrine of his church. For example, over the centuries the Roman Catholic Church has taken a stand against anything that artificially interferes with procreation. Therefore, any method of birth control that uses mechanical or chemical products is unacceptable. Certainly sterilization is not an acceptable alternative. A person who is a member of the Roman Catholic Church might adhere to this standard. Alternatively, another person might decide that he or she does not accept this standard and would use a contraceptive device. In the same way, you will explore your own religious background as you make individual ethical decisions.

Nursing offers a wide variety of job opportunities to the new graduate. Before you accept a position, you may want to consider whether it holds the potential to create conflict with your basic beliefs. Most employers are willing to recognize this as a valid criterion for accepting or

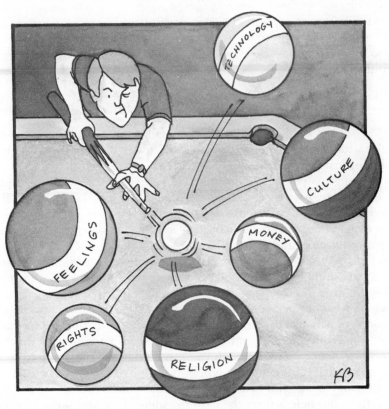

Figure 6–1. Decisions made in relation to one aspect of an ethical situation will affect all other aspects of the problem.

rejecting a position. Certainly you cannot expect to avoid all conflict or problem situations, but you probably would want to avoid working in an area in which there was constant conflict. For example, if you are ethically opposed to abortion, it would be wise to avoid employment on an obstetrical unit where therapeutic abortions are routinely performed.

Similarly, your personal value system might lead you to work in a particular area in which you have identified special needs. The hospices for the dying in England were begun by religious groups who saw value in the life of the person who was dying. Their religious beliefs were and have continued to be part of their approach to care. If you strongly value your own ethnic or cultural approach to health care, you might choose to work in a health care setting where that approach is part of the philosophy.

Codes for Nurses

Some common guidelines have been accepted by the profession as a whole for nurses to use in making ethical decisions. They are contained in the American Nurses' Association's (ANA) "Code for Nurses," which attempts to outline the nurse's responsibilities to the client and to the profession of nursing (Fig. 6–2).

The ANA code is somewhat unique among professional codes because it addresses fairly specific issues and does not confine itself to matters of etiquette or broad general statements. Warren T. Reich, editor in chief of the *Encyclopedia of Bioethics,* was quoted as stating,

---

A. N. A. CODE FOR NURSES

1. The nurse provides services with respect for human dignity and the uniqueness of the client unrestricted by considerations of social or economic status, personal attributes, or the nature of health problems.
2. The nurse safeguards the client's right to privacy by judiciously protecting information of a confidential nature.
3. The nurse acts to safeguard the client and the public when health care and safety are affected by the incompetent, unethical, or illegal practice of any person.
4. The nurse assumes responsibility and accountability for individual nursing judgments and actions.
5. The nurse maintains competence in nursing.
6. The nurse exercises informed judgment and uses individual competence and qualifications as criteria in seeking consultation, accepting responsibilities, and delegating nursing activities to others.
7. The nurse participates in activities that contribute to the ongoing development of the profession's body of knowledge.
8. The nurse participates in the profession's efforts to implement and improve standards of nursing.
9. The nurse participates in the profession's efforts to establish and maintain conditions of employment conducive to high quality nursing care.
10. The nurse participates in the profession's effort to protect the public from misinformation and misrepresentation and to maintain the integrity of nursing.
11. The nurse collaborates with members of the health professions and other citizens in promoting community and national efforts to meet the health needs of the public.

(Reprinted by permission of the American Nurses' Association)

Figure 6–2.

"This is probably the most interesting and responsive code I have ever read."[1] Tentative codes were presented by nurses in the 1920s, the 1930s, and the 1940s. Finally, in 1950, a code of ethics was adopted. It has been revised several times since then, most recently in 1976. Early versions stated that the nurse had an obligation to carry out physician's orders; later versions, however, stress the nurse's obligation to the client. This includes protecting the client from the incompetent, unethical, or illegal practice of anyone.

The International Council of Nurses has also adopted a Code for Nurses (Fig. 6–3) and, in addition, has written a Pledge for Nurses. These can both serve as guidelines for ethical conduct. The International Code for Nurses in its 1973 revision is divided into sections. The introductory portion speaks of the general responsibilities of the nursing profession. Five sections follow, dealing with the more specific concerns of people, practice, society, co-workers, and the profession.

The Patient's Rights

The patient's client's rights are another consideration in decision making. Perhaps we have always recognized this in some ways. As early as 1959 the National League for Nursing formulated a statement regarding patient's rights. However, for many years health care professionals assumed the attitude that they knew best and made many decisions without consulting with or considering the rights of the patient/client. For example, the patient with an enlarged thyroid gland was not offered information about possible alternatives in treatment, although they did exist. The individual physician made the decision regarding which treatment method was preferable, and that was the only one presented to the patient.

As the health consumer movement became more active, greater attention was paid to the rights of the patient. Now patients often expect to be informed of all alternatives for treatment and want to participate in making the decision about type of treatment, including both the possible benefits and the risks of the treatment methods presented.

In 1973 the American Hospital Association published "A Patient's Bill of Rights," which outlines the rights of the hospital patient (Fig. 6–5) and serves as a basis for making decisions about hospitalized patients. Some have criticized this document, saying that it is rather innocuous in that it simply reminds patients of their rights (such as privacy, confidentiality, and informed consent) but says nothing of hospitals that fail to act in accordance with these rights. The heaviest criticism levied against this paper is that "A Patient's Bill of Rights" fails to recognize explicitly the patient's right to adequate medical care.[2]

1973 CODE FOR NURSES

Ethical Concepts Applied to Nursing

The fundamental responsibility of the nurse is fourfold: to promote health, to prevent illness, to restore health and to alleviate suffering.

The need for nursing is universal. Inherent in nursing is respect for life, dignity and rights of man. It is unrestricted by considerations of nationality, race, creed, colour, age, sex, politics or social status.

Nurses render health services to the individual, the family and the community and coordinate their services with those of related groups.

Nurses and People

The nurse's primary responsibility is to those people who require nursing care.

The nurse, in providing care, respects the beliefs, values and customs of the individual.

The nurse holds in confidence personal information and uses judgment in sharing this information.

Nurses and Practice

The nurse carries personal responsibility for nursing practice and for maintaining competence by continual learning.

The nurse maintains the highest standards of nursing care possible within the reality of a specific situation.

The nurse uses judgment in relation to individual competence when accepting and delegating responsibilities.

The nurse when acting in a professional capacity should at all times maintain standards of personal conduct that would reflect credit upon the profession.

Nurses and Society

The nurse shares with other citizens the responsibility for initiating and supporting action to meet the health and social needs of the public.

Nurses and Co-Workers

The nurse sustains a cooperative relationship with co-workers in nursing and other fields.

The nurse takes appropriate action to safeguard the individual when his care is endangered by a co-worker or any other person.

Nurses and the Profession

The nurse plays the major role in determining and implementing desirable standards of nursing practice and nursing education.

The nurse is active in developing a core of professional knowledge.

The nurse, acting through the professional organization, participates in establishing and maintaining equitable social and economic working conditions in nursing.

(Reprinted with the permission of the International Council of Nurses)

Figure 6-3.

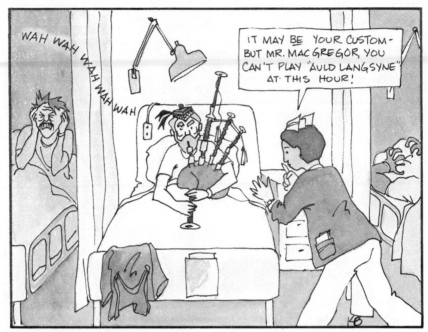

Figure 6–4. The nurse in providing care respects the beliefs, values, and customs of the individual.

Other groups have also formulated statements regarding rights of the health consumer, nurses' associations among them. In some states, rights of the health consumer are being formalized into legal statements.

Basic Ethical Concepts

Four concepts are involved in most ethical situations—beneficence, autonomy, justice, and fidelity. Identifying how they apply to a particular situation and balancing their competing claims often present some of the most difficult dilemmas.

Beneficence refers to the obligation to do good, not harm, to other people. One difficulty arises in who is to decide what is good for a person. In most instances we expect that a person will make her or his own decision. But who decides for the infant, the mentally incompetent, and others who are unable to make decisions? Another problem centers around what is good. Is all life good, or is some life not good? Is it better to sustain life in the face of all disability, or is it better to allow a person to die and have suffering ended?

A PATIENT'S BILL OF RIGHTS

Approved by the House of Delegates of the American Hospital Association February 6, 1973

The American Hospital Association presents a Patient's Bill of Rights with the expectation that observance of these rights will contribute to more effective patient care and greater satisfaction for the patient, his physician, and the hospital organization. Further, the Association presents these rights in the expectation that they will be supported by the hospital on behalf of its patients, as an integral part of the healing process. It is recognized that a personal relationship between the physician and the patient is essential for the provision of proper medical care.

The traditional physician–patient relationship takes on a new dimension when care is rendered within an organizational structure. Legal precedent has established that the institution itself also has a responsibility to the patient. It is in recognition of these factors that these rights are affirmed.

1. The patient has the right to considerate and respectful care.

2. The patient has the right to obtain from his physician complete current information concerning his diagnosis, treatment, and prognosis in terms the patient can be reasonably expected to understand. When it is not medically advisable to give such information to the patient, the information should be made available to an appropriate person in his behalf. He has the right to know by name, the physician responsible for coordinating his care.

3. The patient has the right to receive from his physician information necessary to give informed consent prior to the start of any procedure and/or treatment. Except in emergencies, such information for informed consent, should include but not necessary be limited to the specific procedure and/or treatment, the medically significant risks involved, and the probable duration of incapacitation. Where medically significant alternatives for care or treatment exist, or when the patient requests information concerning medical alternatives, the patient has the right to such information. The patient also has the right to know the name of the person responsible for the procedures and/or treatment.

4. The patient has the right to refuse treatment to the extent permitted by law, and to be informed of the medical consequences of his action.

5. The patient has the right to every consideration of his privacy concerning his own medical care program. Case discussion, consultation, examination, and treatment are confidential and should be conducted discreetly. Those not directly involved in his care must have the permission of the patient to be present.

6. The patient has the right to expect that all communications and records pertaining to his care should be treated as confidential.

7. The patient has the right to expect that within its capacity a hospital must make reasonable response to request of a patient for services. The hospital must provide evaluation, service, and/or referral as indicated by the urgency of the case. When medically permissible a patient may be transferred to another facility only after he has received complete information and explanation concerning the needs for and

(continued)

Figure 6–5.

A PATIENT'S BILL OF RIGHTS *(continued)*

alternatives to such a transfer. The institution to which the patient is to be transferred must first have accepted the patient for transfer.

8. The patient has the right to obtain information as to any relationship of his hospital to other health care and educational institutions insofar as his care is concerned. The patient has the right to obtain information as to the existence of any professional relationships among individuals, by name, who are treating him.

9. The patient has the right to be advised if the hospital proposes to engage in or perform human experimentation affecting his care or treatment. The patient has the right to refuse to participate in such research projects.

10. The patient has the right to expect reasonable continuity of care. He has the right to know in advance what appointment times and physicians are available and where. The patient has the right to expect that the hospital will provide a mechanism whereby he is informed by his physician or a delegate of the physician of the patient's continuing health care requirements following discharge.

11. The patient has the right to examine and receive an explanation of his bill regardless of source of payment.

12. The patient has the right to know what hospital rules and regulations apply to his conduct as a patient.

No catalogue of rights can guarantee for the patient the kind of treatment he has a right to expect. A hospital has many functions to perform, including the prevention and treatment of disease, the education of both health professionals and patients, and the conduct of clinical research. All these activities must be conducted with an overriding concern for the patient, and, above all, the recognition of his dignity as a human being. Success in achieving this recognition assures success in the defense of the rights of the patient.

(Reproduced by permission of the American Hospital Association, © 1975)

Figure 6–5. (continued)

Autonomy refers to the right to make one's own decisions. However, there are limitations on that right. What should those limitations be? Are there instances when those with more background and understanding should make decisions for others? In what instances should the legal system interfere with personal decision making? How does autonomy relate to professionals as well as to patients and their families?

Justice refers to the obligation to be fair to all people. How is fairness defined? Does this mean that people should be treated the same? Does it mean that the government should provide what people cannot provide for themselves? What are the rights of one person when they affect the rights of another?

Fidelity refers to the obligation to be faithful to the agreements and responsibilities that one has undertaken. What are the responsibilities of health care personnel to individuals, employers, the government, and society? When these responsibilities conflict, which has priority?

As we present a variety of ethical concerns, try to relate these four concepts to the problem and identify which of them is presenting the greatest difficulties.

Ethical Theories

It is not our intent to delve with any depth into the writings of early philosophers. However, some of their ethical theories are mentioned frequently enough in the literature that surrounds bioethical issues that some background seems appropriate.

An *ethical theory* is a moral principle or a set of moral principles that can be used in assessing what is morally right or morally wrong. Over the years we have called on the theories of philosophers to guide us in our decision making.

Utilitarian ethics is found most prominently in the works of Jeremy Bentham (1748–1832) and John Stuart Mill (1806–1873). As the name suggests, the basic concept is that an act is right if it is useful in bringing about a desirable or good outcome for the greatest number. This ethical theory would encourage us to act in ways that would produce the greatest balance of good over evil and is sometimes said to be "the greatest happiness principle."

Immanuel Kant (1724–1804) left theories that command attention in discussions today. Kant strongly opposed utilitarianism and espoused an ethical theory in which the moral rightness or wrongness of human action would be considered totally independent of the consequences of the action. Kant's work is complex and some parts are difficult to understand. The fundamental principle of Kant's work is what he called the "Categorical Imperative," a maxim that can be interpreted as universal law. A person, according to Kant's imperative, should be used as an end, never as a means. Kant believed that certain moral commands must be obeyed under all circumstances. It was not the consequences that made an action right or wrong, but the principle on which one acts. Thus two major concepts of Kant's work are its universal application and respect for the person.

The "Natural Law Theory" is found in the writings of St. Thomas Aquinas (1223–1274). The fundamental concept of his theory is that actions are morally right when they are in accord with our nature and end as human beings and are morally wrong when they are not in accord with our nature and end as human beings. Basically this states that good should be promoted, evil should be avoided, and ethics should be grounded in our concern for human good. The word good was not defined in a way that might be clear to all of us, but Catholic theologians conceive of natural law as inscribed by God, endowing all things with potentials that serve to define their natural end.

Rawls proposed a concept of social equity as an approach to justice. He believed that if people of reason were placed in a situation of ethical choice without knowing which position they had in society (a situation he called the original position), they would choose the alternative that supported the most disadvantaged person. Using this approach, the concern of society should be directed toward the most disadvantaged, since they are the ones who are least able to speak for themselves.

SOCIAL FACTORS THAT INFLUENCE ETHICAL DECISION MAKING

Ethical decisions are not made in a vacuum. Many factors exert pressure and demand response as we search for appropriate answers to the dilemmas that face us. All facets of today's world are experiencing change, and nursing is no exception. The "truths" of yesterday are being challenged by the realities and new problems confronting us today.

In studying ethical issues it is important for you to understand the many forces that are operating. These forces are not independent or mutually exclusive, but act and react on one another in a constantly changing milieu, causing evolutionary changes in all segments of society.

Social and Cultural Attitudes

Changes in the attitudes of society as a whole profoundly influence each of its segments. For example, the shifting role of women, attitudes toward marriage and the family, and the changing status of minorities have all required nurses to reexamine their personal feelings and alter their way of providing nursing care.

Ethical concerns are the by-products of a number of factors at work in our society today. The rights of the individual have been increasingly emphasized in all aspects of living and, more recently, in dying. In the health care field this is most pointedly illustrated by the use of the terminology *health care* as opposed to *medical care*. Health care suggests much greater involvement of others and places the person in the center of the activity, whereas medical care places the physician in the key role. The meaning of *consumer unit* is shifting from an individual to a total family, or even a whole community. The focus of care also has changed from one that was primarily disease-oriented to one that is strongly preventive.

The size of the group being affected by ethical decisions has a bearing on the decision-making process. The smaller the group, organization, or society that is involved in the decision making, the easier the process of arriving at an acceptable alternative. Many of our ethical considerations now involve our society as a whole or, in some cases, the world; therefore, solutions are difficult. For example, a couple who already have two children may have little trouble deciding that sterilization is an appropriate birth control method for them. But if we try to extend that same decision to all couples of an entire city block, it becomes more difficult. This is because we believe in each person's right to exercise choice, because of each person's beliefs and conscience, and because of conflicts that arise between and among individuals.

The value a society places on the individual directly impacts on the standard of care. (It is unlikely that kamikazes, who purposefully directed their planes into significant targets, and thereby sacrificed their lives, would ever have developed in a culture that places high value on the individual existence rather than on the glory achieved through sacrificing life for the society.) A culture's religious values and belief in an afterlife directly affect ethical issues. The population, or, more accurately, the overpopulation, of a country may also have a direct bearing on the value placed on life.

Science and Technology

Most significantly, scientific advancement and technology have left us wrestling with concerns that would have been considered science fiction 50 years ago. Before the development of kidney dialysis, we accepted the fact that people with nonfunctioning kidneys would soon die. After machines that would filter body wastes became available, a genuine dilemma arose over which of the many candidates would have dialysis and which would not and would consequently die. More people needed treatment than there were equipment, time, and personnel to treat them.

The advent of machines that could artificially respirate someone challenged the medical and legal professions to examine their definition of life and brought into focus problems of when to turn off the machine.

Heart and lung machines that could adequately perfuse the body while the heart was stopped for surgical procedures have enabled operations to be performed that were unheard of 50 years ago. Fetal monitors, which can be attached to mothers-to-be while they are in labor, provide a continuous readout of the baby's status. Such monitoring has resulted in an increase in the number of babies delivered by cesarean section. The implantation of an artificial heart in a human subject has received worldwide attention. These scientific and technological advances continue to present ethical questions for which there are often no readily apparent answers.

Legislation

Social change and legislation are constantly in flux. Each causes action to occur and reacts to the effects resulting from the other's exercise. Because legislation solidifies action into law, the conflict becomes more acute for those who are opposed to the stand that the law supports.

Legislation may follow changes in society's attitudes, converting new ideas into law. Alternatively, legislation may lead society into change in the way that civil rights legislation did in the 1950s and 1960s. Recent legislative action that speaks to the needs and opportunities available to the handicapped has brought about changes in policies, procedures, and even architecture.

Judicial Decisions

Many ethical issues have legal implications. The judicial system also provides a major avenue for change. We therefore find that more and more issues are taken to court and judicial decisions are made. As you continue this chapter, note that we have often cited a landmark decision that resulted in a change. The process does not stop there, however. Some people may disagree with a judicial decision and continue to oppose it. Judicial decisions may also be overturned by higher courts. Meanwhile, the questions regarding the individual person's role in carrying out a judicial decision remain. For example, although the law in the past forbade abortions, some physicians believed so strongly in the right of the individual to have the procedure done and were so upset by the results of nonprofessional abortions, that they were willing to perform them in spite of the law prohibiting them. These physicians were, of course, liable to prosecution if they were caught, and some were prosecuted for performing illegal abortions.

Funding

The financing of health care represents an area of conflict. The federal government has become more and more involved in providing funds for health care. Some people are asking how much time, money, and energy we should allocate to health care and how should that money be divided. How obligated are we as a society to make some form of health care available to all? What is it that health care can and cannot provide? Which is more important, prevention or cure? Some of that care includes controversial procedures, such as abortions and sterilization. Some taxpayers cannot ethically sanction these procedures and do not want their tax dollars used to fund them. Thus individual decisions can have far-reaching effects.

OCCUPATIONAL FACTORS THAT INFLUENCE DECISION MAKING

By virtue of the positions they hold in the health care system, nurses have special forces acting on them as they try to make decisions. An awareness of these factors may help you as you struggle with personal problems in decision making.

Status as an Employee

Most nurses are not in independent practice, but are employed by hospitals, other institutions, or physicians. Thus there are pressures that divide the nurse's loyalty among patient, employer, and self. You will notice that codes do not speak of responsibilities to the employer, yet certainly there are responsibilities to the one who pays the salary and makes decisions in regard to your work. It is not unusual for an ethical decision to involve conflict between the best interests of the employer and the patient.

When discussing ethical decisions in the abstract, most people say that, of course, the *patient's* best interest should be the only priority. In real situations, however, the issues often are not so clear-cut. If a nurse's decision affects the employer adversely, the result may be job loss, poor references, and severely curtailed economic and career future. It would be desirable if this were not the case, but often it is all too real. As an example, one physician was known to routinely require his patients to sign blank surgical permits on admission to the hospital. One of the staff nurses became upset with this procedure after learning that the patients often did not understand what was being planned. Eventually she discussed the matter with the physician, pointing out that she did not believe that it was ethical to require the patients to sign the blank documents, especially since they were not informed of alternative methods of treatment. The physician became angry and complained to the hospital administration, threatening to take his surgeries elsewhere. This would have created a considerable economic loss for the hospital and, depending on the action of the administrator, the nurse might have been labeled a troublemaker and even discharged in order to placate the physician.

Collective Bargaining Contracts

Collective bargaining contracts can protect nurses in making ethical decisions. By formalizing reasons and procedures for termination of employment and outlining grievance measures so that individual nurses have a mechanism for protecting themselves, the contract may provide greater freedom.

Some people believe that contracts hamper individual freedom. The supervisor who believes that an employee does not deliver optimal care may feel unable to do anything about the situation because the correction and termination process under a contract are so complex. Often many specific steps related to notifying the employee of unsatisfactory work and assistance for employee growth are required before a person can be discharged.

Collegial Relationships

Relationships among nurses who work together (colleagues) in which they support one another, share in decision making, and present a unified approach to others can provide an excellent climate for ethical decision making. All too often such relationships are lacking in hospitals. Nurses feel alone and are not experienced in seeking out and supporting one another. Greater effort on their part in this area might be rewarding.

Authoritarian and Paternalistic Backgrounds

The historically authoritarian and paternalistic attitudes of physicians and hospitals often have relegated nurses, most of whom are women, to dependent and subservient roles. These role differentiations have in the past inhibited nurses from taking independent stands on issues, and they continue to affect relationships in the health care field. Some physicians have been heard to comment that all ethical decisions rest on the physician's shoulders, and that once the physician has made a decision, all other members of the health care team are obligated to acquiesce. This attitude results in people absolving themselves of moral responsibility by simply following orders. An example of a unilateral decision by a physician would be in the case of a patient suffering from terminal cancer. The physician may order that a narcotic be given every half hour by the intravenous line even though the cumulative effect of the narcotic will seriously compromise the patient's respirations, perhaps to the point of stopping them. The nurse would be expected simply to carry out the order.

Today's nurses increasingly are speaking out against such an approach, which leaves them out of the decision-making process. In the case above, nurses of today might expect the physician to discuss the situation with the patient, the family, and the nursing staff. They would expect the nurses' input to be considered and to have a voice in decision making. The result might be an order for a narcotic to keep the patient pain-free yet alert. The patient might be able to express his or her needs, and the nurse would have orders that provided liberal guidelines as to amount and frequency for the narcotic. The nurses would be expected to make careful assessments and to function in light of the overall decisions made during the conference.

Consumer Involvement in Health Care

The widespread consumer movement has become a significant factor in health care. Consumers are demanding a greater voice in all aspects of their own health care delivery. Part of this involvement is at the decision-making level.

Many hospitals have had ethics committees for years. Such committees were traditionally composed of physicians and were for the purpose of monitoring the behavior of physicians. They were called on to act when a physician's inappropriate behavior, such as arriving at the hospital intoxicated, was reported to them. Today the scope of ethics committees has enlarged considerably. They may consider the appropriateness of procedures to be done, what patient should receive treatment, and when treatment should be withdrawn. Membership has grown, and, increasingly, members of the hospital administration, the community, and other health care disciplines are being represented. When nurses participate they are provided with a formal mechanism to share in ethical decision making.

If a nurse makes an ethical decision on the basis of the patient's best interest but contrary to the physician's or hospital's interest, public support may be forthcoming. The public increasingly sees health care as big business and tends to support those who champion consumer interests that conflict with the institution's interests. This support may be short-lived and therefore should not be relied on for protection against the adverse consequences of an ethical decision.

With consumers involved in decision making, nurses again may face a situation in which they are expected to take action or no action based on the conclusions of others. Modern-day nurses may find this as problematic as action based on a physician's decision. For example, an obstetrical patient who has hemorrhaged severely may refuse blood transfusions because of religious beliefs. The nurse, recognizing the benefit of the transfusion, may have difficulty maintaining effective communication and rapport with the patient and family because of her own convictions that a transfusion is the best treatment.

SPECIFIC ETHICAL ISSUES RELATED TO THE PROFESSION OF NURSING

Some of the ethical issues that are of concern to nurses relate specifically to the nursing profession, others relate to bioethical issues confronting all of society. Here we will discuss the areas facing nursing through commitment to the patient, commitment to personal excellence, and commitment to the nursing profession as a whole. Bioethical issues that relate to the whole society are discussed in Chapter 7. We present a definite viewpoint regarding ethics in the nursing profession. We feel strongly about the individual's responsibility for nursing practice and place high value on personal integrity in professional relationships.

Commitment to the Patient/Client

Nursing has a strong history of being commited to the well-being of the patients and clients who need care. Both the ANA Code for Nurses and the 1973 Code for Nurses clearly point out the obligation that the nurse has in fulfilling this commitment. This obligation has been used to try to persuade nurses that they must not be concerned for self, working conditions, salaries, or other aspects of the employment situation. This is not realistic, and may even be counterproductive to the development of effective autonomous nurses. However, rejection of a handmaiden philosophy does not require rejection of a basic philosophy that identifies nursing as a profession focused on providing patients and their families with support for growth to maximum health and well-being.

Patients/clients can never become objects for nursing but must be approached as unique individuals who deserve concern, respect, and the best we have to offer.

Recommending a Care Provider

Clients and other people of your acquaintance may ask you to recommend a physician or other type of care provider because they believe that, as a nurse, you have special expertise in such matters. In the past, nurses were admonished not to express opinions about care providers and were simply to direct clients to the yellow pages, directories, or hospitals that referred patients to staff physicians on a rotating basis. If you indeed have no personal knowledge about the requested information, then this would be a reasonable approach. But if you do have knowledge, it seems inappropriate to sidestep the issue. You could recommend several competent persons, pointing out characteristics of each that might be factors in personal choice. For example, if asked to recommend an obstetrician, you might recommend three. You could then further state that Drs. A., B., and C. are all board-certified specialists in obstetrics. You might add some information about their practices: Dr. A. is an older physician with a more traditional approach to childbirth; Dr. B. is a young and innovative physician who strongly advocates father participation and the natural childbirth method (also known as Lamaze method); Dr. C. is new in the community but appears to allow patients a great deal of choice in their approach to childbirth. The client can further research these physicians and make a choice.

If you are specifically asked about a physician whose care you believe to be less than satisfactory, you are faced with a different dilemma. Making severely critical statements might leave you open to a legal charge of slander by the physician (see Chapter 5). However, to say nothing is ethically a problem because you are not acting to protect the client. A safe approach is to state, "I personally would not choose Dr. X. as my physician. Instead I would prefer to see Dr. N. or Dr. O." If pressed to give reasons, you are legally securer if you indicate that you would prefer not to discuss specifics.

You do need to be careful that any recommendations are not based on hearsay or gossip. If you do not have solid information on which to base a referral, do not be drawn into making one.

Dealing with Poor Care

The day has passed when nurses could be expected to provide unwavering support of all members of the health care team, whatever their actions or the outcomes for the patient. Concern for the welfare of patients requires that nurses acknowledge the existence of poor care or unwise practice and work toward change. We see the issue in terms of the form and extent the involvement should take, rather than whether the nurse should become involved.

The first step in any situation in which you believe poor care or unwise practice to exist is for you to collect adequate, valid information. Do not make decisions based on gossip, hearsay, or a single isolated instance. If you do, you may find yourself creating problems for yourself as well as for others rather than solving problems for the patient. Sometimes a single incident is serious enough that you want to act, but before taking action, be sure of your facts.

Your second step is to be certain you understand both the official and the unofficial systems of authority and responsibility within your facility. You need to know which people have the authority to make decisions and changes, what the official prescribed route of change is, and what the hidden priorities of the institution might be. For example, the official lines of authority may provide the physician who has been elected chief of staff with authority within the medical group. Your knowledge of the informal system may reveal that a certain respected physician who does not have an official position actually is able to exert more influence for change. Within the nursing chain of responsibility, you may be aware that the head nurse of your unit, although officially having authority, in reality refers all decision making to the supervisor.

The most commonly recommended initial action is that you take your concerns to your immediate supervisor. If you do this, your legal responsibility, if there is one, usually is satisfied. Many people would also say that this fulfills your ethical responsibility. If the system always worked effectively, your supervisor would carry the concern onward within the organizational structure, and each person contacted would forward the concern to the next appropriate person until it reached the individual or committee with the authority and duty to act.

However, the system does not always work. Your concern may be dropped or ignored at any one of many points. You may never learn what was done. Occasionally results are identified only much later, when a change in procedure and policy occurs.

Sometimes an alternative initial approach is more appropriate to the situation. You may volunteer to serve on committees such as those that deal with peer review. If there are no such committees, you may work to have them established, perhaps through a bargaining unit. This route of action will require a considerable investment of your own time and effort. The cry of "Why doesn't somebody do something?" may often be answered "Because nobody takes the time." This is a very real constraint on action.

Another initial approach is to use the informal system within the facility. You may discuss your concern with a trusted person who has influence within the system. You may learn that you are not alone in your concerns, that efforts toward change are being made, and that your input of data is welcomed. Be careful when using informal systems; they can backfire. If your immediate superior learns that you went over his or her head with your concerns, he or she may direct anger at you.

If your initial approach is not effective, one formal route for seeking further change would lead you through the official lines of authority within your facility. After discussing your concern with your immediate supervisor and receiving no satisfactory response, you would tell the supervisor formally that you intend to carry your concern to the next higher authority. Technically you could proceed in this manner until you reached the administrator or even the board of directors.

Another formal route for seeking further change is through designated committees or procedures within your facility. This might require a carefully written documented report explaining your concern. You might then be called to answer questions that the committee has.

You might also decide to return to the unofficial power system within the facility. You might seek out other health professionals whom you believe would be interested, and secure support for change in this way.

A final alternative is to offer your resignation if the change is not made. Continuing to exist in an environment in which poor practice exists may place you in conflict with your ethical standards and values.

If you decide to pursue any of these routes, you need to be fully aware of the possible consequences. You may be labeled a trouble-maker, or worse. You may lose the opportunity to be promoted because you are seen as being antagonistic to the system. It is even possible that you could lose your job for creating too many waves. Officially this should not happen, but in reality it can and does. We do not mean to be unduly discouraging, but we want to warn you that the role of change agent is not easy, and you should be aware of and weigh the consequences before you decide to act.

Commitment to Personal Excellence

In order to meet the commitment to the patient/client, each individual nurse must be committed to personal excellence. Basic to moving toward personal excellence is a willingness to engage in self-evaluation and assume responsibility in the work setting.

Self-evaluation

Self-evaluation is discussed throughout this text in relationship to personal career goals, legal concerns, and continuing education. There also exists a strong ethical responsibility for the health care professional to practice self-evaluation. You are the one who is best able to identify your weaknesses and practice deficits as well as your strengths. Your careful self-evaluation is the patient's best protection against poor or inadequate care.

Self-evaluation is not always an easy or pleasant task. If we are truly honest with ourselves, we will be likely to uncover areas we wish were not there. Remember, done informally, these do not have to be shared with anyone; that is one of the beauties of self-evaluation. On the other hand, do not hesitate to ask for assistance if you think you need it. One is seldom criticized for trying to do a better job. Many institutions are now

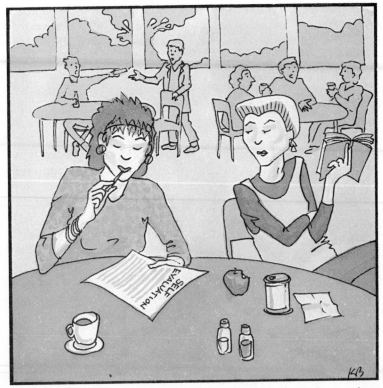

Figure 6–6. One of the advantages of self-evaluation is that it does not have to be shared.

including self-evaluation in the formal evaluation of employees. If this is the case, you may be asked to prepare a written self-evaluation that will be shared with at least your immediate supervisor.

One avenue of approach to self-evaluation is the use of the nursing process format. Begin by a thorough *personal assessment* (see Fig. 6–7). To do this you will have to gather data about your own performance. This requires a level of objectivity that is not easy. You might outline areas in which you want to gather data and actually keep notes on yourself.

After data has been collected, you will need to give yourself time to reflect on it and analyze it thoroughly. The self-assessment outline includes questions you would ask yourself, however, the criteria that you use to determine whether your answers reflect the quality of performance you want to attain are not included. Those specific criteria must be individualized to the setting in which you work and the nature of your role in that setting. The breadth of data that represents excellent practice for the nurse in the emergency room differs from what would represent excellence for the nurse working in a rehabilitation setting. The amount of decision making in which the patient participates differs between the recovery room and the outpatient clinic.

Your analysis can reveal strengths, weaknesses, and areas for growth or improvement. Congratulate yourself on the strengths identified and then clearly identify those areas in which you want to change. As in nursing care planning, clearly identifying and stating the problems or growth needed helps you to plan more effectively.

SELF-EVALUATION PLAN

Assessment of Patients

1. Do I gather enough breadth of data about patients and families, including both strengths and deficits?
2. Do I gather data in great enough depth?
3. Do I listen closely to the patient and attend to what is being said?
4. Do I regularly use all available sources for information about my patients? (patient, family, other staff, chart, Kardex, and so forth.)
5. Have I recognized problems quickly so that they did not become worse through inattention?
6. Do I recognize physiological, social, and psychological problems?

(continued)

Figure 6–7.

SELF-EVALUATION PLAN (continued)

Planning for Patient Care

1. Do I routinely seek more information on which to base decisions about patient care?
2. Do I include the patient in decision-making whenever possible?
3. Do I consult with others on the health care team when planning?
4. Are my written plans clear, concise, and reasonable to carry out?
5. Do I take into account the realities of the situation when planning care?
6. Are my plans for care sound and appropriate to the individual patient?
7. Do I employ principles from the biological and social sciences in planning?

Intervention

1. Is my work organized and finished on time?
2. Do I maintain optimum safe working habits?
3. Do I perform technical skills in an efficient and safe manner?
4. Do I communicate clearly and effectively with patients, family, and staff?
5. Do I use therapeutic communication techniques appropriately and effectively?
6. Do I use teaching approaches appropriate to the individual patient and family?
7. Do I keep accurate and complete written records?
8. Do I understand and perform any administrative tasks which are my responsibility? (ordering supplies, planning for laboratory tests, and so on.)
9. Do I make the effort to learn about new techniques and procedures?

Evaluation

1. Do I routinely evaluate the effectiveness of the nursing care I give?
2. Do I effectively assist in evaluation of the patient's response to medical care and to ordered therapies?
3. Do I encourage the patient to participate in evaluating both the process and the outcomes of care?
4. Is self-evaluation a planned part of my activities?
5. Do I use data collected during evaluation for the improvement of my own functioning and patient care?

Personal Growth and Relationships

1. Have I established a sound trust and working relationship with co-workers?
2. Do I support and assist my co-workers when possible?
3. Do I communicate effectively with others on the health care team?
4. Have I sought opportunities for learning and personal growth?
5. Is my attitude helpful and productive?
6. Do I have sound working habits? (appearing on time, limiting coffee and lunch breaks to the correct time, and so forth)
7. Is my appearance appropriate to the working environment?
8. Do I use appropriate channels of communication within the institution correctly?
9. Do I handle criticism constructively?
10. Am I doing my share in overall professional activities such as serving on committees or assisting with development projects?
11. Am I honest with myself, being neither too harsh nor too easy going?

Figure 6–7 (continued).

After you have identified your problems, it is appropriate to establish a plan of action. The plan is more helpful to you if it contains clearly defined goals. What is a realistic expectation for yourself? When is an appropriate time to reach that expectation? As part of realizing these goals, you might find it helpful to establish criteria you will use to identify your progress. Once the goals are set, you are better able to plan appropriate action to meet them. You might consider such things as requesting in-service education, taking continuing education courses, consulting with colleagues, and doing independent reading and study. Some plans would need to include specific things that you will be doing in your daily nursing care for improvement. To do this you may want to request assignments that will provide opportunities for practice of skills.

All this planning must not go to waste. *Implementing* this plan will require you to remain focused on what you are trying to accomplish. Keeping records on yourself is often helpful.

Periodic evaluation of your progress is necessary so that you do not become discouraged. Any records you have kept will be valuable for this purpose. Sometimes it is hard to identify gradual change. You might even plan rewards for yourself for improvement that occurs. Try not to become discouraged if you do not see the improvement you desire. Remember, that just as in patient-care planning, a reassessment and a new or revised plan are often necessary, so may it be in the self-evaluation process. Keep in mind that your overall goal is personal excellence in nursing practice.

Responsibility for Supplies

Pilfering is stealing in small amounts or stealing objects of little value. In fact, many people who are otherwise scrupulously honest do not recognize that taking small items from a place of employment is indeed theft. Hospital employees often take home a thermometer, adhesive bandage strips, and other such objects so routinely that they do not even consider whether this is right or wrong. With the large number of employees in a modern hospital, this constant petty theft may total thousands of dollars. The cost of this must be passed on to those who pay the bills—the patients. As a leader in the care setting, the registered nurse is often in a position to clearly communicate to all employees that pilfering is unacceptable and to serve as an example of careful stewardship of the hospital supplies.

Commitment to the Nursing Profession

Commitment to the nursing profession requires that each individual nurse be concerned not only about personal performance, but also

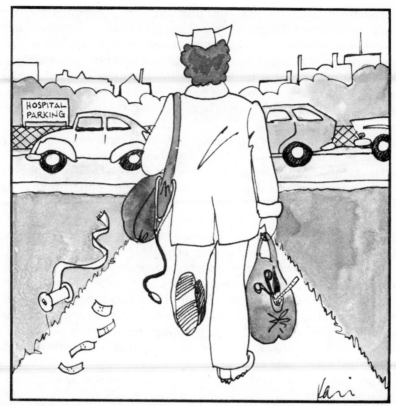

Figure 6–8. Many people who are otherwise scrupulously honest do not recognize that taking small items from a place of employment is theft.

about how nursing is practiced. This involves participation in peer evaluation, formal evaluation of nursing care, dealing with poor care, and identifying the impaired nurse.

Evaluating Peer Performance

Nurses always have evaluated one another in both formal and informal ways. Some people think that evaluation implies noting error or deficiency. Good evaluation is much broader than this. The main purpose of peer evaluation is to maintain consistent high-quality nursing care. This is an ethical, professional obligation.

Informal Evaluation. The methods of evaluation vary. An important component of peer evaluation is actual observation of the performance of others. Often co-workers are the ones who are best able to observe a nurse's performance. Watching other nurses will also help you to grow in your own practice. When you observe co-workers, you need to strive for objectivity. A common mistake is to let personal feelings, likes, and dislikes influence our observations so that we see only what we want to see. We may view a close friend only in a positive light, whereas we see only the negative aspects of a nurse with whom we have a poor personal relationship.

Another important aspect of evaluation is examining results or outcomes of care. Two nurses may use different approaches or techniques in similar situations, but both may achieve positive results.

Evaluation is not negative. As you observe behavior and outcomes in nursing practice, you will most often see good nursing care. Do not hesitate to commend others and share your positive feelings. Everyone benefits from positive reinforcement of skill. Doing this would help nurses to create a good climate for personal growth and sharing.

An ethical dilemma arises when you observe a colleague practicing what you think is poor patient care, such as poor sterile technique. A variety of avenues of action are available to you. What you choose to do depends on the seriousness of the situation you have observed. We suggest the following pattern for action as one that may assist in correcting a problem and at the same time maintain positive working relationships.

Usually the simplest and most effective answer to any problem is to go directly to the person involved and state: "I observed this specific incident and it seemed to me that it was not in the best interest of the patient because . . . How do you feel about it?" This does not level accusations of good and bad nursing and does allow the nurse to give rationale for the action taken. When you understand the situation more fully, you may have a different point of view also. If you disagree and the situation is not critical, you might want to simply state that you do differ. Sometimes just calling an incident to the attention of the person will result in a change in behavior, even if there is no open agreement that a change is needed.

If you observe poor care another time, you might again approach the person. State what you have seen, and note that it is the second time. If the person still disagrees that a problem exists, state that you feel obligated to discuss this with your immediate superior because it is not in the best interest of the patient. You should then follow through on this.

When you approach a supervisor, you need to give specific information with dates, situations, and the action you took. You should not indulge in generalities or sweeping statements, but should stick to specific observed instances. Let the supervisor know that you have talked with the person under discussion and have informed the person that you would speak with the supervisor. It is important to specify the action you would like to see occur. You might ask the supervisor to discuss the matter with both of you to clarify the correct nursing procedure. Or you might ask that the supervisor talk about the matter with the other nurse or observe the nurse. A vague declaration of "You should do something about this!" is not helpful.

If your focus has been on enhancing the welfare of patients and you have been quick to praise the good care provided by others, your action in response to poor care will be more readily accepted. Remember that your attitude when approaching another nurse is crucial. Facial expressions and tone of voice as well as words need to be considered. If you are perceived as friendly and caring, your comments probably will be accepted in a far different manner than if you are seen as being negative and critical.

But you cannot always count on this. Many nurses feel threatened by the idea of evaluation or have had bad experiences in which evaluation only involved pointing out deficiencies. These nurses may be angry and upset with any colleague who deems evaluation to be part of the colleague role. There is a great deal of pressure in these situations to close your eyes to what is happening around you and concentrate only on your own care.

If you observe an incident that has the potential for serious danger to the patient (such as an unreported medication error) or one that has legal ramifications (such as falsifying narcotic records), you would have a legal as well as an ethical responsibility to go immediately to a supervisor with your information. In a situation that has the potential for legal involvement, it is prudent to keep an exact personal record of your observations and actions. Your record should include times and dates of the incident and of your reporting efforts (see Chapter 5).

Formal Evaluation. Formal evaluation of nursing is occurring in most settings under the title of quality assurance. Quality assurance is a planned program of evaluation that includes ongoing monitoring of the care given and of outcomes of care. It includes a mechanism for instituting change when problems or opportunities for improvement are identified. Quality assurance programs are required by the Joint Commission on the Accreditation of Health Care Organizations and by Medicare.

The first aspect of nursing care that is usually evaluated is whether the nursing actions taken were complete and appropriate for the situation. Criteria developed to evaluate this aspect are called *process criteria.* One basis for developing process criteria is the "Standards for Nursing Practice" developed by the ANA. There are general standards that refer to all settings, and more specific ones for gerontological, maternal-child, community health, and psychiatric-mental health nursing.[3]

Another basis for formal evaluation is the use of outcome criteria for patient care. *Outcome criteria* are specific, observable patient behaviors or clinical manifestations that are the desired result of care. They usually are established by nurses working in groups. Nursing literature is consulted so that appropriate criteria are established.

A number of methods have been used to evaluate both the process and the outcomes of nursing care. *Conferences* designed to discuss the matter to be evaluated are personal and flexible but may lack objectivity. Simple *interviews* with either patients or staff also lack objectivity, although valuable insight and direction may be gained from them. *Direct observation* of patients provides an excellent means of evaluation if specific criteria are set up before the observation, but it is time-consuming. The method that is gaining wider acceptance in nursing is the *audit* based on review of the patient's record. If information does not appear in the record, then, for the purposes of the audit, the observations were not done or the action was not taken. This may come as a shock to nurses who reply, "But we *always* do that!"

All types of evaluation first call for establishing specific criteria to be used in the evaluation. These criteria may refer to process, to outcome, or to both. The creation of the criteria is a professional nursing responsibility. The chart review involves comparing the patient record with the criteria. Often medical records personnel may do this. The accuracy of the review depends on the adequacy of the charting. This is just one of the reasons why you must recognize the importance of your charting and make sure that you maintain a high standard in written records. If audits are being done at your institution, you should become familiar with the criteria being used. These criteria can serve as guidelines for you in evaluating your own care and in record keeping.

This kind of review has raised some serious concern and often results in increased attention to charting, and even revision of charting systems in some areas. Once the information has been gathered, nurses again take the initiative in determining the meaning of the data and what the next step should be. Because the goal is improvement of patient care, it is hoped that the audit will result in plans to enhance patient well-being. Changes in policies and procedures and in in-service education classes are some of the approaches that have been used. Once remedial action has been taken, reevaluation is done to determine its effectiveness. Formal evaluation of nursing care is successful only if all nurses recognize their individual responsibility and accountability for practice and are willing to learn and grow in order to enhance patient care.

The Chemically Impaired Nurse

The *chemically impaired nurse* is a term used to describe that person whose practice has deteriorated because of chemical abuse, specifically the use of alcohol and drugs. There is a strong possibility that each of you, if you remain active in the profession, will at some time find yourself working with a chemically impaired colleague.

One would like to believe that nurses, who have studied the physiological effects of alcohol and drugs on the system, would avoid the chances of such abuse. This is not the case. There are approximately 40,000 alcoholic nurses in the United States, and it has been estimated that narcotic addiction in nurses parallels that of physicians (30 to 100 times greater than it is in the general population.)[4] From September 1980 to August 1981 the National Council of State Boards of Nursing collected data on disciplinary actions from its member state boards. Of the cases reported during that period, it was determined that 67 percent of the disciplinary proceedings involving nurses were related to some form of chemical abuse.[5] That figure is somewhat higher today.

Why are so many nurses affected by this problem? Factors that lead to chemical dependency include the stress that one encounters in the nursing profession, particularly in intensive care units and emergency rooms. Frequent shift changes and staffing shortages add to the situation. Unrealistic personal expectations, frustration, anxiety, and depression contribute to the problem. Once the problem exists, denial is a big part of the disease.

Jefferson and Ensor provide the following information about addiction:

> Addiction is an insidious process that occurs as the result of a) prolonged intake of a chemical, b) processes going on within the individual (including genetic, psychological, and chemical), and c) processes external to the individual (that is, the actions and reactions of family, friends, co-workers, supervisors, and society). . . . Addiction is present any time a chemical interferes with any aspect of a person's life and that person keeps using the chemical.[6]

In 1981 the ANA appointed a Nursing Task Force on Addiction and Psychological Disturbance to develop guidelines for treatment and assistance for nurses whose practice is impaired by alcoholism, drug abuse, or psychological dysfunction. The guidelines were designed for use by state nurses' associations.

The concerns for the chemically impaired nurse are twofold. The first is on a personal level for the nurse who is afflicted: the illness may go undetected and untreated for years. The second concern is for the patient, whose care is jeopardized by the nurse whose judgment and skills are weakened.

Because nurses, by virtue of their education, are socialized into caring roles, they have not always dealt with the problem in a head-on fashion. The impaired nurse was often protected, transferred, ignored, and in some instances, promoted. None of these actions helped the problem.

What are some of the behaviors you will notice in a chemically impaired colleague? Some similar behaviors will be seen in the nurse impaired by either alcohol or drugs. They include the following:

- Increased absenteeism
- Inability to meet schedules
- Tendency to shrink from new and challenging assignments
- Changes in personality and mental status, mood swings
- Changes in behavior
- Illogical and sloppy charting
- Excessive errors
- Unkempt appearance
- Decreased ability to concentrate
- Poor to inaccurate recall
- Medication "errors" that require many changes in charting
- Arriving on duty early or staying late for no valid reasons

In addition, the nurse who is consuming alcohol while working may have alcohol on the breath, have slurred speech and an unsteady gait, and have a flushed face.[7]

Problems related to drug abuse are complicated by the fact that the nurse usually is obtaining drugs from the supply available on the hospital unit and is therefore in violation of the Controlled Substances Act. Some of the factors that may indicate a problem with a particular nurse include increased charting errors, increased incidents of dropped or wasted medication when that nurse is on duty, and complaints of little or no relief from pain medication from patients assigned to that nurse. (This may occur because the nurse takes all or part of the medication prescribed for the patient and gives the patient distilled water, saline, or diluted narcotic.) Eventually you may notice that the nurse in question makes frequent use of the bathroom, and you may find used syringes and bloody cotton balls left there. Nurses who abuse narcotics also usually prefer to work alone, may express a desire to work on a night shift (where there is less contact with others), or may express a preference for areas of the hospital where many narcotics may be given with less surveillance because of patient short-stay (*e.g.,* emergency or delivery rooms).

What should you do if you suspect that a colleague has this problem? First of all, you need to be sure that a problem exists. Collect data and document it, including dates and times. Do not confront or accuse the person whom you suspect. There are at least two good reasons you should not confront the person whom you suspect at this time. First, the person may become more secretive about the behavior because of the danger of being caught. This will make collection of data more difficult, if not impossible. The suspected person may ask for a transfer to another shift or to a different part of the hospital, or, if truly threatened, may seek employment in another hospital.

We have already alluded to the second reason you should not confront the suspected person at this time. You are still collecting data and documenting it. You cannot be sure from a single observation that a problem exists. There are often reasons why things are not the way we initially perceived them. Once you are certain that a definite problem exists, it is a good idea to have a second person present to validate your observations. This might appropriately be the supervisor or, if that is not possible, another colleague. Once you are sure of the facts, do not hesitate to enlist the assistance of your head nurse or supervisor, or, if necessary, the director of nursing service. Usually once you have notified your supervisor, he or she will assume responsibility for the problem but may need your continued assistance with data collection.

Once adequate information has been gathered, hospital administrative personnel will notify the State Board of Nursing, and the State Board of Pharmacy if drugs are involved. More investigation will be carried out; records will be examined. If a problem exists, actions appropriate to the situation will be taken and referrals for help will be provided. In some states the disciplinary code of the state practice act mandates that such behavior, once it has been determined to exist, be reported. The worst thing you can do if you suspect a problem is to ignore it or help a colleague "cover" for inadequacies. The problem will not get better if it is not recognized and treated. The longer the delay, the greater the chance that an innocent patient will be placed in jeopardy. Fortunately help and rehabilitation are being made available to those who need it.

CONCLUSION

Understanding the basic concepts related to ethics sets the stage for approaching a wide variety of concerns in the nursing position specifically and in society as a whole. Here we have tried to help you understand the many forces that impinge on an ethical decision maker and the factors that make each situation so complex. Specific ethical issues in the profession were presented from a definite viewpoint of the nurse's obligation and commitment to the patient/client, to personal excellence, and to the profession of nursing as a whole. We encourage each prospective nurse to examine these issues and his or her own response to them.

REFERENCES

1. New encyclopedia of bioethics includes A.N.A. code. Am J Nurs 77:8, Aug 15, 1977
2. Kroeger – Mappes EJ: Ethical dilemmas for nurses: Physicians' orders versus patient's rights. In Mappes TA, Zembaty JS (eds): Biomedical Ethics, 2nd ed, p. 127. New York, McGraw-Hill, 1986
3. American Nurses' Association: Standards for Nursing Practice. Kansas City, American Nurses' Association, 1973
4. Jefferson LV, Ensor BE: Confronting a chemically impaired colleague. Am J Nurs 82:574, Apr 1982
5. Help for the helper. Am J Nurs 82:572, Apr 1982
6. Jefferson LV, Ensor BE: Confronting a chemically impaired colleague. Am J Nurs 82:574, Apr 1982
7. Jefferson LV, Ensor BE: Confronting a chemically impaired colleague. Am J Nurs 82:576, Apr 1982

FURTHER READINGS

Ecklund V. Is there a chemically dependent nurse on your staff? Professional Nurses Q 1:22, Winter 1986

Gaskin J: Nurses in trouble. Can Nurse 82:31 – 34, Apr 1986

Lachman VD: Why we must take care of our own — drug and alcohol abusers in our own profession. Nursing 86:41, Apr 16, 1986

Levine ME: Nursing ethics and the ethical nurse. Am J Nurs 77:845 – 847, May 1977

Naegle MA: Educational and clinical perspective in alcoholism. In Perspective in Nursing 1985 – 87: Based on Presentations at the 17th NLN Biennial Convention. NLN Pub. 1985 #41-1985 124 – 129

New ANA Task Force will seek answers for impaired RNs. Am J Nurs 82:242, Feb 1982

Rinaldi L, Kelly B: What to do after the audit is done. Am J Nurs 77:268–269, Feb 1977

Romanell P: Ethics, moral conflicts, and choice. Am J Nurs 77:850–855, May 1977

What the SNA's are doing: Ensor BE: In Maryland. Dilday RC: In Georgia. Harakul BM: In Ohio. Heins M, Bowman RA: In Tennessee. Am J Nurs 82:581–584, Apr 1982

What are your ethical standards? Nurs 74, 29–33, Mar 1974

7 | Bioethical Concerns in Nursing Practice

Objectives

After completing this chapter, you should be able to

1. *Define the term* **bioethics.**
2. *Discuss some of the various positions with regard to family planning practices.*
3. *Outline the major arguments for and against abortion.*
4. *Discuss reasons genetic screening and sterilization are of concern to some people.*
5. *List some of the possible ethical and legal problems associated with the practice of employing a surrogate mother.*
6. *Discuss the problems associated with determining the death of a person.*
7. *Identify major concerns associated with organ transplantation.*
8. *Define* **active euthanasia** *and* **passive euthanasia.**
9. *Identify at least three patient's rights with regard to informed consent and treatment.*
10. *Discuss reasons we have difficulty establishing firm rules regarding the treatment of the mentally ill.*

Bioethics is the study of ethical issues that result from technological and scientific advances, especially in biology and medicine. This area of study may also be called biomedical ethics because of its association with medical practices. It sits as a subdiscipline within the larger discipline of ethics, which, as discussed in Chapter 6, is the philosophical study of morality. This chapter should be read, studied, and discussed considering all the information concerning ethical decision making that was provided earlier. Perhaps even more than before you will be looking to judicial rulings, legal mandates, and social standards to assist in resolving some of the concerns with which you will be faced. You have had some exercise in looking at what is right or wrong with regard to your personal professional practice. This chapter examines those issues that apply to the bioethics of patient care.

The bioethical issues surrounding the delivery of health care are numerous and multifaceted. And it may be more than just a philosophical musing to observe that most of the truly serious debates are related to birth, death, or the processes that bring a person to either point. There are other bioethical issues with less serious consequences, but the ones that cause the most concern, questioning, and challenge often involve the creation of life and the processes under which it occurs, or looking at the circumstances that allow for peaceful and timely death.

Entire textbooks have been devoted to bioethical considerations. Initially most of these were written for medical students, but recently a number have been directed toward the nursing student. Centers for research in bioethics have emerged, most notably the Institute of Society, Ethics, and the Life Sciences, located in Hastings-on-Hudson, New York (often called The Hastings Center), and the Kennedy Institute Center for Bioethics, located at Georgetown University in Washington, D.C. Journals such as the *Hastings Center Report* and the *Journal of Medicine and Philosophy* have come into being and an encyclopedia, *The Encyclopedia of Bioethics,* has been published.

Most of the bioethical issues with which we wrestle were not a concern 20 years ago. They are a product of the technological advances that have occurred in medical practice and research. Twenty years ago we were not doing heart-lung transplants. Therefore, there was no need for donor organs or critical decisions with regard to the life status of the possible donor. We were not able to fertilize ovum outside the human body and reimplant the fertilized egg in a woman's uterus. Lifesaving machines, such as respirators, and miracle drugs, such as some of the chemotherapeutic agents used today, were not available to offer extension of life. Concerns related to the quality of life were often more clear-cut. As advances occur in medical practice, so must we challenge ourselves to think through our own beliefs and feelings with regard to these practices.

It is our intent in this short section to share with you some of the major bioethical issues confronting the new graduate today. Through exposure you will have opportunity to gain information, explore philosophical and religious issues, and integrate your own beliefs into your concept of the nurse's role.

BIOETHICAL ISSUES CONCERNING BIRTH

Family Planning

The modern birth control movement probably can trace its beginnings to the writing of a minister in the Church of England. In 1798 Thomas Malthus, in an essay titled "On Population," expressed deep concern about a population that was growing faster than were the resources to support it. To offset this problem he advocated late marriage, no marriage, or abstinence in marriage. No forms of contraception as we know them today were available, although women may have had homemade devices that they developed in an effort to prevent pregnancy. Most commonly these devices were sponges dipped in various herbs and other substances that, when inserted in the vagina, soaked up semen.

Those starting life in the United States during its early development were no more enlightened, and some of the controversy related to the issue of birth control has its roots in early legislation that was passed in the United States. In 1873 Congress passed the Comstock Act prohibiting the sale, mailing, or importation of any drug or article that prevented conception. It was not until 1965 that a clear, legal concept of planned parenthood was developed, when the Supreme Court of the United States established the right of the individual to obtain medical contraceptive advice and counseling in the case of *Griswold and Buxton vs the State of Connecticut*.[1] But certain restrictions still existed. Currently there is considerable controversy about the advertising of contraceptives in the media.

Additional controversy over birth control is related to theological teachings of some religious groups. According to their beliefs, interference with procreative powers is wrong. Orthodox Judaism has specific rules about when sexual intercourse may or may not occur; these rules are geared toward multiplication of the race. The Orthodox Jewish population is so small, proportionately, to other groups that the impact is not significant. Encyclicals from popes of the Roman Catholic Church from very early to the present have forbidden the use of artificial birth control. The Catholic Church believes strongly that the natural use of reproductive powers assures the propagation of the race and that anything that impedes attainment of the purpose for which these organs were created (*i.e.,* reproduction) is immoral. We see high birthrates in countries that are predominantly Catholic. The members of the Church of Jesus Christ of Latter-Day Saints (Mormons), although less adamant in their teachings, also discourage the use of artificial birth control under normal circumstances.

In instances in which the individual's personal beliefs prohibit the use of artificial birth control, the nurse must be knowledgeable about natural methods of family spacing that will meet the patient's need, regardless of any personal views the nurse may have.

Of the methods of birth control available to those who have no religious sanction against their use, not all methods are acceptable to all people. For example, some find the intrauterine device (IUD) unacceptable because they believe that interfering with a fertilized egg should be viewed as abortion. (Researchers are not entirely sure how the IUD works, but believe that it prevents the fertilized egg from implanting in the wall of the uterus.) The other extreme is represented by those who find abortion an acceptable method of family spacing.

Central to all discussions of contraception is the issue of freedom to control one's body. This immediately raises a second question: who has that right? Is it the woman's right because it is her body? Avid feminists would answer with a resounding yes. What if the partners disagree about family planning practices? Does one have more say than the other? What if one partner wants to have a family and the other does not? It is not within the scope of this chapter to explore the ramifications of all these concerns, but nurses working in this area need to be aware of the many issues that can come to bear. Largely because of personal values, there is disagreement over how contraception should be practiced, by whom, and at what age. In general, it is assumed that adults are capable of giving free and informed consent. The ability to procreate precedes what is generally considered legal age, however, and we find ourselves grappling with problems related to age of consent and its definition.

Problems of Consent and Family Planning

In legal terms, the *age of consent* is "the age at which one is capable of giving deliberate and voluntary agreement, especially to marriage or to unlawful sexual intercourse."[2] Implied in this is physical and mental power and free action. Before reaching the age of consent parents are required to give consent for care of their children. Implicit in this is the assumption that the parents have the best interests of the child at heart, and that they are better qualified than the child to make decisions in the child's best interest. The authority to give consent goes along with the understanding that the parents are responsible for the care and education of the minor, including medical costs. However, trends of today cloud the issue, and legislators and concerned citizens continue to struggle with legislating "rights" through arbitrary points such as age. In former times the age of 7 was felt to be sufficient because by that age children were expected to know right from wrong and to have reached the age of reason. Although few of us would feel that this is an age at which a child should be responsible to give consent for medical treatment, guidelines of the Department of Health and Human Services (formerly the Department of Health, Education, and Welfare) have allowed that it is sufficient to *refuse* consent, despite parental opinion.[3]

For many years the general opinion was that any treatment of a minor without parental permission could constitute battery. Although there is not one reported case in which a doctor was successfully sued for treating a minor 15 years of age or older without parental consent, public opinion did serve as a strong deterrent.[4] Likewise, no cases have been reported in which a doctor was held liable for providing medical examinations and family planning to any minor 14 or older.[5]

The trend has recently been toward the concept of the "emancipated minor." Although *emancipation of a minor* legally "means the entire surrender by the parents of the right to care, custody, and earnings of such a child as well as renunciation of parental duties," it is done with the agreement of the parents. Both parents and child agree that the child is able to care for self, may leave home, may earn a living, and may pay for cost of health care. This usually does not take place before the age of 16, but it may. Most states recognize some form of emancipation of minors.[6]

Another term we often hear is *mature minor,* a relatively new concept. This term is applied to "youths who are sufficiently mature and intelligent to understand the nature and consequences of a treatment that is for their benefit."[7] Under this definition, a minor who wants birth control devices because he or she is sexually active demonstrates ability to make a mature decision, although the parents may not agree with the decision. This definition also allows minors to consent to therapy for venereal disease and drug abuse as well as pregnancy care, and health workers have no legal obligation to inform parents of the treatment. The most liberal legislation applies to the treatment of venereal disease and is endorsed by most states. Minors of any age can consent to diagnosis and care for venereal disease.

Many parents strongly oppose this position. They believe that this undermines their parental role and sanctions sexual activity between young people. To illustrate this viewpoint let us consider the case of an 11-year-old girl who sought treatment for gonorrhea. At her insistence the physician promised to honor her legal right to confidential health care and not to inform her parents. Later a public health nurse who was working with the girl learned that the child was being repeatedly sexually assaulted after school by a 16-year-old neighbor while her parents were still at work. The nurse also felt bound to a pledge of confidentiality but was able, with modest encouragement, to get the child to discuss this with her parents and enlist their support. In this instance the statute that protected the "rights" of the child may have led health care professionals to become involved in activities that did not serve the best interests of the child.

In 1973 the American Academy of Pediatrics developed the Model Act, which addresses the issue of consent of minors for health care. This act recommends that minors be allowed to give consent for health services when they are pregnant or afflicted with reportable communicable disease, including venereal diseases, or drug and substance abuse, including alcohol and nicotine. It is generally accepted that the age of the patient is not to be considered for some treatments, but that parental consent is automatically required for other treatments if the patient is under 18. Certainly there will be times when physicians' ethical and moral convictions will prevent them from complying with adolescents' requests for care. This occurs most commonly with requests for contraceptive pills and abortions. In such cases the physicians often discuss their beliefs with the adolescent and frequently refer the patient to a medical colleague for assistance.

A major controversy exists around the role of the school in the sex education of high school students and the dispensing of contraceptives. Those who are concerned about the rising incidence of teenage pregnancies and sexually transmitted diseases argue that the information must be disseminated, regardless of who does it. Conservatives think that this is an erosion of the role of the family, and worry that the indiscriminate dispensing of contraceptives encourages promiscuity among teenagers.

Abortion

What has been said about contraception becomes an even greater issue when related to abortion. In medical terms abortion is the termination of the pregnancy before viability of the fetus, that is, any time before the end of the 6th month of gestation. An abortion may occur spontaneously, that is, as a result of natural causes; pregnancy may be interrupted deliberately for medical reasons (*therapeutic*), or for personal reasons (*elective*). It is these last two classifications that induce bioethical debate, especially the latter. The debate entails two schools of thought about the nature of the fetus. One believes that new life occurs at the moment of conception. The other contends that human life does not exist until the fetus is sufficiently developed biologically to sustain itself outside the uterus.

The legal aspects of abortion were clarified on January 22, 1973, when the U.S. Supreme Court ruled that any state laws that prohibited or restricted a woman's right to obtain an abortion during the first 3 months of pregnancy were unconstitutional. In the case of *Roe vs Wade* it was ruled that the decision to have an abortion is to be left to the medical judgment of the pregnant woman's physician, and that the state may not intervene.[8] "Jane Roe" was the fictitious name Norma McCorvey used when two young attorneys, both female, filed her lawsuit. A pregnant, divorced waitress, a victim of a gang rape and beating, Jane Roe sued the state of Texas because she could not obtain a legal abortion in that state and was too poor to travel to New York or California, where abortion was legal. Without access to abortion, she had the baby, whom she placed for adoption. Four years later the Supreme Court struck down the laws that prevented her seeking abortion. Justice Blackmun, in writing an opinion that met with agreement from six other justices, decided that a woman's decision to terminate a pregnancy was encompassed by the right to privacy, up to a certain point in the development of the fetus. Justice Blackmun contended that the state had a legitimate interest in the health of the mother up to a certain point.[9] It was established that this interest lasted until the end of the first trimester. After the first 3 months the state could regulate the circumstances under which the abortion could be performed and, in the interest of a viable fetus, after the age of viability the state could proscribe abortion except when necessary to save the life of the mother. More recently, the federal government has sanctioned abortion through the 6th month of pregnancy. In a June 1986 ruling on a Pennsylvania case, the Supreme Court affirmed the *Roe vs Wade* decision. However, the court's vote was 5 to 4, a much narrower vote than the 7 to 2 ruling in 1973.

Although this certainly assists with the legal aspects of the abortion issue, it does little to deal with the bioethical concerns. Many people view termination of life at any point after conception as murder. The Second Vatican Council's *Pastoral Constitution on the Church in the Modern World* emphasizes that from the moment of conception, life must be regarded with greatest care, and that abortion and infanticide are crimes. Pope Paul VI, in his 1968 encyclical, again excluded abortion for any reason, including therapeutic, as a licit means of regulating birth. This was reiterated in November 1974, when the Vatican's Sacred Congregation for the Doctrine of Faith issued a Declaration on Procured Abortion. Each year on the anniversary of the *Roe vs Wade* decision, anti-abortion groups picket abortion clinics and carry out other activities to bring the public's attention to this issue.

Others believe that although abortion is a distasteful procedure, there may be certain circumstances that would make it justifiable, for example, in the cases of rape or incest or in instances where amniocentesis indicates that a fetus would be born retarded or genetically defective. Still others think that early termination of the pregnancy could be acceptable, but any termination after the 4th month would not be desirable.

Those who argue for abortion state that "respect for privacy is the basis for the concern that the pregnant woman maintain control over her own body."[10] They emphasize that quality of life is equally as important as right to life and suggest that the quality of life of an unwanted child may be minimal — not to mention the quality of life of a child who will be born with a deformity or genetic defect. Interesting and challenging cases have emerged with respect to this concept. They are generally known as "wrongful birth" cases, which are based on the principle that it is wrong to give birth to a child whose life will not have the same quality as that of other children, as in the case of children with birth defects or limitations that can be diagnosed or anticipated before birth.

As a nurse, you may find it easier to assist with an abortion done as a dilation and curettage (D and C) at 10 weeks' gestation in a doctor's office or clinic than to assist with a saline abortion carried out at 5½ months' gestation in a hospital labor room. The products of conception aborted at 10 weeks have little that is lifelike in their appearance. The fetus aborted at 5½ months appears much like a premature infant. Certainly, as a nurse, you have the right to refuse to be involved in abortive procedures or the care of patients seeking abortion. However, employment in a given area, for example, labor and delivery room, may rest on the nurse's willingness and ability to assist with abortions and to give conscientious care to the patient who has had the abortion. Some religiously affiliated hospitals have opted to close their labor and delivery suites rather than perform abortions.

Attention has been focused on events in which an abortion was attempted toward the end of the 5th or 6th month of gestation, and the fetus was born showing signs of life. Is the doctor or nurse obligated to try to keep the infant alive? Is the doctor or nurse guilty of malpractice, or even murder, if he or she does anything to hasten the infant's death? Should this infant be considered a human being? Does the infant have "rights"? Does the mother have legal possession of and responsibility for the child if, in fact, she attempted to abort the fetus? This issue, like so many others, probably will be settled in a court of law while we continue to debate it ethically.

The abortion issue is also complicated by consent problems. Many states have recognized the special problems related to parental consent and to health care involving pregnancy and have legislated special exceptions.

Perhaps there is no right or wrong answer to abortion other than the one each person reaches for herself or himself. Certainly the legal entanglements become more complex with each court ruling and seem to be limited only by someone's willingness to challenge another aspect of the question.

Amniocentesis, Prenatal Diagnosis, and Genetic Screening

A major breakthrough in our ability to detect genetic abnormalities before birth occurred in the 1970s with the development of techniques to carry out amniocentesis. An amniocentesis is done between the 14th and 20th weeks after the last menstrual period. With this test, a 4-inch needle is inserted through the pregnant woman's abdomen and uterus and about 20 ml of amniotic fluid is removed and analyzed. From these cells a number of genetic problems can be diagnosed prenatally, among them such conditions as Down's syndrome, hemophilia, Duchenne's muscular dystrophy, Tay–Sachs disease, and problems related to the brain and spinal column (*e.g.,* anencephaly and spina bifida). *Down's syndrome* (also called *mongolism*), a condition occurring with predictable frequency in mothers in their later thirties and older, is the most common reason for seeking amniocentesis. This procedure can also tell us which sex the child is.

One obvious outcome of amniocentesis is that the woman who knows she is carrying a baby who is defective has the option of seeking an abortion. People who are against abortion may be against the performance of this procedure. In some instances women have sought amniocentesis strictly for determination of the sex of the unborn and may elect an abortion if the sex of the unborn child is not what is desired. Those who would condone the abortion of a defective fetus may not support the abortion of a fetus who is the "wrong" sex.

Some couples request amniocentesis if they are in an "at-risk" group but state that under no circumstances would they abort the fetus. They believe that the additional 5 months will give them time to adjust to the fact before the baby is born. Usually doctors are reluctant to do an amniocentesis under these circumstances because the risk, although small, does not seem justified.

Some people are concerned about this procedure because of where it will end. Is mass genetic screening a possibility? Ethicists have expressed concern about the government's making diagnostic amniocentesis and abortion of all defective fetuses mandatory. Karp believes that this is unlikely and sums it up by stating, ". . . if our government does indeed reach the stage of being able to mandate abortion, then I suspect that will be one of our lesser problems."[11]

Still others argue against genetic counseling and amniocentesis because of the stress it places on the marriage of the couple and, in cases in which it can be determined, the guilt that is placed on the partner carrying the defective gene. Their argument is that there are some things we are better off not knowing. Genetic screening also may result in at least one of the partners, often the carrier, seeking voluntary sterilization to prevent pregnancies with less than favorable outcomes.

There are some positive aspects of amniocentesis. Prenatal diagnosis, for example, may save more fetal lives than it terminates. Many women carrying high genetic risk fetuses might resort to abortion if the diagnostic techniques were not available. Such women, unwilling to take a chance, would rather abort a healthy fetus than risk bearing a defective one.

The advent of amniocentesis has heralded the development of yet another medical specialty, that of prenatal surgery. Although the specialty is still in its infancy, some corrective surgery is being done on infants while they are in their intrauterine environment.

Sterilization

For years surgical operations that have resulted in permanent sterilization of the patient have been performed for purposes of therapy. Examples of this could include removal of reproductive organs to halt the spread of cancer or other pathological processes. Although problems may arise for the patient and his or her family as a result of such surgeries, usually they are resolved without serious ethical debate, depending on the family's religious values, the patient's body concept, family plans, and personal values.

With increasing frequency, voluntary sterilizations have been requested by couples for purposes of terminating reproductive ability.

These surgical procedures, performed on either the man or the woman, should, for all intents and purposes, be considered permanent and irreversible. It has been estimated that approximately 3 million American couples of childbearing age have chosen to be sterilized, half by vasectomy and half by tubal ligation. For those who have the number of children they desire, sterilization may pose few problems. In those cases, full and informed consent generally is obtained from both husband and wife, and the surgery is performed. Although many people see this as the prerogative of the individuals, others find any type of sterilization in conflict with their religious and moral beliefs. A few states still have laws forbidding voluntary sterilization for contraceptive purposes, although in fact these laws may not be enforced.

Eugenics

Of greatest controversy is any type of sterilization performed for eugenic purposes, especially if there is any question about the procedure being voluntary. *Eugenics* is the movement devoted to improving the human species through the control of hereditary factors in mating. The practice of eugenics is not new. The idea of improving the quality of a race is at least as old as Plato, who wrote on the topic in his *Republic.* The modern eugenic movement is thought to have started in the 19th century. Charles Darwin's theory of evolution was advanced by his cousin Francis Galton, who created the term *eugenics.* Keyed to this were philosophical beliefs of certain 18th-century thinkers about the notion of human perfectibility. When Mendel's law provided an explanatory framework about the transmission and distribution of traits from one generation to another, the eugenics movement took hold. Organizations focusing on eugenics were created around the world.

The center of the eugenics movement in the United States was the Eugenics Record Office at Cold Spring Harbor, New York, and its leader was geneticist Charles Davenport. Up to the early 1930s the eugenic movement grew. Eugenicists presented a two-part policy. *Negative eugenics* advocated the elimination of unwanted characteristics from the nation by discouraging "unworthy" parents. As may be expected, this included such approaches as marriage restriction, sterilization, and permanent custody of "defectives." Many of the eugenicists were geneticists and were active in a variety of other timely causes, including prohibition, birth control, institutionalization of defectives, and bills that would outlaw miscegenation (marriage between two persons of different races, especially between white and black in the United States). During this time states passed compulsory sterilization bills. In 1907 Indiana passed the first such bill, which required compulsory sterilization of state institution inmates who were insane, idiotic, imbecilic, or feeble-minded. The bill was extended to cover certain convicted rapists and criminals. By 1931, 30 states had adopted similar legislation, some of which greatly increased the range of who were considered "hereditary defectives."

Also passed at this time was the Immigration Restriction Act of 1924. This bill dramatically limited the immigration of people from southern and eastern Europe on the grounds that they were "biologically inferior."

Positive eugenics encouraged the increase of desirable traits in the population by urging "worthy" parents. "Superior" couples were encouraged to have more children.

The eugenics movement grew in Germany as well as in the United States. In 1933 Hitler sanctioned as law the Hereditary Health Law, or the Eugenic Sterilization Law, which assured that the "less worthy" members of the Third Reich did not pass on their genes. It also provided for the mass murder of millions of other "undesirables."

By the late 1930s eugenics in the United States began a tremendous decline. Americans became concerned about the concept of a "master race." At the same time psychologists and anthropologists were conducting research that indicated that culture and environment also had great influence over human development.

When the eugenic movement was rekindled in the 1960s, it had a different focus—one related to genetic counseling and genetic research. Today a couple who gives birth to a defective child or who realizes that one of them is carrying a genetic trait that could result in a defect in the child might voluntarily seek genetic counseling and possibly opt for sterilization of one of the partners. Again, this approach may offend the religious and moral values of some, but generally it is viewed as the couple's prerogative.

Problems are created when the concept of eugenics is applied to minors or to institutionalized people. Problems also arise in the language of laws in certain states that would include "epileptics, habitual criminals, and moral degenerates" among those eligible for compulsory sterilization.[12] Some states have expanded compulsory sterilization to include those who might become wards of the state.[13] In the case of epileptics, modern medical advances have changed our understanding of the role of heredity in the disease and our attitudes toward people who are affected. The trend in recent years has been for states to either modify or repeal their eugenic sterilization laws.

In states that still permit compulsory eugenic sterilization, questions can be raised as to who would request the sterilization, who would sign the consent, and who would fund the procedure. A recent court decision forbids the use of federal monies for this purpose.[14] However, the taxpayer contributes to the costs of institutionalization for people who are not capable of existing independently in today's society and for the care of those with severe illnesses and disabilities. Therefore, it is not only a personal concern but also society's concern.

Test Tube Conception

We have already addressed the prevention of conception and the early termination of the products of conception. Another interesting issue involves the creation of life or, more correctly, the conditions under which it may occur. In 1978 in England attention was directed at the birth of a child who was conceived in a test tube. Owing to a blockage in the mother's fallopian tubes, conception in the tubes was impossible.

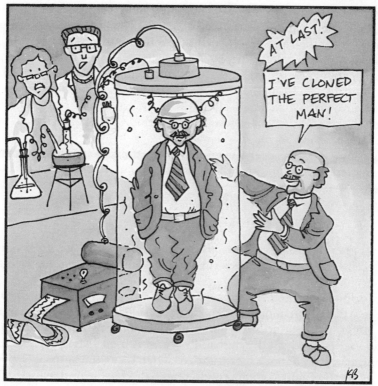

Figure 7–1. Another interesting issue involves the creation of life or, more correctly, the circumstances under which it may occur.

The ovum was removed from the mother, united with the father's sperm in a laboratory test tube, and then implanted into the mother's uterus, where it grew to term and was delivered by cesarean section.

Many heralded this as one of medical science's great advances. Others thought that this was going too far, that there are already too many risks involved in the birth process, and that we are only asking for more complications. The Rt. Rev. Msgr. Robert Deegan, director of the department of health and hospitals for the Catholic Archdiocese of Los Angeles, stated: "We believe it disrupts the relationship between the procreative, or life-giving, and the unitive, or love-giving, aspects of human sexual intercourse . . . that it is tinkering with nature and circumvents the natural way."[15] Others expressed concern about the ethics of using tax dollars to fund this type of research.

Despite the objections that have been raised against test tube conception, it is now recognized as a viable alternative for many couples who would otherwise be childless (at least as far as natural parenting is concerned). Reproductive problems often stem from blocked fallopian tubes in the female. By means of a laparoscope, mature eggs are obtained from the female. These are then fertilized with the husband's sperm. A number of fertilized ovum are then allowed to develop. Approximately three to five of the fertilized ovum are then implanted in the woman's uterus in the hope that at least one will survive the procedure (a process that has resulted in some multiple births). The remainder are discarded. Once again a bioethical concern is raised if one believes that life begins at conception.

More recent concern has focused on the practice of employing surrogate mothers to carry the fertilized ovum. This issue is discussed later in the chapter.

Artificial Insemination

Other discussions revolve around the topic of *artificial insemination,* which is the planting of sperm in the woman's uterus to facilitate conception.

Although we tend to think of this as a fairly new procedure, the first time artificial insemination is said to have been used was in Philadelphia in 1884.[16] There are two different kinds of artificial insemination: *homologous,* in which the husband's sperm is used (AIH); and *heterologous,* in which a donor's sperm is used (AID). Using the husband's sperm is by far the most common and creates the fewest problems legally, ethically, and morally. In some instances the sperm from the husband

and the sperm from a donor with similar physical characteristics are mixed together.

Although few concerns arise if the husband's sperm is used, that is not true with a donor sperm. If the wife is artificially inseminated with donor sperm without the knowledge and consent of her husband, the problems are multiplied. One of the major questions that is raised is that of adultery, which is considered a criminal act in most states. If conception occurs and the child is not biologically that of the husband, can one say that adultery has occurred? In at least one instance the wife was found guilty of adultery after being artificially inseminated with donor sperm.[17] Others question whether the child should be legally adopted by the husband, an act that, to some extent, helps to clarify issues of inheritance, child support (if the couple should later divorce), and the legitimacy of the child.

Surrogate Mothers

Other problems arise with surrogate mothers, a practice by which a woman agrees to bear a child conceived through artificial insemination and to relinquish the baby at birth to others for rearing. What if the child is born defective, as occurred with a New York couple in 1982? The man who paid a woman to be artificially inseminated with his sperm and carry his child rejected the infant, who was born with microcephaly, stating that he could not be the father. The surrogate mother and her husband also did not want to accept the responsibility for parenting the child. How are these dilemmas to be solved? What will eventually become of the child?

More recently problems associated with surrogate mothering have centered around the surrogate mother's unwillingness to give up the child after birth, as in the case of "Baby M," as the court calls her. This baby was born to a surrogate mother after she was impregnated with the sperm of a man for whom she agreed to bear the child. This man's wife, a pediatrician, believed that she could not bear a child because she had multiple sclerosis. Although signed agreements existed, the surrogate mother broke the contract within days of the baby's birth and asked for custody of the child.

Other individuals who champion the rights of the downtrodden and disadvantaged object to surrogate mothering because it could result in a "caste" of women who serve only as "breeders" or "carriers" within our society. Regardless of the ethical and legal questions, thousands of surrogate births have occurred in the United States.

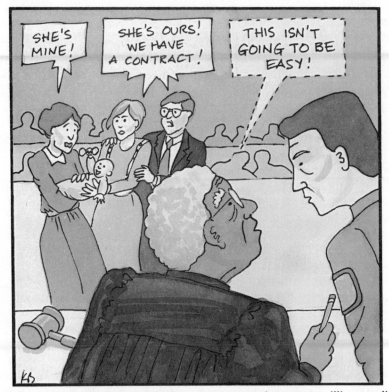

Figure 7–2. Complexities arise when surrogate mothers are unwilling to relinquish the infant after birth.

Single Parents

Another ethical issue has arisen as our society has granted greater acceptance to single-parent families. More single women are trying to adopt children, and some see artificial insemination as a logical solution. In some instances these women have also professed to being lesbians. Providing a parenting option to lesbians is totally unacceptable to many people. Aside from the additional emotion that the issue of a lesbian life-style may introduce, there is the argument against artificial insemination of any single woman on the basis that the traditional two-parent family is in the best interest of all children.

Sperm Banks

Another aspect of the artificial insemination issue is the issue of sperm banks. Sperm banks have been established in different parts of the United States for various reasons. Men who want to have a vasectomy may contribute to a sperm bank "just in case" they change their minds at some future time. People who are to be exposed to high levels of radiation or other harmful substances that might result in sterility or mutation of genes also have had sperm stored. In most cases the sperm banks are established by the medical community so that sperm is available for artificial inseminations. In California a sperm bank was started that contains sperm of only outstanding and brilliant men. The idea was to create children with this sperm who will be genetically endowed with greater intelligence and creativity. Many find this unacceptable because it brings up the issue of creating a superrace.

BIOETHICAL ISSUES CONCERNING DEATH

One of the most important areas of ethical debate involves the topic of death and dying. As mentioned earlier, the advent of lifesaving procedures and mechanical devices has required redefinition of the term *death,* has caused us to examine the meaning of "quality of life," and has created debates about "death with dignity."

Death Defined

Until recently the most widely accepted definition of death was from *Black's Law Dictionary,* which defines death as the irreversible cessation of the vital functions of respiration, circulation, and pulsation.[18] This traditional view of death served us well until the development of artificial respirators, pacemakers, and other advances in medical science made it possible to sustain these functions indefinitely. We also have learned that various parts of the body die at different times. The central nervous system is one of the most vulnerable areas, and brain cells can be irreversibly damaged if deprived of oxygen, whereas other parts of the body will continue to function.

Newer definitions of death have been built around the concept of *human potential,* in other words, the potential of the human body to interact with the environment and with other people, to respond to stimuli, and to communicate. When these abilities are lacking, there is said to be no potential. Because this potential is directly related to brain function, the method most generally used to assess capability is electroencephalography (EEG). Brain activity, with few exceptions, is said to be nonexistent when flat EEG tracings are obtained over a given period of time, often 48 hours.[19] At this point the person may be considered dead, although machines may be supporting the vital functions of respiration and circulation. Many institutions now accept this definition of *cerebral* death and use it as a basis for turning off respirators and stopping other treatments.

In some instances the family has sought court orders to have extraordinary life-support measures discontinued. Such was the case of Karen Quinlan. This young woman, who suffered severe brain damage as a result of drug overdose combined with medication, was reduced to a vegetative state. She was placed on a respirator, and her physicians thought that she would live only a short time if removed. Her parents requested that the respirator be discontinued, but since she continued to manifest a minor amount of brain activity, they were turned down. After previous petitions to the Supreme Court of New Jersey had been rejected, a final decision, rendered March 31, 1976, held that Karen's father had sufficient legal interest in the matter to make him a proper guardian.[20] Acting in her behalf on the basis of right of privacy, he had the respirator discontinued. Much to everyone's surprise, Karen continued to live after the respirator was stopped, although she never emerged from her comatose condition; she died in 1986.

Organ Transplantation

Developments in the area of organ transplantation have also necessitated a clearer definition of death. The supply of organs that can be used for transplantation has not been able to keep up with the demand. This is due in part to the larger number of organs that are being transplanted today. It is also due in part to the decreased availability of organs as a result of modern technology's saving more lives. Conflicts between the interest of the potential donor and the person receiving the donor organ are easy to anticipate. Certainly no one would want to remove an organ from a donor as long as that person had any potential for recovery. On the other hand, it is imperative that donor organs be removed soon after the death of the host, before the organ to be removed is rendered unusable.

Although there is lack of uniformity in the definition of death throughout the 50 states, it is generally accepted that organs can be removed from donors who have a flat EEG.[21] This action is based on the 1975 definition of death, which states: "For all legal purposes, a human body with irreversible cessation of total brain function, according to usual and customary standards of medical practice, shall be considered dead."[22]

The idea of consent again comes into play when we talk about organ transplantation. It is more desirable if the consent can be obtained from

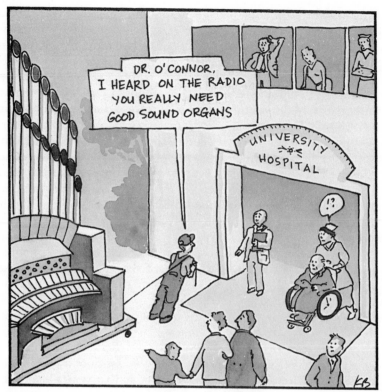

Figure 7–3. The need for organs that can be used for transplant has become greater, and obtaining these organs has become more difficult.

the donor. This has been facilitated in many states by the *Uniform Anatomical Gift Act,* which was drafted by a committee of the National Conference of the Commissions of Uniform State Laws in July 1968 and adopted in all American jurisdictions in 1971.[23] People who are willing to donate parts of their bodies after death may indicate the desire to do so in a will or other written documents or by carrying a donor's card. Many states now provide a space on driver's licenses where the person can authorize permission for organ donations.

The spouse or the next of kin can also grant permission for the removal of organs after death. However, the time factor is crucial; the deaths are often accidental, and the relatives are often so emotionally distressed at the time that the process of obtaining permission may be difficult. Most medical personnel have at least some initial hesitancy in requesting permission for donor organs at this critical time.

In response to the inadequate supply of organs to meet societal needs—a situation labeled *scarce medical resources*—some states have passed legislation that requires that donor organs must be requested of the family when it is apparent that the patient has no chance for survival. This brings forth other problems. Who is to be responsible for approaching the family and requesting the organs? Must it be the family's physician? Would critical time be saved if it were the emergency room nurse or hospital social worker? Policymaking groups within the American Hospital Association are currently wrestling with this problem, and protocols are being developed in hospitals.

Other problems arise with regard to organ transplantations, especially because there are more people who need organs than there are organs available. The skill of modern technology has resulted in the development and transplantation of artificial organs such as the heart. Such technological advances were once viewed as science fiction, but the transplantation of artificial organs now occurs frequently enough that it no longer attracts the attention of the media. Historic cases receive a great deal of publicity, but slowly the procedure becomes more and more refined and media coverage is discontinued. The general public has little awareness of the number of satisfactory cases conducted each year.

How will it be determined who will receive a donated organ? Is there any "elitism" in their distribution, that is, does a white-collar worker have a better chance to receive an organ than does a blue-collar worker? Most insurance policies, and certainly Medicare, refuse to pay for the cost of an organ transplant. Transplants are expensive procedures, often running into several hundreds of thousands of dollars. If money is required "up front," as it sometimes is, where can the needy person procure such funds? Other questions involve both donor and recipient. Should the donor or the donor's family be able to say who will receive the organ? How can one "get in line" for an organ, and how can that need be made known?

In 1982, the father of a child dying because of the need for a liver transplant made national news when he made an impassioned plea before a meeting of the Academy of Pediatrics for them "to keep their eyes and ears open" for a donor for his child. Several days later he received a donation from a family in Salt Lake City, Utah. But his approach has been criticized because his daughter lived while others who needed liver transplants died. Who shall decide?

Much has been written about the problem of selecting recipients for organ transplantation when the number of applicants exceeds the number of available organs. Many criteria have been suggested, and as one might anticipate, these criteria have received arguments both pro and con. The criterion requiring medical acceptability is probably the only exception. Many transplants require that compatibility exist in the tissue and blood type of donor and recipient. It would not be logical to give a much needed organ to a person whose body would automatically reject it.

The criterion of the recipient's social worth is probably one of the hardest to defend, although it was used in the Pacific Northwest to decide who should be allowed to live by kidney dialysis. Social worth, both of past and future potential, was considered, and even such factors as church membership and participation in community endeavors were considered.[24]

Others suggest some type of random selection once the criterion of medical acceptability has been met. This could be either a natural random selection of the first come, first served variety or an artificial selection process such as a lottery. A criticism of this method is that it removes rational decision making from the process.[25]

We offer no suggestions to solve this problem but merely demonstrate the difficulty it presents. Even the issue of who should serve on the decision-making committee can be touchy. The problem of personal biases is one big concern.

In an effort to gather donations and disseminate information about people who need various organs, an Organ Procurement Program has been started in Pittsburgh, Pennsylvania. This program hopes to facilitate the matching of donor with recipient and provide a central listing agency for those in need of transplants.

Euthanasia

Another bioethical consideration facing us today is that of euthanasia. *Euthanasia,* meaning "good death," may be classified as either negative or positive.

Negative Euthanasia

Negative, or *passive, euthanasia* refers to a situation in which no extraordinary or heroic measures would be undertaken to sustain life. The concept of negative euthanasia has resulted in what are called no-codes in hospital environments, a condition in which hospital personnel do not resuscitate those persons on a no-code status.

This again raises the question of consent. Often the person receiving the care is unconscious or unable to give consent. Does the responsibility for action, or the lack of action, then fall to the physician, the family, or the nurse? In an attempt to gain greater control over the area of dying, many people are now signing living wills. By signing a *living will* the person requests that no extraordinary procedures be implemented to sustain life. Although the living will is not necessarily considered legal consent, it does reveal the desires of the person under consideration (see Fig. 7–4).

It is also difficult to describe what constitutes extraordinary measures and on whom they should or should not be used. Is it one thing to

**TO MY FAMILY, MY PHYSICIAN, MY LAWYER, MY CLERGYMAN
TO ANY MEDICAL FACILITY IN WHOSE CARE I HAPPEN TO BE
TO ANY INDIVIDUAL WHO MAY BECOME RESPONSIBLE FOR MY
HEALTH, WELFARE OR AFFAIRS**

Death is as much a reality as birth, growth, maturity and old age—it is the one certainty of life. If the time comes when I, _____
can no longer take part in decisions for my own future, let this statement stand as an expression of my wishes, while I am still of sound mind.

If the situation should arise in which there is no reasonable expectation of my recovery from physical or mental disability, I request that I be allowed to die and not be kept alive by artificial means or "heroic measures". I do not fear death itself as much as the indignities of deterioration, dependence and hopeless pain. I therefore, ask that medication be mercifully administered to me to alleviate suffering even though this may hasten the moment of death.

This request is made after careful consideration. I hope you who care for me will feel morally bound to follow its mandate. I recognize that this appears to place a heavy responsibility upon you, but it is with the intention of relieving you of such responsibility and of placing it upon myself in accordance with my strong convictions, that this statement is made.

Signed _____

Date _____

Witness _____

Witness _____

Copies of this request have been given to _____

_____

_____

_____

Figure 7–4. The Living Will.

defibrillate a 39-year-old man who is admitted to an emergency room suffering from an acute heart attack, and quite another to defibrillate the 90-year-old whose body is riddled with terminal cancer and whose heart has stopped? Often people who are involved in giving medical and emergency care develop an almost automatic response to lifesaving procedures and have difficulty accepting dying as an inevitable part of the life process. It is difficult to know when it is permissible to omit certain life-supporting efforts, or which efforts should be omitted. If the 90-year-old who is dying of terminal cancer were to also develop pneumonia, should the physician prescribe antibiotics? This brings us to a distinction between stopping a particular life-supporting treatment or machine, as discussed earlier in the chapter, and not starting a procedure in the first place.

Other issues may be raised over how far one should go with the concept of negative euthanasia. A historic case occurred in 1963, when a couple on the East Coast gave birth to a premature infant who was diagnosed as having Down's syndrome, with the added complication of an intestinal blockage. The intestinal blockage could be corrected by surgery with minimal risk; without the surgery the child could not be fed and would die. The Down's syndrome, however, would result in some degree of permanent mental retardation. The severity of the retardation could not be determined at birth but would usually run from very low mentality to borderline subnormal.

The mother of the infant was a nurse, the father an attorney; they had two normal children at home. The mother believed that it would be unfair to the other children to raise them with a child with Down's syndrome and refused permission for the corrective operation on the intestinal blockage. Her husband supported her position. Although it was an option, the hospital staff did not seek a court order to override the decision. The physician thought that it was unlikely that the court would sustain an order to operate on the child against the parents' wishes when it was a situation in which the child had a known, serious mental abnormality and would be a burden to the parents financially and emotionally, and perhaps to society. The child was put in a side room (an interesting action) and was allowed to starve to death, a process that took 11 days. When confronted with the possibility of giving medication to hasten the infant's death, both doctors and nurses were convinced it was clearly illegal.[26]

The situation above stimulates some interesting ethical and legal questions. Would the approach have been the same if the infant had not been mentally retarded? Would the staff have been guilty of murder if the infant had been given medication? If a court decision had been requested and granted to proceed with the surgery, who would have been responsible for the costs incurred? What are the rights of the child?

On March 22, 1983, federal regulations went into effect that required a sign to be conspicuously posted in nurseries, neonatal intensive care units, and pediatric and maternity wards alerting people to the fact that handicapped infants are accorded protection in the Rehabilitation Act. This act states that no person can be discriminated against on the basis of handicap. Any violation of this act was to be reported to the Department of Health and Human Services (DHHS) for immediate investigation of hospital records. The address and 24-hour hot line telephone number of the DHHS were also to be posted.

The legislation, popularly called the Baby Doe rule, was the result of an Indiana case in which an infant was born afflicted with Down's syndrome and a digestive tract blockage. The parents refused to authorize treatment, although the blockage could have been surgically corrected. Nothing could be done about the Down's syndrome. The hospital sought court guidance. After widespread publicity, President Reagan sent the secretary of the DHHS a memo, reminding him of the Rehabilitation Act. The ruling resulted.

The ruling was challenged by the American Academy of Pediatrics and several other medical groups. After the refusal of a Long Island hospital to allow examination of a baby's medical record and a government suit to obtain the records, a federal judge struck down the regulation. The 98th Congress then attached an amendment to anti-child abuse legislation that required that handicapped infants receive treatment when, in the physician's judgment, such treatment would probably correct or lessen the severity of the child's health problem. It did not require treatment of infants whose condition was irreversible or when care would be futile. Responsibility for monitoring such problems was placed with the state.

Positive Euthanasia

Positive, or *active, euthanasia* occurs in a situation in which the physician would prescribe, supply, or administer an agent that would result in death. In the case mentioned earlier in which the parents chose to let a newborn with Down's syndrome and an intestinal blockage die, positive euthanasia would have been used if the doctors had hastened the infant's death with medication. There may well be more instances of positive euthanasia than we know about publicly. In the strict sense of the law, neither the imminence of the death nor the evidence of the patient's suffering would provide a legally effective case, and the courts could find the doctor guilty of murder. However, in two known cases where American physicians were tried for positive euthanasia, the jury acquitted the accused in both cases.[27]

The issue of positive euthanasia is cloudy. On some occasions the physician will prescribe strong narcotics for a terminal patient and will request that the medication be given frequently enough to "keep the patient comfortable." Nurses often are reluctant to administer a medication that they realize has a potentially fatal effect when given in that dosage. If this should happen, a ward conference with an oncology specialist or with a nurse skilled in the area of death and dying will help the staff to clarify values and deal with individual feelings.

Truth-Telling and the Medical Field

Although the issue of to tell or not to tell may not carry the emotional and bioethical impact that one experiences with concerns such as euthanasia, it is one that is frequently encountered in the hospital environment. Despite the fact that informed consent has forced a more straightforward approach between physician and client, the problem of having the patient fully understand the outcome of care still exists. Sometimes the question about the outcome of care results from a request made by a close relative, but most of the time it results from the persistence of past medical practices.

In such instances the physician operates in a paternalistic role in relation to the patient. Under this model of care, the locus of decision making is moved away from the patient and is now with the physician. "Benefit and do no harm to the patient" is the dictum often cited as the ethical basis for this approach. It rationalizes that complete knowledge of his or her condition would place greater stress on the patient. More recent discussions of medical ethics explore the rights of patients, particularly their right to make their own medical decisions. These discussions emphasize that in our pluralistic society, which has also fostered medical specialization to keep up with advances in knowledge and technology, physicians may be unable to perceive the "best interests" of their patients and act accordingly.

Physicians do not agree on how much patients should know about their condition. We usually experience the major controversy relating to this issue when the patient has a terminal diagnosis such as cancer. Because, ideally at least, physicians are committed to protecting their patients from potential harm, both physical and mental, many have difficulty sharing bad news that will result in unhappiness, anxiety, depression, and fear. These physicians are concerned that if the patients know they are suffering from a terminal illness, they will give up. After all, medical science might be wrong, or research may develop new cures that would change the course of the disease.

Physicians who argue the other side of the issue state that there exists a common moral obligation to tell the truth. They believe that the anxiety of not knowing the accurate diagnosis is at least as great as knowing the truth, especially if the truth is shared in a humane manner. These physicians also argue that one needs to have control over one's life and, if the news is bad, to have time to get personal affairs in order.

Still other physicians choose to deal with the problem in a quasi-truthful manner. Such approaches would include the selection of language that would avoid the word cancer or telling the truth in such a complete and scientific way that the patient would not understand what had been said. For example, if the patient were to be told that he or she has "a neoplasm with the characteristics of leiomyosarcoma with possible secondary metastatic growth," the medical jargon would leave most patients uninformed.[28]

Although to tell or not to tell is a problem that exists between patient and physician, nurses often become involved in it. First of all, the nurse may have definite personal feelings one way or the other. For example, if the physician has decided not to tell the patient, or to delay sharing this information until later and the nurse believes that the patient has the right to be informed, the nurse may be in a frustrating situation and may even be angry with the physician. Because the nurse is in contact with the patient for a more extended period of time, he or she may be put on the spot by the patient's questions. The nurse may feel that by hedging on a response there is a compromise of the ethics of nursing practice. In such instances a ward conference, whether formal or impromptu, that would involve the physician, nurses, and other appropriate members of the health team, may help everyone deal with the situation. The nurse who is new to the nursing role in the health care system should realize that anyone can instigate a ward conference, although appropriate channels of communications should be followed in organizing it.

So far we have discussed situations in which information regarding a terminal illness is shared with the patient and family. At least one other circumstance that involves telling the truth is worth mentioning, although there are many examples that could be included. One that we often see in the obstetrical area of the hospital deals with sharing information with the parents of a newborn who is critical or who has a malformation. Sometimes physicians may want to spare the mother unpleasant news until she is stronger. This occurs frequently enough for obstetrical nurses to have labeled it the *spare-the-mother syndrome.* In other instances the physician may want to delay giving information until suspicions can be validated. If the doctor is waiting for the return of laboratory tests to confirm suspicions of genetic abnormalities, several days may be required. Again, if good communication exists between nurse and physician, so that the nurse is well informed, the nurse can often do much to comfort and meet the patient's need for information. Once again, a team approach usually is advocated.

THE RIGHT TO REFUSE TREATMENT

A final bioethical concern that should be considered focuses on the patient's right to refuse treatment. We discussed some of the outer parameters of this issue in the section on the right to die, but there are some other aspects that can create even bigger problems for the nurse.

The moral, if not legal, precedent for refusing treatment occurred in 1971. Carmen Martinez was dying of hemolytic anemia, a disease that destroys the body's red blood cells. Her life could be maintained by transfusions, but her veins were such that a "cut-down" (a surgical opening made into the vein) was necessary to accomplish the transfusions. Finally Martinez pleaded to have the cut-downs stopped and to be "tortured" no more. The physician, fearful of being charged with aiding in her suicide, asked for a court decision. The court ruled that Martinez was not competent to make such a decision and appointed her daughter as her guardian. When the daughter also asked that no more cut-downs be performed, the compassionate judge honored the daughter's request. He decided that although Martinez did not have the right to commit suicide, she did have the "right not to be tortured." She died the next day.[29]

People working in the health care field are frequently confronted by such dilemmas. Cases in which a patient refuses to have a leg amputated, although it is evident that not performing the surgery will undoubtedly result in death, frequently make the news. When children are involved, it is even more newsworthy. In such cases the courts usually are involved. A case in Illinois in 1952 is typical. Eight-day-old Cheryl suffered from erythroblastosis fetalis (Rh incompatibility). Her parents, Jehovah's Witnesses, refused to authorize the administration of blood that was necessary to save her life. The judge in the case ruled that Cheryl was a neglected dependent and overrode the parents' refusal. In such instances the child is usually made a temporary ward of the court, and legal documents are attached to the chart authorizing the

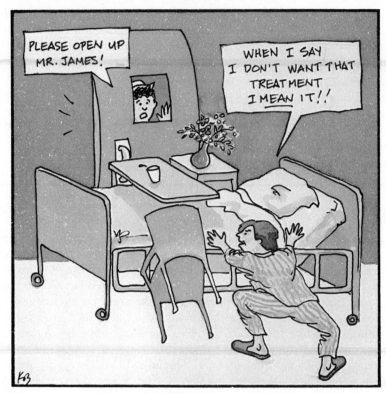

Figure 7–5. People working in the health care field are frequently confronted with the dilemma of patients who may wish to refuse treatment.

needed treatment. Such court decisions usually have been based on the premise that the right to freedom of religion does not give parents the right to risk the lives of their children or to make martyrs of them.[30]

In some cases in which time is not a factor, the court will recommend that treatment be delayed until the child is 15 or 16 and can make a decision for himself or herself as an older minor. Other judges will rule just the opposite, deciding that it is cruel to place the burden of the decision on this older minor. Such was the case of Kevin, whose parents' refusal of a blood transfusion made the surgery to correct a deformity of his face and neck too risky to consider. The family court judge ruled against the delay and against letting Kevin participate in the decision on the basis that it would cause him psychological harm if he had to choose between his parents wishes and his own.[31]

Situations like the above are always difficult for those involved. Because they have the most contact with the patient, nurses in particular must examine their own feelings and attitudes. They must recognize that patients also have the right to attitudes and beliefs. If the nurse decides that his or her own feelings are so strong that they may interfere with the ability to give compassionate care, it would be wise for the nurse to ask to be assigned to other patients.

Ethical Concerns and Behavior Control

Before leaving this discussion of bioethical issues, we should say a few words in relation to behavior control. Many people experience extreme discomfort when contemplating research into human behavior. Although it may be one thing to work with atoms, molecules, and genes, it seems quite another to look at the science of human behavior.

Some of the problem seems to center around the fact that people define "acceptable behavior" in different and sometimes conflicting ways. When is behavior deviant? When is the patient mentally ill? An excellent example is that of homosexuality, which at one time was listed by the American Psychiatric Association as a mental illness. Although many people may not approve of homosexuality, they would not classify all homosexuals as being mentally ill. Increasingly, society looks on sexual orientation as a personal matter.

The world has benefited from the work of many people whose behavior might not be looked on as being normal. Van Gogh cut off his ear; Tchaikovsky had terrible periods of depression; Beethoven was known for his uncontrollable rages. Some have suggested that Florence Nightingale's flights into fantasy could better be described as schizophrenia. Should this behavior have been changed, and by what methods?

We can now change behavior by a variety of methods. Certainly one of the most common methods in which nurses will be involved is the administration of pharmacologic agents. Tranquilizers are now one of the largest classifications of drugs in the United States. Other chemicals, such as alcohol, marijuana, cocaine, and LSD, also change behavior. Some of these are considered socially acceptable, whereas others are not. Some are socially acceptable to some people or to some whole cultures, while unacceptable to others.

Electric shock therapy (EST), also called *electroconvulsive therapy* (ECT), has been used for years to alter depressive characteristics. Although tranquilizers are used more frequently today, few nurses who had their first psychiatric experiences in the 1950s escaped from some time assisting with EST. Opponents of this form of therapy are becoming an organized political force.

Psychosurgery, for example, frontal lobotomy (portrayed in *One Flew Over the Cuckoo's Nest*), has been used since the 1930s. This is undoubtedly one of the most criticized of treatment modalities because of its effect on the person. Its use has greatly decreased.

Psychotherapy can change other behavior. This technique includes verbal and nonverbal communication between the patient and the therapist. Although psychotherapy requires considerable time, it is widely used.

When are any of these methods justified? Who makes the decision? What behavior is beyond the realms of acceptability? Who determines this? How does behavior control mesh with our beliefs about the autonomy of the individual, or with concepts of self-respect and dignity? The issues of power and coercion pose a concern at this point. Problems related to involuntary commitment have moved this from the arena of ethics to that of legal determinants.

Halleck has defined behavior control as treatment "imposed on or offered to the patient that, to a large extent, is designed to satisfy the wishes of others. Such treatment may lead to the patient's behaving in a manner which satisfied his community or his society."[32] Halleck goes on to point out that the question of behavior control has become more critical because newer drugs and new behavior therapy (such as aversive therapy and desensitization) make it possible to change specific behavior more rapidly and effectively. Traditional psychotherapy, which works slowly, offered the patient time in which to contemplate the change and reject it if it was unacceptable.

Dworkin has proposed a set of guidelines that preserve autonomy in behavior control. Briefly stated here, these guidelines include the following:

- We should favor those methods of influencing behavior that support the self-respect and dignity of those who are being influenced.
- Methods of influence that destroy or decrease a person's ability to think rationally and in his or her own interest should not be used.
- Methods of influence that fundamentally affect the personal identity of the person should not be used.
- Methods of influence that deceive or keep relevant facts from the person should not be used.
- Modes of influence that are not physically intrusive are preferable to those that are (such as drugs, psychosurgery, and electricity).
- A person should be able to resist the method of influence if he or

she so desires, and changes of behavior that are reversible are preferable to those that are not.

- Methods that work through the cognitive and affective structure of a person are preferable to those that "short-circuit" his beliefs and desires and cause him to be passively receptive to the will of others.[33]

CONCLUSION

There are no easy answers to many of the issues we have presented, and we have only scratched the surface of concerns that face us. In many instances the courts have been asked to help the public make decisions. In some instances the churches have also been asked to assist with ethical issues. Other times the profession as a whole has developed codes of conduct. Many times the decision is made at the individual level. It is not to be anticipated that the issues will grow smaller in number or easier in terms of decisions: just the opposite should be expected.

As you consider all the many issues presented in this chapter, we hope that you will endeavor to keep an open mind toward all points of view. You will, of course, make your personal decision, but do not let that blind you to the factors in someone else's life that may bring her or him to another decision. There is an old saying that we cannot really understand what it is like for another person until we have "walked a mile in his moccasins." This is especially true with ethical issues. Nurses must strive to remain open to other people if they are to function most effectively in their professional role.

REFERENCES

1. Hayt LR: Medicolegal Aspects of Hospital Records, 2nd ed, p 397. Berwyn, Illinois, Physicians' Record Company, 1977
2. Thomas CL (ed): Taber's Cyclopedic Medical Dictionary, 13th ed, p A-44. Philadelphia, FA Davis, 1977
3. Hellegers AE: Bioethical debates in gynecology and obstetrics. In Romney SL et al: Gynecology and Obstetrics: The Health Care of Women, p 36. New York, McGraw-Hill, 1975
4. Hellegers AE: Bioethical debates in gynecology and obstetrics. In Romney SL et al: Gynecology and Obstetrics: The Health Care of Women, p 46. New York, McGraw-Hill, 1975
5. Holder AR: Minors and contraception. JAMA 71:2059 Jun 21, 1971
6. Mancini M: Nursing, minors, and the law. Am J Nurs 78:124, Jan 1978
7. Mancini M: Nursing, minors, and the law. Am J Nurs 78:126, Jan 1978

8. Rothman DA, Rothman NL: The Professional Nurse and the Law, p 57. Boston, Little, Brown, 1977

9. Blackmun Justice H: Majority opinion in Roe vs Wade. In Mappes TA, Zembaty JS (eds): Biomedical Ethics, 2nd ed, p 480. New York, McGraw-Hill, 1981

10. Fenner KM: Ethics and Law in Nursing: Professional Perspectives, p 132. New York, Van Nostrand, 1980

11. Karp LE: The prenatal diagnosis of genetic disease. In Mappes TA, Zembaty JS (eds): Biomedical Ethics, 2nd ed, p 502. New York, McGraw-Hill, 1981

12. Hayt LR: Medicolegal Aspects of Hospital Records, 2nd ed, p 389. Berwyn, Illinois, Physicians' Record Company, 1977

13. Hayt LR: Medicolegal Aspects of Hospital Records, 2nd ed, p 389. Berwyn, Illinois, Physicians' Record Company, 1977

14. Hellegers AE: Bioethical debates in gynecology and obstetrics. In Romney SL et al: Gynecology and Obstetrics: The Health Care of Women, p 36. New York, McGraw-Hill, 1975

15. Louise's birth comes at a time of raging debate, p C-12. The Seattle Times, Aug 18, 1978

16. Fromer MJ: Ethical Issues in Health Care, p 140. St. Louis, CV Mosby, 1981

17. Hayt LR: Medicolegal Aspects of Hospital Records, 2nd ed, p 401. Berwyn, Illinois, Physicians' Record Company, 1977

18. Rothman DA, Rothman NL: The Professional Nurse and the Law, p 133. Boston, Little, Brown, 1977

19. Rothman DA, Rothman NL: The Professional Nurse and the Law, p 134. Boston, Little, Brown, 1977

20. Rothman DA, Rothman NL: The Professional Nurse and the Law, p 140. Boston, Little, Brown, 1977

21. Rothman DA, Rothman NL: The Professional Nurse and the Law, p 137. Boston, Little, Brown, 1977

22. Capron AM: Death, definition and determination of: Legal aspects. In Reich WT: Encyclopedia of Bioethics, Vol 1, p 300. New York, The Free Press, 1978

23. Hayt LR: Medicolegal Aspects of Hospital Records, 2nd ed, p 412. Berwyn, Illinois, Physicians' Record Company, 1977

24. Alexander S: They decide who lives, who dies. In Hunt R, Arras J (eds): Ethical Issues in Modern Medicine, p 415. Palo Alto, Calif, Mayfield Publishing, 1977

25. Childress JF: Who shall live when not all can live. In Mappes TA, Zembaty JS: Biomedical Ethics, 2nd ed, p 611–620. New York, McGraw-Hill, 1986

26. Gustafson JJ: Mongolism, parental desires, and the right to life, p 529. Perspect Biol Med, Summer 1973

27. Sterns N, Copelon R, Capron A: Legal considerations, in Romney SL, et al: Gynecology and Obstetrics: The Health Care of Women, p 50. New York, McGraw-Hill, 1975

28. Veatch RM: Death, Dying and the Biological Revolution, p 223. New Haven, Conn, Yale University Press, 1976
29. Veatch RM: Death, Dying and the Biological Revolution, p 116. New Haven, Conn, Yale University Press, 1976
30. Veatch RM: Death, Dying and the Biological Revolution, p 125. New Haven, Conn, Yale University Press, 1976
31. Veatch RM: Death, Dying and the Biological Revolution, p 151. New Haven, Conn, Yale University Press, 1976
32. Halleck SL: Legal and ethical aspects of behavior control. In Mappes TA, Zembaty JS (eds): Biomedical Ethics, p 268. New York, McGraw-Hill, 1981
33. Dworkin G: Autonomy and behavior control. In Mappes TA, Zembaty JS (eds): Biomedical Ethics, p 278. New York, McGraw-Hill, 1981

FURTHER READINGS

Bardman EL: The dilemma of life and death: Should we let them die? Nurs Forum 17:118–132, 1978

Calderaro P: A time to die. Am J Nurs 77:861, May 1977

Cawley M: Euthanasia: Should it be a choice? Am J Nurs 77:859–860, May 1977

Christensen RA: When each extra day counts. Am J Nurs 77:853–855, May 1977

Churchill L: Ethical issues of a professional in transition. Am J Nurs 77:873–875, May 1977

Fowler MD: The role of the clinical ethicist. Heart Lung 15:318–319, May 1986

HHS stands by "baby doe" policy despite court's ruling on regs. Am J Nurs 83:851, 868–869, Jun 1983

Hunt R, Arras J: Ethical theory in the medical context, in Hunt R, Arras J (eds): Ethical Issues in Modern Medicine, pp 1–48. Palo Alto, Calif, Mayfield Publishing, 1977

Johnson P: The gray areas: Who decides? Am J Nurs 77:858–865, May 1977

Kaserman I: A nursing committee and the code for nurses. Am J Nurs 77:875–876, May 1977

Lestz P: A committee to decide the quality of life, Am J Nurs 77:862–863, May 1977

Levine ME: Nursing ethics and the ethical nurse. Am J Nurs 77:845–847, May 1977

Nursing ethics. Nurs 74:34–44, Sep 1974

Malecki MS: A personal perspective: Working with families who donate organs and tissues. AD Nurse 2:12–14, Jul/Aug 1987

McGuire MA: Have you ever let a patient die by default? RN 40:56–59, Nov 1977

Mitchell C et al: Code gray: Ethical dilemmas in nursing. NursLife, Pt 1, 6:18–

23, Jan/Feb 1986; Pt 2, 6:26–30, Mar/Apr 1986; Pt 3, 6:50–54, May/
Jun 1986; Pt 4, 6:26–30, Sep/Oct 1986

Newscaps: States must monitor care for "baby does." Am J Nurs 84:1535, Dec
1984

Panel says patient has right to end life. Am J Nurs 83:700, May 1983

Pence T: Ethics in nursing: An annotated bibliography, pt 2. NLN Publ 1986
#20-1989 1-255

Regs on impaired newborns spark lawsuit vs. HHS. Am J Nurs 83:706,727,
May 1983

Romanell P: Ethics, moral conflicts, and choice. Am J Nurs 77:850–855, May
1977

What are your ethical standards? Nurs 74:29–33, Mar 1974

Yeaworth RC: The agonizing decisions in mental retardation. Am J Nurs
77:864–866, May 1977

The Health Care Delivery System

8

Objectives

After completing this chapter, you should be able to

1. *Define the term* **primary health care provider.**

2. *Outline some of the problems related to the use of the nurse practitioner and the physician's assistant as primary health care providers.*

3. *Differentiate between the terms* **technologist** *and* **technician; therapist** *and* **therapy technician.**

4. *Discuss the rationale given for and against credentialing of all individual health care practitioners.*

5. *Compare and contrast licensure and certification as credentialing methods*

6. *List the major recommendations for credentialing of health occupations made by "A Proposal for Credentialing Health Manpower."*

7. *Describe the various agencies and institutions that provide health care to the community.*

8. *Identify problems related to the distribution and supply of private care providers.*

9. *Discuss the reasons for people using other than*

> *the conventional health care system to meet*
> *health needs.*
>
> 10. *Describe the distribution of power in the*
>   *health care system.*
> 11. *Discuss the impact of cost containment on*
>   *health care delivery.*
> 12. *Define prospective payment and discuss how*
>   *diagnosis-related groups are used in*
>   *relationship to prospective payment.*

We speak of the health care system as if it were an organized entity, with each part relating to another in a systematic way. The reality is often more like a nonsystem of many diverse people and organizations, each going in its own direction. There is no central authority in the U.S. health care system, no setting of overall priorities, and no general planning for the use of resources. There are private components and governmental components, nonprofit sectors and profit-making sectors, individuals and groups all performing independently.

Although this nonsystem is chaotic, it has produced some of the most significant advances in medicine and health care ever seen. At the same time there is a maldistribution of the benefits of those advances as attested to by the high infant mortality rate in the United States, which exceeds that of many other major industrialized nations. Some people receive outstanding health care in the most modern of settings. Others receive no health care.

In order to look at some of the concerns regarding the health care delivery system, we will first introduce people in the system and then organizations. Issues and trends related to each of these areas will be discussed as they arise.

COLLEAGUES IN HEALTH CARE

Many groups deliver health care both within and without what we usually see as the conventional health care system. All of these providers exist because they meet needs of our society. Some of these groups are believed to be valuable, but others are the subject of considerable debate.

More than 230 types of health care workers have been identified within the United States. It is not within the scope of this book to discuss each of these occupations individually, but we will attempt to outline the general categories with which you may be working.

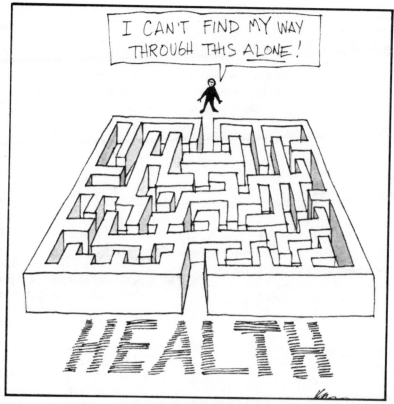

Figure 8–1. Clients often need assistance in finding their way through the modern health care system.

Primary Health Care Providers

The primary health care provider furnishes entry into the health care system. This person is consulted by the patient for routine health maintenance, as well as for care of episodic illness. This health care provider has traditionally been a medical doctor, osteopathic physician, or dentist. These professionals are licensed in all states and are authorized to treat illness, including the prescribing of drugs.

Medical Care Providers

Traditional medical doctors (also called *allopathic* physicians) and osteopathic physicians have a similar educational background. Undergraduate education may vary in focus, but a strong science background is required. This is followed by 4 years of medical school. During this time formal education is stressed, with patient contact occurring most often at the latter part of the program; however, some medical schools are beginning to provide patient contact earlier in the educational process. After completion of medical school, licensing examinations are taken. Once a person is licensed as a physician, he or she then participates in a 1-year internship program. These programs are developed by hospitals and primarily focus on patient care. At the end of the internship, the physician is able to practice independently. Specialty training, such as for surgery, is done after the internship (or even after a period spent in independent practice) and varies in duration according to the specialty. After specialty training is completed, the physician is ready to write examinations to become certified in the specialty. These examinations are prepared and administered by the specialty physician's organizations. The person who successfully passes the specialty examination is termed "board-certified." It is not *legally* required that a physician be board certified to practice in a specialty area.

There are also subspecialties in medical practice. A subspecialty of surgery might be chest surgery. Subspecialty training takes place after completion of specialty training.

The differences between osteopathic medicine and allopathic medicine are becoming less distinct. Historically, the philosophy of care and remedial techniques of osteopathic physicians included more treatments such as back manipulation and nutritional counseling, while fewer drugs were prescribed and less surgery was performed. Osteopathic physicians and allopathic physicians practiced entirely independently of each other and used separate hospitals; a visible antagonism between the two groups was often apparent. Recently the move has been toward greater cooperation, with physicians from both traditions practicing side by side in many hospitals. The osteopathic group is considerably smaller, has far fewer specialists, and fewer resources for research, and is less well known.

Podiatrists (formerly called *chiropodists*) are educated in the care and surgery of the foot. They care for corns, bunions, and toenails, prescribe and fit corrective shoes and arch supports, and perform surgery on the feet, such as correction of deformities, removal of bunions, and removal of small tumors. A podiatrist does not prescribe systemic medication or care for any generalized disease condition.

As demands on the system have increased, additional people have been added to the group of primary care providers. Nurses working in specialized roles as primary care nurses or *nurse practitioners* are one example. These nurses have obtained education in addition to that required for basic licensure, and in some instances they have earned certification in a particular specialty. Nurse practitioners may work with a physician in an office or clinic, or they may function independently in a nurse clinic. At least one state grants nurse practitioners who meet state guidelines the authority to write prescriptions. This type of authority is the subject of heated debate in other states.

Another primary caregiver is the physician's assistant. This person, also called the *medex*, has medical and emergency training, such as from the military service or other health occupations, and has completed a university program (most often 1 year in length). Baccalaureate programs also can prepare physician's assistants. These people are all trained to care for and treat routine problems so that the physician with whom they work is free to deal with the more complex problems. They must work under the direction of a physician.

The use of physician's assistants is controversial. Some patients think that they are receiving less than quality care if they are treated by a physician's assistant. Within the health care team, the appropriateness of physician's assistants writing prescriptions and orders on the charts of hospitalized patients has been questioned. Nurses have been concerned because their own licensure laws state that they can administer medications only on the order of a licensed physician, osteopath, or dentist, and they are being asked to give medications on the order of a physician's assistant before the order has been countersigned by a physician. In the state of Washington a court decision stated that nurses should not give medications ordered by a physician's assistant until those orders are countersigned by a physician.

Another area of concern has been whether nurses working in expanded roles should be classified as physician's assistants. Some nurses have enrolled in and completed the regular physician's assistant programs and are working in this capacity. Other nurses feel strongly that the role of the nurse is an independent one and that the nurse in primary care should not be considered a physician's assistant, but rather an independent nurse. The American Nurses' Association (ANA) has supported the view that the nurse in primary care is more than a physician's assistant and should not be included in that classification.

Physicians, dentists, and others who maintain offices in the community are an important part of the health care system. One of the problems is maldistribution of private care providers. Within large cities, care providers are concentrated in more affluent areas. Many programs that would provide an incentive to establish a practice in an area that is insufficiently served have been attempted. Some of these programs include financial loans that are forgiven or cancelled if the person works in a needy area after completion of the course of study. In other instances schools have tried to recruit students from needy areas, hoping that after graduation the student would return home to practice. Some schools incorporate into their programs learning experiences in rural or poorly served areas in the hope that graduates may be attracted to the area and return later to work.

Despite these efforts, the problem still exists for several reasons. Physicians prefer to practice where there is access to specialized medical centers and where opportunities for consultation are readily available. Another factor that deters physicians from practicing in rural areas is the tremendous physical strain involved in being the only care provider.

The large number of specialists compared with the number of physicians in general practice is another problem. The current emphasis on

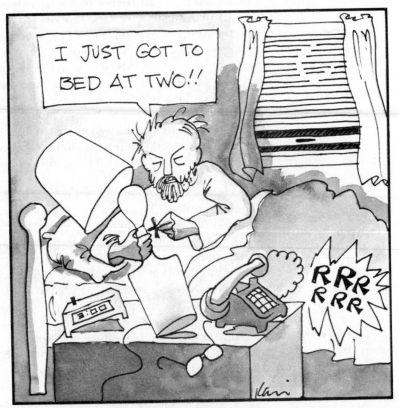

Figure 8–2. The demands on time and energy help to deter the independent physician from practicing in rural areas.

family practice in many medical schools and the increase in family practice as a specialty area are helping to alleviate this situation.

The trend in private medical practice is toward group practices. Several specialties may be represented within the group. Although patients may have a private physician, they may easily receive care from other members of the group. Group practice assures the individual physician of more time for personal and family life.

Care in private practice usually is based on predetermined fee schedules, although some physicians may attempt to make adjustments for those with less ability to pay. Insurance may pay for some outpatient care, and it funds most of the care given during hospitalization.

Other Primary Care Providers

Social workers and *clinical psychologists* frequently perform a primary care role in that they provide the person's entry into the mental health care system, serve as the supervisors of care, and furnish referral as needed. Because they are not able to treat physical problems, they often work in cooperation with psychiatrists or other physicians who are able to manage this aspect of care.

Optometrists provide vision testing and prescribe glasses, contact lenses, and corrective exercises for eye problems. They have a general background in assessment of eye disease so that they can screen and refer patients to an *ophthalmologist* (a physician who specializes in eye disease) when diagnosis and treatment are needed. Because ophthalmologists offer some of the same services as optometrists, there is some disagreement between the two groups over scope of practice.

Dentists provide for primary care of the teeth and mouth. Many dentists are beginning to include general health screening, such as taking blood pressure, as part of their overall plan of care. The patient is referred to a physician if an abnormality is noted. Dentists have an educational background similar in length to that of the physician, 4 years of baccalaureate education followed by dental school. There is no internship period, and dentists begin independent practice after passing state licensing examinations. Dentists are empowered to prescribe medication in addition to providing care for the mouth and teeth. There are specialty areas in dentistry, such as *orthodontics* (the application of devices to change the occlusion of the teeth), just as there are in medicine. Education for specialities takes place in universities that have dental schools. After the student is graduated, his or her diploma indicates competence in the speciality. There is no legal requirement for advanced education to practice a dental specialty, although there are strong professional constraints.

Allied Health Workers

This term refers to the various people employed in health care who are not in one of the traditional health professions. Sometimes the term is used to describe all those who are not physicians. Allied health workers are categorized in many ways. Frequently the term *technologist* is used to refer to those with baccalaureate preparation, and *technician* is used to identify those with 2 years of education or less. The term *therapist* usually denotes a higher level of functioning than *therapy technician*. Most of the allied health professions provide services that are prescribed by the physician or are supportive to other health professionals.

Laboratory and Diagnostic Services

Included in the laboratory and diagnostic group are those who work in the clinical laboratory, such as the medical laboratory technologist and technician, as well as those who work in all the specialized diagnostics fields, such as nuclear medical technician, electroencephalograph technician, and radiologic technician. They assist with all of the tests that are now used to diagnose and monitor progress in illness.

Administrative and Business Aspects

As health care facilities have become more complex, the administrative and business aspects have multiplied rapidly. Many people are needed to maintain and retrieve information from the medical record. These workers include the medical record administrator, the medical record technician, and the medical secretary. Many jobs are filled by people who have conventional business education, but the posts of hospital administrator and assistant administrator require specialized knowledge. Many universities offer graduate programs in health care administration.

Community Health Care

As a growing field, community health has required an increasing number of workers. The major focus of community health care is the promotion of health rather than care of illness. Some workers, such as the health educator and community health visitor, work directly with individual clients. Others, such as the sanitarian, are engaged in assisting the community as a whole toward better health through maintenance of standards related to cleanliness and infectious disease control.

Makers of Prosthetic and Assistive Devices

With technological advances, the number of different types of prostheses and assistive devices increases. Those who make and fit devices such as eyeglasses, braces, and artificial limbs need specialized education. They do not have licenses. Most are employed by health care institutions, although some (*e.g.*, dispensing opticians who make eyeglasses) may be in private business.

Dietary Services

The dietitian spends a large percentage of time planning for the special dietary needs of patients as a group, that is, determining the menu for those on a diabetic diet, a low-salt diet, or any other special diet provided by the facility. In addition, dietitians work with individual patients in planning appropriate diets and teaching nutrition. Registered dietitians have 4 years of college plus an internship. Dietetic technicians have a 2-year associate degree education.

Respiratory Care

Those who provide direct care related to respiratory treatments and the use of respiratory devices are called respiratory therapists, respiratory technicians, and inhalation therapists. Many are educated in associate degree programs. Some have on-the-job training only. Others have baccalaureate degrees. They are employed by hospitals and may provide patient teaching, as well as specific treatments in respiratory care.

Pharmacy Services

The pharmacist has a baccalaureate degree. In many universities preparation for this includes clinical work in a hospital or other patient care setting. Although pharmacists are principally involved with dispensing medications, they also provide drug therapy consultation to physicians and nurses and directly teach patients how to comply with their drug regimens. Many pharmacies also employ on-the-job trained pharmacy technicians to complete certain routine tasks in the pharmacy.

Physical Therapy

The physical therapist is educated in a 1-year postbaccalaureate program or a 4-year baccalaureate program. The focus of physical therapy is the restoration of normal function of large muscle groups, bones, and joints. Treatment includes exercise, heat and cold therapy, electrical stimulation, and the use of other physical agents. The physical therapist also teaches the patient to use crutches, prostheses, and other devices. There is a strong movement within the physical therapy profession that advocates the master's degree as the requirement for practice. Physical therapy technicians are educated in 2-year associate degree programs and work with registered physical therapists in carrying out planned exercise regimens.

Occupational Therapist

The occupational therapist focuses on restoring fine motor skills and the ability to accomplish activities of daily living. Treatment includes exercise, the making of splints and assistive devices, and identifying ways to modify the environment to make the performance of daily living activities possible. Meaningful activities such as crafts and games are often used to provide needed exercise. Occupational therapists also provide diversional activities that are appropriate to the patient's strength, ability, and interest, or that are designed to achieve psychosocial goals for the patient. Occupational therapy technicians have associate degrees and carry out plans for therapy that have been established by the registered occupational therapist.

Other Specific Therapies

Many health occupations involve the provision of specific types of therapy. The speech pathologist and radiation therapy technician are among these. Also included in this group, but more rarely seen, are the music therapist, the bibliotherapist, and the art therapist.

Only a few of the many different health occupations have been mentioned here. Table 8-1 outlines some of the more frequently encountered health occupations and identifies the educational level and credentialing of each.

Nursing Care Providers

Nursing care may be provided by practical nurses and nursing assistants as well as by registered nurses. Educational preparation for practical nursing was discussed in Chapter 2. The scope of practice for

(Text continues on p. 253)

Table 8–1. Occupations in Health Care with Corresponding Level of Education and Type of Credential

Occupational Group	Educational Requirement					Credentialing		
	Less Than 1 Year	1 Year	Associate Degree	Baccalaureate	Post-bacca-laureate	Professional Certification or Registration	Legal License	None
Primary Care Providers								
Clinical psychologist					4 yr plus		X*	
Dentist					4 yr		X	
Doctor of medicine					5 yr plus	X	X	
Doctor of osteopathy					5 yr plus	X	X	
Doctor of podiatry					3–4 yr		X	
Nurse practitioner			X ————		1 yr		X	
Optometrist			X	plus	4 yr		X	
Physician's assistant		X ————		X		X	X*	
Administrative and Business								
Hospital administrator					1–2 yr			
Medical records administrator				X ————	1–2 yr	X		
Medical records technician			X			X		

(continued)

249

Table 8–1. *Occupations in Health Care with Corresponding Level of Education and Type of Credential* (continued)

Occupational Group	Educational Requirement					Credentialing		
	Less Than 1 Year	1 Year	Associate Degree	Bacca-laureate	Post-bacca-laureate	Professional Certification or Registration	Legal License	None
Medical transcriptionist	X		X			X		
Medical secretary		X				X		X
Medical assistant	X					X		
Ward manager	X		X					X
Laboratory and Diagnostic Services								
EEG technician	X		X			X		
EKG technician	X		X			X		
Cytology technician						X		
Medical technologist				X				
Medical laboratory technician			X			X		
Radiologic technologist			X	X				

Direct Care Services

	1	2	3	4	5	6	7	8
Registered nurse			X———X					
Practical nurse		X						X
Nursing assistant	X							X
Dietitian						X	X	
Dietetic technician		X		X				X
Emergency medical technician	X							
Paramedic		X———X						

Specific Therapies

	1	2	3	4	5	6	7	8
Child life worker (play therapist)						X		
Occupational therapist						X		X
Occupational therapy technician		X						
Pharmacist				X			X	
Pharmacy technician	X							
Physical therapist			X———X 1 yr					X
Physical therapy technician		X						
Speech pathologist						X		X
Radiation therapy technician				X				
Recreation therapist	X———X							
Respiratory therapist	X							X

(continued)

Table 8 – 1. Occupations in Health Care with Corresponding Level of Education and Type of Credential (continued)

Occupational Group	Educational Requirement					Credentialing		
	Less Than 1 Year	1 Year	Associate Degree	Bacca-laureate	Post-bacca-laureate	Professional Certification or Registration	Legal License	None
Makers of Prosthetic and Assistive Devices								
Prosthetist				X				
Prosthetics technician			X					
Optician	X————		X			X	X*	
Community Health								
Health educator				X				X
Community health worker	X							X
Environmental technologist				X				X
Environmental technician			X					X

X——— X indicates that preparation varies between categories marked.
*Licensure in some states, not all.

practical nurses varies widely. In some settings, especially those delivering long-term care, the practical nurse may even assume charge of patient care units.

Nursing assistants typically receive little or no formal education, although a few states do have a minimum number of required instruction hours. Most frequently all training, both classroom and job experience, is conducted by the health care facility. Because these positions are demanding and low-paying, turnover tends to be high.

The most common employment areas for nurses are institutional settings such as hospitals and long-term care facilities. Home health agencies also employ many nurses, and an increasing number of nurses are working in noninstitutional settings.

Nurses often are employed in private practice to provide supportive nursing services to those patients being seen by the physician. In some settings nurses are establishing a more autonomous role by offering health counseling and patient and family teaching in the physician's office. Some nurses have independent private practices. Most of these are nurse practitioners who deliver primary care in rural areas. Some nurses are setting up nurse clinics to provide direct nursing services related to health maintenance and patient and family teaching.

EDUCATION AND CREDENTIALING OF HEALTH CARE PROVIDERS

Just as there are different types of credentials in nursing, the credentials for other health care occupations may also vary. Some people want to know why credentials for all health occupations are necessary. We return to the same arguments used many years ago in relationship to nursing. The public may suffer through receiving care from less competent people if there is no clear way to identify competence. Furthermore, those who are engaged in careers in health occupations want to be assured that they will not be replaced by people with less educational preparation who would be willing to work for lower wages.

Those who oppose credentialing of additional individual groups of health care workers believe that modern-day employers are able to assess workers and differentiate between them on the basis of competence and that reliance on formal credentialing procedures limits career mobility and adds to the cost of health care. Because individual health care consumers seldom contract with individual health care workers, the consumer can rely on the institution's judgment regarding the health care workers' competence. Some of those who oppose credentialing of individual health occupations believe that licensing the institution that hires the employees would be an adequate safeguard for the public.

Diplomas and Certificates of Graduation

Those who have formal education of some kind, whether it be a 6-week program for a nursing assistant or 12 years for a surgeon, receive a diploma or certificate attesting to that educational attainment. This may be the only credential the person possesses.

When only a diploma or certificate is available, it is necessary to know about the educational program itself to evaluate the person's abilities. Education for the various health occupations may vary widely. For groups such as physicians, the program is standardized across the nation. For some of the new allied health workers, such as respiratory technicians, the course of study may not be standardized. Methods of accrediting these programs also vary.

The Kellogg Foundation funded a project titled the "Study of Accreditation of Selected Health Educational Programs." This project hoped to provide a clearer picture of the health occupation programs and accreditation methods in existence and to make recommendations for the improvement of the system.

Certification

For some groups there is an additional credential available. This may be in the form of certification provided by a nongovernmental authority. Workers with this type of credential are referred to as "certified" or as "registered." This type of credential should not be confused with a legal credential. Certification usually is granted on completion of an educational program and the passing of a standardized examination, both of which are prescribed by the professional organization.

Some professional organizations provide certification for related occupational groups as well as their own. One such organization is the National Association of Medical Records Administrators, which examines and *registers* medical records administrators and examines and *certifies* medical records technicians.

In some fields a separate, independent organization has been formed with the sole purpose of credentialing in a particular field. The National Accrediting Association for Clinical Laboratory Sciences is such a group. At one time the American Society of Clinical Pathologists was responsible for credentialing people in the laboratory sciences; however, in an attempt to make the credentialing system more independent and as objective as possible, a separate organization was formed for that purpose. Members of the various professional groups involved cooperated in setting up this accrediting association. The organization is incorporated as a private, voluntary entity and is *not* a governmental institution or department. Many states have made certification by this body the required criterion for practice in clinical laboratory sciences. It is recognized by all groups in the field of laboratory science as a professional credential.

Some other bodies that currently accredit are investigating the possibility of setting up independent national entities with the sole purpose of credentialing. One reason for this action relates to the current consumer movement. In general, the public has not trusted the objectivity of people in professional groups. The creation of an independent credentialing body would ensure that those currently practicing a profession would not be the sole arbiters in determining who enters the field. A second reason for this move is financial. By setting up a separate organization, which must be self-supporting through fees for its services, the professional groups are relieved of the financial liability that can result when an accrediting program grows rapidly and costs escalate. A third reason is to provide a broader-based support for the credentialing process. The board members of these organizations commonly include representatives from the profession, the educational setting, the public, and related professions. A fourth reason relates to the complex federal laws governing nonprofit organizations and their tax-exempt status.

Licensing

Licensing is a legal credential conferred by a governmental agency (see Chapter 4). Many different health occupations are licensed in different states. Most states restrict licensing to those who have more direct contact with patients or clients. Physicians, dentists, pharmacists, and nurses are licensed in all states. The licensing of other occupational groups varies.

Qualifications required for licensure and the testing for competence also differ greatly from state to state. The uniform licensing examination system available to registered nurses is unique in health care. Most licensing laws specify completion of a state-approved educational program and require in addition the successful completion of a written examination prescribed by the state. In some states the licensing laws require continuing education to maintain competence. The trend toward including this provision in licensure laws is growing. In many states pharmacists have been one of the first groups required to pursue continuing education. Perhaps this relates to their ability to demonstrate new knowledge about drugs to the public.

The Future of Credentialing in Allied Health Care

Numerous new health care occupations related to new procedures and processes in medical care are developing. This has created pressure to license each new occupation. Educational programs vary and a considerable amount of overlapping has occurred between occupational groups, creating a complex situation. In response the Department of Health, Education, and Welfare (now called the Department of Health and Human Services) was asked to study and make recommendations in relation to licensing and credentialing of health personnel.

One recommendation of the initial report was for a moratorium on new legislation regarding licensure of health occupations. The first moratorium lasted from 1971 to 1973 and was then extended several times.

The study on licensing and credentialing of health occupations was completed, and in 1976 "A Proposal for Credentialing Health Manpower" was drafted and distributed to professional organizations and state agencies. The final report, published in 1977, recommended directions and paths for change. It suggested that the role of the Public Health Service in credentialing was to assist others and that the responsibility for credentialing should remain with the state government or private organizations, such as the professional groups or credentialing bodies previously discussed.[1]

Other major recommendations included in the report are as follows:

- That there be a national voluntary system for allied health certification
- That national standards (as opposed to individual state standards) for credentialing be adopted
- That criteria be developed by states for deciding whether licensure laws should be enacted
- That improved procedures for state licensing be developed to strengthen accountability and effectiveness of licensure boards
- That all processes of credentialing use some form of competency measurement rather than simply educational qualifications
- That continued competence be mandated and support be given to mechanisms that will provide continued competence.

No organized effort has been mounted to implement these recommendations, but as licensure laws and credentialing processes are reviewed by the appropriate bodies, changes have occurred that reflect some of the recommendations. Credentialing in the various health occupations will remain an important concern.

AGENCIES AND ORGANIZATIONS PROVIDING CARE

Many different institutions are involved in providing various types of health care within our communities. It has been estimated that there are over 7,000 hospitals, 19,000 long-term care facilities, and 4,000 community health agencies in the United States.

Acute Care Hospitals

The traditional hospital is changing in many ways because of the demands of modern health care. More and more the hospital is used only for those in need of acute care, a situation that is largely due to the increasing cost of care in hospitals. These costs reflect the vast amount of specialized equipment that is used, the number of laboratories needed, the specialized operating rooms and treatment facilities, and the many people employed in the modern hospital. For each hospitalized person, more than five persons are employed. This includes maintenance, kitchen, and office workers as well as health care personnel. Although at one time hospital workers were poorly paid in comparison with the rest of the community's workers, collective bargaining has changed this. Hospital workers are no longer willing to subsidize the cost of health care by receiving substandard wages.

After World War II health care moved more and more into hospitals and large medical centers. The diagnostic and treatment methods used required a high degree of skill, and everyone was in favor of using the best technology. Within the past 10 years there has been increasing concern that this concentration of care in acute hospitals is expensive and frequently not essential to individual care. The result has been the increasing move of stabler or more convalescent patients to early discharge to home or to long-term care facilities and the provision of more services on an outpatient or ambulatory care basis. The acute care hospital of today is becoming a center for delivering specialized care to a severely ill population.

Through financial support for building hospitals and regulations regarding the use of federal funds, the federal government has gained a great deal of control over the operation of the acute care hospital. The demands of accrediting bodies, state governments, third-party payers, and patients have all helped to shape today's hospitals.

Each hospital must be licensed by the state in which it is located. The licensure requirements vary among states. In addition to the required state licensure, almost all hospitals adhere to national standards through seeking voluntary accreditation by the Joint Commission for the Accreditation of Hospitals (JCAH). Many third-party payers, such as Medicare and Medicaid, require that a hospital be JCAH-accredited in order to receive reimbursement for care provided. The JCAH has been effective in influencing hospital construction, operation, and evaluation by means of the criteria that have been set for this national accreditation. The Joint Commission is composed of members of the American College of Surgeons, the American Hospital Association, the American Society of Internal Medicine, and the American Medical Association. A consumer representative also serves on the board of the Joint Commission. Although nursing is a major focus of hospital care, there is no nursing representation on the Joint Commission. The ANA has tried many times to become part of the JCAH but has repeatedly been refused. Nurses have testified about nursing practice standards and have been employed individually by the JCAH in a variety of positions related to accrediting. Continuing efforts are being made by both consumer and professional groups to broaden the representation on the JCAH.

Public hospitals are those owned by state or local governmental agencies. These hospitals often provide low-cost or free care to those without financial resources. The federal government also operates hospitals for specific groups, such as veterans, the military and their dependents, and certain Indian tribes. These hospitals are administered through different branches of the federal government. Private hospitals include both proprietary (profit-making) and nonprofit hospitals. Private nonprofit hospitals may actually make a profit on operations, but any profit must be used for hospital purposes.

Policy and direction for a hospital are usually provided by a governing board. In the public hospital this may be elected officials or a group of people appointed by elected officials. Federal hospitals do not have individual governing boards, but are directed by the rules and regulations of the federal agency responsible for their function. Proprietary hospitals are directed by the board of the corporation owning the hospital. Nonprofit hospitals often have boards composed of influential members of the community. In many areas consumers are seeking greater representation on hospital governing boards.

The actual functioning of the hospital is directed by a chief administrator, or executive officer, and a wide range and diversity of divisions and departments and their administrators. The medical board of a hospital, composed of those primary health care providers with authority to admit patients, governs medical practice within the facility and consults with and advises the administration in regard to other concerns.

Long-term Care Facilities

The majority of long-term care facilities are nursing homes and convalescent centers. These institutions traditionally provided care for people — most of whom were elderly — who had stable problems and needed custodial, rather than highly skilled, care. The situation has rapidly changed with the decreased lengths of hospital stays and the increasing emphasis on not using the acute setting for anything that can be accomplished elsewhere. Nursing homes may have as patients people who are still receiving chemotherapy for cancer, or long-term ventilator support, as well as the traditional residents. Our understanding of the needs and problems of the elderly has expanded, and we are beginning to recognize that skill in care involves not only technical procedures but also skill in perceiving a person's unique needs and planning care that supports continued independence and prevents deterioration whenever possible.

One development in the area of long-term care has been centers for developmentally disabled young adults. These centers allow young people who are physically or intellectually disabled to live in community-type surroundings with other young people who have similar problems. Efforts are made in these settings to increase independence and foster self-care. Other long-term care centers have been established to offer rehabilitative services to those who have had strokes or spinal cord injuries. In these centers it is possible to provide the kinds of comprehensive coordinated services that achieve the best results.

The area of long-term care continues to grow rapidly for several reasons. More people are surviving acute illnesses, injuries, and congenital problems that would have been fatal a decade ago. Many of these people need care for a long period of time. Advances in nutrition and health care contribute to longer life spans, and many very old people who have disabilities require care and support. Social changes have made it more difficult for families to provide care at home, and an alternative setting for care is sought. Because of its rapid growth, long-term care offers many opportunities for nurses.

Standards for long-term care have been constantly rising. Many of the facilities are now accredited by state or national groups and therefore meet established criteria for sound care. Some provide exceptionally fine care. Unfortunately there are some long-term care facilities that still provide minimal or marginal care. This is often related to funding difficulties.

Funding for long-term care is a serious concern within the health care community. Many elderly and dependent people who need permanent total care in nursing homes have minimal financial resources. Few insurance companies cover long-term care. Medicare coverage of such care is limited to specific and narrowly defined situations and conditions and is also limited in the length of time that coverage is available. Many people must rely on government assistance programs administered by the states for financial support of long-term care needs. With increasing pressure on budgets from taxpayers and from inflation, dependent people in long-term care have often not had a strong enough voice to make an impact on decision makers. Those involved in long-term care delivery constantly strive to inform the public of the need and seek the funding necessary to provide high-quality care.

COMMUNITY HEALTH CARE AGENCIES

Within each community there are many organizations, groups, and individuals who offer health care. Some of these are funded publicly, and others are funded privately. Within the past few years there have been severe cuts in the federal funding of all community social and health services. In addition, many states have had to severely curtail spending and social and health services have had diminished funding from the state. This has created a situation in which demand for services has often been greater than the ability of agencies to meet the need. More funding is being sought from private sources, but many groups are seeking support from the same sources. It is often difficult for nurses when they find that there is no source of health care for a particular client's needs.

Community Mental Health Centers

Community mental health centers have been established in many areas to allow those with emotional problems to remain in their own communities. There is strong evidence to support the belief that those who remain in their communities on an outpatient basis, with family and community ties intact, have more successful treatment outcomes. For those who must be hospitalized, the community mental health center provides a resource so that early discharge from the hospital setting is possible. Another advantage is that people seek help more readily when it is available within the community. These centers usually employ a variety of mental health workers including psychiatrists, clinical psychologists, social workers, marriage and family counselors, psychiatric nurses, and community workers. Services may include individual counseling and therapy, group or family counseling, evaluation, and referral.

In actual practice, community mental health centers have not been adequately funded to meet the many and varied needs of those with mental health problems. The mentally ill are often not eligible for care that can maintain their health, but only eligible when they have again become acutely ill. Some people are not eligible for help because of the complex rules and regulations governing funding. Still others do not continue with prescribed treatment, and thus become acutely ill again. The entire area of community mental health has many problems and challenges.

Day-Care Centers for the Elderly

These centers were established to allow elderly people to remain outside of institutions as long as possible. A variety of maintenance and rehabilitative services are usually available, including exercise classes, medication education and supervision, recreational activities, mental health care, and an opportunity to interact with other people. Some of these centers provide "drop in" or intermittent services for those who need one aspect of the program. Others provide care each day for those who need continuing supervision while other family members are at work or school.

Public-Health Departments

Public health departments usually have the responsibility of maintaining the health of the community as a whole. This involves such diverse duties as inspecting restaurants for sanitation, licensing food handlers, providing for immunization programs, and treating venereal disease and tuberculosis. The exact responsibilities are specific to the laws and funding of each community. Some public health departments also provide nurses, who make home visits to offer a variety of supportive services. These services usually are directed at health maintenance through assisting with well-child management, teaching people how to manage their own care, or following up on communicable disease treatment. Some public health departments also provide direct-care services. Care through public health departments is usually free or provided at cost. Many of the services are delivered by nurses.

Home Health Care Agencies

Home health care is growing dramatically. Individuals and their families may need assistance with direct care, supervision of health status, and education related to self-care. With early discharge, intensive support may be needed for a period of time. Increasingly, these agencies employ a variety of personnel, ranging from nurses for skilled care to home health aides who can cook and clean. Personnel assignments are based on the client's needs. These agencies may be either nonprofit or profiting making. In the nonprofit agency, fees may be based on the client's ability to pay. In profit-making agencies, payment usually is based on a preset fee schedule.

Health Maintenance Organizations

Health maintenance organizations (HMOs) have been in existence in the United States for more than 30 years, but their growth in numbers was slow until the federal government provided the impetus to start new HMOs through legislation passed in 1972 and 1974. Although HMOs differ from one another in the extent of care provided, they have many similarities. Fees are paid on a flat rate per month. This fee usually covers routine health care and hospitalization and, in some instances, is designed to cover prescription costs, long-term care, and other items. Primary health care providers often are employees of the organization and receive a salary that is not related to the specific services provided. In other instances a group of primary health care providers contracts with the HMO to provide services for a preset fee. HMOs also employ many other health care workers, including nurses. In some HMOs clients have a choice of care providers, in others they do not. Because the HMO receives the same income regardless of whether the client requires extensive care, there is a built-in incentive to emphasize preventive care and avoid costly hospitalization.

The Kaiser Permanente Health Care organization in California and Oregon is one type of HMO Kaiser owns and operates its own hospitals. The physicians are members of a group that contracts with the organization to provide medical services. The fee for membership provides for almost all health care costs, including both outpatient and inpatient costs.

Group Health Cooperative of Puget Sound, located in Washington State, is a consumer-owned and -operated, cooperative that owns and operates its own hospitals and clinics and employs physicians. People who join the cooperative as members pay an entry fee as their share in the capitalization of the program and thereafter pay a monthly fee for comprehensive health care, which includes both outpatient and inpatient services. Members have a vote in the operation of the cooperative. In addition, Group Health Cooperative contracts with employers to provide comprehensive, prepaid coverage for employee groups. Members of the employment groups do not pay a capitalization fee and are not voting members of the cooperative. Their monthly fees may be paid by the employer or the employee.

Preferred Providers

In an attempt to contain costs, some insurance companies have negotiated with individual and organizational providers of health care to provide certain kinds of care at an agreed on, usually lower price. The insurance company then provides an incentive for clients to use these "preferred providers." This incentive may involve the waiver of co-payments by the insured or coverage of additional conditions or situations. PPOs are preferred provider organizations, which may be corporations employing care providers or groups of care providers who have joined together in order to negotiate more successfully with insurance companies for these special contracts. The advantage to the provider is the assurance that all bills will be paid in full and that a greater number of patients will be cared for. In a time of competition in health care, this may be a significant advantage. Each PPO operates independently and is not regulated by the government, therefore the exact structure and contractual arrangements are individual.

Nontraditional Ambulatory Clinics

A phenomenon that arose during the 1960s is the nontraditional community clinic for ambulatory care. Some provide a wide range of outpatient services; others are specifically for women's health care, well-child care, or care for the elderly. Most of these clinics are characterized by informality and acceptance of all people. Some of them began as community movements to seek better and more responsive health care for people residing in a certain area. Others were started in order to provide an alternative to conventional health care systems for those whose life-style or philosophy was incompatible with the current highly organized structure of modern health care. Funding for many of these clinics has been a continuing difficulty. Clients usually are asked to pay what they can afford. Many of the clinic workers may be volunteers or work for minimal salaries. A large number of the paid staff are usually nurses. Private contributions may be one source of funding. Federal grants have been used by many, but this source of funding has been unstable. Some established clinics have been short-lived, but the ones providing a needed service and having sound management and planning have survived to become an important part of the health care delivery system.

Commercial Ambulatory Care Centers

The number of profit-making corporations moving into the health care arena has been increasing. One fast-growing field is ambulatory

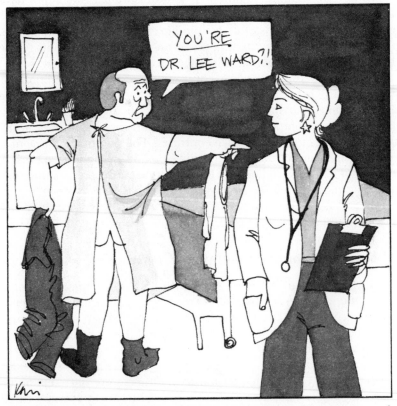

Figure 8–3. Clients are often uncomfortable receiving care from persons who do not meet their personal expectations.

care. These ambulatory care centers (sometimes called emergency-centers) are staffed by salaried physicians and nurses. They provide walk-in care for minor accidents and commonly occurring illnesses. They advertise the speed and convenience of their services. Locations are often in or near shopping malls or on major thoroughfares. Some people think that their presence has added choices for consumers and that they have introduced much needed competition into health care. Others believe that they are draining off the profitable segment of ambulatory care and leaving emergency rooms with only the most expensive critical care. This creates more financial concerns for the acute care hospital. Some physicians have also expressed concern that people will not have a stable primary health care provider and that this may lead to a lower quality of care.

Alternative Health Care Resources

Professionals in health care often ignore the many alternative avenues of health care that people use. When they consider them at all, they often dismiss them as quackery, with little recognition of why people turn to these resources. One of the reasons for the appeal of these alternative health care routes is the caring and personalized response that clients often receive. To the person who has felt intimidated by a very businesslike clinic and who was made to feel unimportant by an impersonal professional, the warm, concerned, accepting atmosphere of the nonconventional setting may meet many personal needs. If you understand the major role that stress and anxiety play in any health problem, you may understand why many people are helped by therapies that may or may not be based on sound scientific knowledge.

The health food movement in the United States is very popular. There are countless books written and innumerable products produced for this market. One of the appeals of this approach to health care is that it focuses on the normal and natural, as opposed to science and technology. The reality is that many people are helped by paying attention to good nutrition. In addition, some may benefit from using food and vitamins in therapeutic ways. Often it is possible to work with clients who rely on this approach to health care by accepting what they believe helps them, as long as it is not detrimental to their well-being. When you are willing to acknowledge their philosophy and values, they may be willing to consider what you have to say about health care.

Many people seek medical help from chiropractors, who are licensed in most states. *Chiropractic* is a method of treatment that is based on the theory that disease is caused by interference with nerve function. It uses manipulation of the body joints, especially the spinal vertebrae, in seeking to restore normal function. The chiropractor may also use a variety of other treatments commonly associated with physical therapy, such as massage and exercise. There are definite differences among chiropractors. One group recognizes that there are illnesses that they are not competent to treat and do recommend that clients seek medical care. Another group believes that all illnesses may be treated by chiropractic methods and do not refer clients for medical care. Many people with joint and muscle strain and tension find that chiropractic treatments relieve discomfort. The major concern is for those who have more serious illnesses that may be missed altogether or not recognized in time to be given optimal medical attention.

Naturopathy gets its name from the natural agents used in treating disease, such as air, water, and sunshine. The naturopath treats people by recommending changes in life-style, diet, and exercise. For many this is successful. The danger lies in the possibility of delaying treatment of more serious disorders. Naturopathy is licensed in some states.

The herbalist treats illness by prescribing a wide variety of natural herbs. Many of the herbs are imported from around the world. Herein lies one of the difficulties. Rules and regulations regarding labeling and content purity may not be as strict in some countries as in the United States. In one reported situation in California an herb that was being prescribed for backaches was found to actually contain a potent medication, phenylbutazone, which has many side-effects. We do know that plants often may have active ingredients that do affect the human body. Digitalis, for example, was originally a dried leaf of the fox-glove plant. It was indeed effective when used as an herb, but dosage was not accurate, and there was little scientific information regarding its effects at that time. It is wise to recognize the potential problems inherent in the use of herbal medicines. Patients taking such products should be encouraged to share this information with their physician.

Ethnic Health Care Traditions

Native Americans, Chicanos, Asian Americans, and many other ethnic groups have traditional health care resources that are still used by many. Often termed *folk medicine,* these traditions usually are handed down by word of mouth and relate to treating common health problems. Treatment often involves the use of herbs and foods as well as traditional ceremonies. Little is understood about many of the herbs used, but some have demonstrated therapeutic effects. Within the ethnic group there may be people who are designated as healers or people of special knowledge and ability in regard to illness. The advice of such a person may be seen as more appropriate than that of a physician because this person knows the patient well and is trusted.

Those who support the conventional, official methods of health care have long ignored or repudiated the value of these nonorthodox health care traditions. It is important that we recognize that the traditions have persisted because people have found them to be valuable. Acknowledging these health care methods usually is much more productive than trying to oppose them.

POWER IN THE HEALTH CARE SYSTEM

In trying to understand any system it is important to examine the sources of power and authority within it. These sources are those who have ultimate authority to decide who may enter and leave the system, to regulate the right to be part of the system or practice within it, or to control funding.

Regulatory Agencies

The primary regulatory agencies are governmental bodies. These agencies administer licensing laws that govern who is allowed to practice. There are also agencies that approve or accredit institutions that educate personnel for health care and those that provide services. Through regulation these agencies have a profound effect on how institutions operate.

Nongovernmental agencies such as the JCAH have a great deal of power. For example, although nursing experts had taught for years that individualized nursing care plans were important for patients, they were often not written. When, however, the presence of nursing care plans was required by JCAH standards, hospitals began putting time, energy, and money into the education of staff and the evaluation of systems for keeping care plans up to date.

Third-Party Payers

Because they represent the financial interests of large groups of people and control payments for services, third-party payers have the power to demand changes in the system. When initially established, these agencies did not see their role as anything beyond a financial relationship; however, as health care costs rose these agencies began to look for ways of controlling costs to maintain their competitive place in the insurance market. They have increasingly set rigid criteria for payment for services. The standard rates set for payment for procedures have tended to keep the fees for those procedures within a moderate range (although actual fees often are slightly ahead of payment schedules). By determining whom they will pay for services, those who do not wish to find their care outside of their insurance have their choices reduced. Third-party payers thus have power with institutions and individual care providers than an individual has.

Physicians

Physicians have historically had almost unlimited power within the health care system. They determined who entered and when, decided if and when all other services and personnel would be used, and determined when someone would leave the system. Whereas other agencies and individuals have obtained some power or independence, the overall power of the physician has diminished. As a whole, physicians have opposed changes that would disperse power in health care, arguing that they are the most educated and knowledgeable of all health care providers and that their professional judgment should be accepted. Those favoring increased distribution of power have argued that increased competition, increased choice for consumers, and judgments of others will make the system more balanced and more responsive to the individual consumers. Despite changes, physicians are still very powerful in the health care system as a whole. For example, although the consumer through a third-party payer may pay the costs of health care, the physician is the "customer" whom the facility tries to please by providing those services, supplies, and schedules preferred by the physician.

Consumers

Consumers do have rights in the health care system. These are stated in different ways by different institutions and groups, but all revolve around the recognition of the health care consumer as an adult with the ability and right to be self-determining. As a general rule, consumers are not aware of these rights and even when aware may be reluctant to demand them. The consumer is in a particularly vulnerable place in the health care system. Because he or she depends on those within the system for life itself, there is often a reluctance to complain or request changes for fear of offending those on whom one depends. When consumers try to exert power within the system, they may be met with resistance and comments such as "Well, you really do not have the background to understand this issue." Consumers are most often effective in exerting power in the system by working in groups and through established committees and agencies.

Nurses

Nurses have historically had limited power in the health care system, a situation that has roots in many aspects of nursing. Most nurses were women, employees of institutions, and economically unable to take risks. In addition, nursing education did not prepare nurses to try to affect the system, but rather to function within it. However, things are changing in nursing. Nursing education programs try increasingly to educate nurses into a role as patient/consumer advocate and agent of change. Nursing organizations are working to provide nurses with a voice at higher decision-making levels in health care. Collective bargaining has provided nurses with a mechanism for demanding recognition of the importance of their role and for being participants in the decision-making processes. Nevertheless, change does not occur rapidly and nurses are often frustrated because of their inability to influence the system. Many new graduates are especially distressed to learn that, as individuals, they cannot affect the system. Somehow they expected that if they spoke with a voice of reason and acted in the patient's best interests, others would respond positively. By understanding the political realities and the ways in which decisions are made, and by working together to speak with a united voice, nurses are gradually increasing their power within the system. Mechanisms for this are discussed in Chapter 10.

ECONOMIC INFLUENCES IN HEALTH CARE

The cost of health care for the nation as a whole has risen at a faster rate than has the general inflation. A wide variety of factors has been responsible for this phenomenon. Much effort and attention have been given to cost containment.

Causes of Cost Increases

One important factor in cost increase is the cost of new technology. New and more sophisticated diagnostic and treatment devices are being invented each year. Machines such as those used for magnetic resonance imaging (MRI) may cost millions of dollars for initial purchase and hundreds of thousands of dollars for maintenance and operation. Although they allow more precise diagnosis without danger to the patient, they also increase the overall cost of care. This type of cost is found in every area of the health care field. Cardiac care units have computerized monitoring systems. Labor and delivery units have fetal monitoring equipment; laboratories have complex machines that are capable of

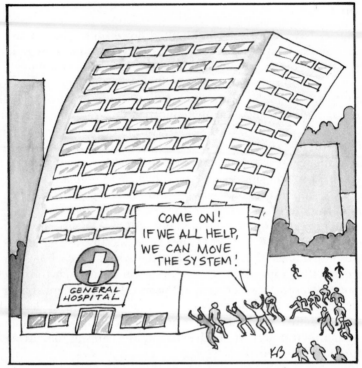

Figure 8–4. In order to have power and exert influence in the health care
system, it is essential that nurses develop effective group action.

doing many tests on one blood sample. Even such a common procedure
as temperature measurement is now done with electronic thermome-
ters. All advances provide for better care but at an increased cost.

Another area contributing to rising costs has been the construction
of new care facilities. An increasing population needs additional facilities, but in addition, the nature of facilities has changed. More space is
needed for each patient unit because of increased equipment that must
often be brought to the bedside. Oxygen, compressed air, and suction
are piped in. New knowledge about infection control has led to changes
in heating, ventilating, and plumbing systems, and the location of facilities. Fire regulations are more stringent and require complex smoke
and fire detection systems. Patients are no longer willing to be placed in
large wards with little privacy. We know that the stress, noise, and lack
of sleep associated with large wards is not conducive to the restoration
of health. It has been determined that when the standard room avail-

able is a single room, insurance companies will pay that cost, with the result being that more and more hospitals, and new wings added to existing hospitals are being built with all private rooms. The increased number of staff in a modern acute setting requires more working space. Additional storage space must be allotted for all of the equipment. Conference rooms are essential for the many committees involved in policy and decision making. Each new type of therapy requires additional space. All of these factors combine to make the cost of new hospital construction per bed enormously high.

The average hospital stay for standard diagnoses has been steadily decreasing. The average patient in today's hospital is rapidly discharged to convalesce at home or in a long-term care facility, leaving behind only the very acutely ill. Many patients who would have died quickly in years past are saved but require long and intensive care. These include the distressed neonate, the burn victim, the trauma victim, and those with respiratory failure. All of these factors make the acuity level of a patient today much greater. This in turn requires more intensive observation and care and the use of more specialized equipment.

The population as a whole is growing older and, statistically, the elderly have an increased incidence of all chronic illnesses. Thus a greater percentage of the population requires health care on a regular basis and may be dependent on medications, treatments, and therapies for continued functioning.

As mentioned earlier in the chapter, salaries of health care workers (except physicians) have been far below that of the general society. To remedy this, for a time health care salaries rose more rapidly than the general inflation. Physicians have also had an increase in income greater than the relative inflation rate, resulting in their being among the most highly paid professionals in the country.

Companies that manufacture health-related devices and drugs have reported among the highest profits in industry. This has been justified by them as being appropriate to the relative risk and cost involved in their research and development activities; however, some critics think that they have taken advantage of the public's dependence on their products.

Lack of competition in the health care field is a factor that has been included in some discussions as contributing to higher costs. Physicians have remained primary gatekeepers in the system. The advent of other primary care providers, such as nurse practitioners, has offered alternate and less costly care for many routine problems or normal life processes, such as pregnancy and childbirth. There has been opposition to allowing these practitioners to operate in collaborative rather than dependent or subsidiary roles. One attempt to allow for the availability of alternative care has been the effort to obtain legislation requiring that government agencies and third-party payers (*e.g.*, insurance companies) pay for covered services directly to the person providing the service, such as the nurse practitioner, rather than requiring that payment always be directed to a physician, who then pays the provider. In some areas this has occurred, but in many others physicians are still the only ones with access to third-party payment for primary care.

Cost Containment

In an attempt to slow the rapidly increasing costs of health care, the various governmental agencies have established rules, regulations, and procedures aimed at decreasing the rate of inflation in health care. There has been no expectation of cost reductions or even of cost maintenance, but rather the aim has been to control the *rate* of increase. This effort is termed *cost containment*.

To add new high-cost equipment or additional patient care facilities, a health care institution may be required to apply for a certificate of need. This establishes that there will not be unnecessary duplication of services in an area and that a need for them exists. For example, if each hospital were to purchased CT scan equipment and it was used to only one fourth or one third of capacity, the cost per use would have to be higher to cover the investment and maintenance costs than if the device were used to capacity.

Nonprofit hospitals must make application for rate increases. In their applications, they must document all the factors contributing to the increase. Hearings are held, and permission for rate increase is given only when there is evidence that all possible economies are being taken.

Within facilities, personnel are being asked to become cost-conscious. This includes such ordinary things as being conservative with telephone line use, canceling meal trays when patients are discharged, and using expensive supplies with care. Physicians are being asked to carefully judge the necessity of diagnostic studies and costly procedures. Many physicians are upset about these cost-containment measures because they may interfere with the physician's independent decision making. Hospitals with a high population of extra-risk patients (*e.g.*, the very elderly or poor) have expressed concern that discharging a patient for convalescence in a home with a caring family, good food, and a clean environment is very different than discharging a person to a poverty environment, and that this should be considered in the decision to discharge. The proponents point out that these measures have contributed to shortening hospital stays, and thus to containing costs.

The federal government has sought to control costs for Medicare and Medicaid by establishing higher deductibles that the person must pay and by limiting the fees that the government will pay. Because the elderly or the poor often are unable to pay these deductible amounts, they become liabilities that health care providers must meet from higher fees collected from those who do pay their bills.

Statistically, HMOs have shown lower costs for health care than the conventional fee for service systems; therefore, the federal government has subsidized the creation of new HMOs and has encouraged employers to offer an HMO as an alternative to a traditional health insurance plan. This has speeded the development of new HMOs. Another purpose in subsidizing HMOs is to help contain costs in all health plans as a result of the competition.

All of these efforts at cost containment certainly have had effects on the health care system in many areas beyond costs. They have affected decision-making processes, power structures, the kind of care provided, and the practice of individual health care providers. It is important to recognize the impact that cost containment has had.

Diagnosis Related Groups and Prospective Payment

A major change in the method of payment for health care services began at the end of 1983, when the federal government introduced a prospective payment system for Medicare using diagnosis-related groups (DRGs) to determine the payment level. This change was designed to stop the spiraling costs of Medicare and to correct the inequities in which the costs of care in one facility were very different from the costs in another facility.

A prospective payment is not determined by the actual services rendered, but is a predetermined reimbursement and is paid without regard to specific costs. If the costs are less than the prospective reimbursement, the hospital will make a profit, and if they are more, the hospital will lose money. This is designed to be an incentive for hospitals to control costs. Hospitals had previously been paid by Medicare on a retrospective system, in which they were able to bill for each item of care independently; thus there had been a reverse incentive — the more care items, the more the hospital received.

DRGs, the method chosen to determine the rates to be paid in the prospective system, were a result of a computerized analysis of the costs that had been billed in the past. Categories of diagnosis — 463 in all —

were formed. In addition, a decision was made to increase the payment if certain other conditions, called co-morbidities, were present. These were factors such as heart failure in the person with a fracture. Hospitals also receive an additional amount for cases that are determined to be "outliers." An outlier is a case in which the patient stay significantly exceeds the average. The number of days that qualify a case to be considered an outlier is predetermined. For example, if an average stay is 6 days, the stay might have to reach 35 days to be considered an outlier. Some costs are still being paid to the hospital in addition to the DRG reimbursement. These include costs for nursing education, medical education, and research. These areas will be reevaluated in the future. The goal is to include all aspects of cost in one reimbursement figure. Physician costs are also being paid separately, and some suggestions have been made that eventually these should be included in the single rate.

The changeover to the DRG system was not made all at once. A gradual phase-in was instituted in which hospitals were assigned to receive DRG payment based on when their fiscal year began. In addition, the first payments were based on a combination of national, regional, and local statistics. Each year the combination has been revised to reflect a more national perspective; eventually, hospitals are planned to be on an entirely national standard.

Most of the controversy surrounding DRGs has not been an argument with the basic aim of providing incentive for cost control, or even with the prospective reimbursement system itself, but with how the payment amount is determined and how the system is being administered. There are conflicting studies regarding whether or not the DRGs adequately reflect the intensity of nursing care required.[2,3] Another concern is that patients are reported to be discharged after much shorter stays and needing more care (the "quicker and sicker" concern). It is expected that some alterations and modifications of the system will be made, but that the basic prospective plan will remain in place.

There are a variety of implications for nurses in the current DRG system. The importance of charting that will reflect the acuity level and multiple problems of the patient when records are audited for compliance has been emphasized.[4] The need for discharge planning is always present but is more critical as the length of stay becomes shorter. Added length of stay is a crucial component in increasing the costs to the hospital; therefore nursing actions that prevent complications, that avoid inappropriate scheduling, and that facilitate early discharge are important. Nurses in home health agencies and long term care facilities have identified that they are caring for patients with complex nursing needs. A major concern is whether the DRG reimbursement provides adequate funds for quality nursing care to be delivered and whether hospitals, in their attempt to cut costs, will cut quality of care as well.

At the time of the first annual report of ProPAC, Medicare's Prospective Payment Assessment Commission, in April 1985, 21 recommendations for revisions in the DRG payment system were made. Among the recommendations were annual adjustments for inflation and increasing technology costs. The commission also made recommendations regarding the use of the most current data in calculating DRGs and the need to adjust payments to hospitals with a large volume of low income patients. They identified areas that would need study in the future.

In addition to the patients currently covered by Medicare, many states are considering similar systems, and some private insurance carriers are looking at ways the basic concepts could be used in their cost control efforts. Therefore, this will continue to be an issue of concern to nursing.

Patient Acuity

Patient acuity describes the relative severity of a person's current health problem. A variety of ways of measuring acuity in both general hospitals and psychiatric settings have been devised. Most consist of categories that reflect the kind of care needed. These categories are then assigned numerical values. All applicable category values are then summed and compared with a standard. For example, an acuity measuring system might have one category reflecting the need for assistance in personal hygiene. As the person needs more assistance, more points are assigned. Another category might reflect the amount of time needed for monitoring vital signs. The more time that is required, the more points are assigned. Each category is assigned appropriate points and the total is computed. The points identified for the individual patient are then compared with a standard and the patient is assigned an acuity level. Those with the least points are level 1 and require the least care. Those with the most points are level 4 and require the most care. Each system in use has its own scale for determining acuity. These measures are also called "intensity measures" because they reflect the intensity of care needed.

In some settings acuity levels or intensity measures are being used as a mechanism for determining the staffing needs of a patient care unit. This has its limitations because patient turnover and changes in patient condition may drastically alter acuity levels, even within the same shift and it is usually not possible to alter staffing on an hour-by-hour basis. However, through use of averages many facilities believe that a much more realistic staffing pattern is possible than could be done with only a reference to numbers of patients.

Acuity levels have also been used as a means of billing for the level of nursing care needed, rather than have nursing be a constant part of the room charge for the patient. It has also been suggested that prospective reimbursement might be based on acuity level rather than on medical diagnosis because acuity level more closely reflects the real impact on resources than the medical diagnosis does.[5]

The state of New Jersey pioneered in the use of relative intensity measures (RIMs) as a mechanism for determining the cost of providing care.[6] In long-term care settings similar systems have been used for determining costs for billing. In New York a system called resource utilization groups (RUGs) has been developed for this purpose.[7]

FUTURE CONCERNS

In 1984 a large study funded by the American College of Hospital Administrators was reported in which a large number of experts in the health care field were polled as to what they expected to be true of health care in the 1990s.[8] Six groups of experts were consulted: hospital leaders, physicians, other providers, legislators and regulators, suppliers, and payers. Nurses were not separated out, but included in the "other providers" category. They looked at social philosophy relative to health care, governmental regulations in health care, payment systems, competition and marketing, human resources, corporate structure, and finance. Some of the changes they identified are actually occurring. In addition to identifying concerns, they also identified strategies that may emerge to cope with those concerns.

Some changes they saw were the move toward defining a minimum level of health care that is a right. This could lead to a two-tiered system in which those who are able to pay, either through insurance or private means, receive a high level of care and those who are unable to pay receive a minimum level of care. They believe that there will be increasing governmental regulation in health care and that PPOs and HMOs will provide an increasing share of care. They identified increasing competition and marketing of health care services. No health care occupations will have a shortage of personnel; there may actually be a surplus of physicians, leading to changes in the way physicians work.

There will be an increasing number of profit-making health care agencies and much greater business skills will be demanded of all those associated with health care. The emphasis will be on providing ambulatory services, and the hospital share of the health care will decrease. Although no prediction system can be relied on, this study provides food for thought and is worth thorough study by those who have an interest in how the system is changing.

The Arthur Andersen Company, a multinational accounting firm that conducted this study, plans to update it because the company believes that change has been even more rapid than originally predicted. Some nurses have suggested that a panel of nursing leaders be added to the study to increase the breadth of coverage.

During 1987 it became apparent that a nursing shortage was present and that nursing supply was going to continue to fall further behind the demand. Many large hospitals began offering recruitment bonuses and bounties to attract nurses and to increase salaries.[9] Several bills designed to assist in alleviating the nursing shortage were introduced into Congress in 1987. Senate bill S.1402 authorized demonstration projects and also designated $5 million to support five regional nurse recruitment centers.[10]

CONCLUSION

The health care systems of today are complex. When even the professionals cannot keep all the parts of the system organized, is it any wonder that the public is completely baffled when dealing with health care? Part of the role of the nurse is to assist consumers in finding a way through this maze so that they can make informed and careful decisions about personal health care.

REFERENCES

1. Credentialing Health Manpower. Public Health Service Publication No. (05) 77-50057. Washington, D.C., U.S. Department of Health, Education, and Welfare, 1977
2. McKibbin RC et al: Nursing costs and DRG payments. Am J Nurs 85:1353–1356, Dec 1985
3. Halloran E et al: Exploring the DRG equation. Am J Nurs 85:1093–1095, Oct 1985
4. Hoke JL: Charting for dollars, Am J Nurs 85:658–660, Jun 1985
5. DRG's reflect nursing resources: ANA study. *Hospitals* 59(19):56, Oct 1985

6. Joel LA: Relative intensity measures (RIMs) and the state of the art of reimbursement for nursing service. In Shaffer FA (ed): DRGs: Changes and Challenges. New York, National League for Nursing, 1984
7. Mitty E. Prospective payment and long-term care: Linking payments to resource use. Nurs & Health Care 8 (1):14–21, Jan 1987
8. Arthur Andersen & Co., Health Care in the 1990's: Trends and Strategies. Chicago, American College of Hospital Administrators, 1984
9. Some hospitals offer higher salaries to attract RN's. Am Nurse 19:12–13, Jun 1987
10. Morrissey KL: Congress turns attention to nursing agenda. Nurs and Health Care 8(7):378–379, Sep 1987

FURTHER READINGS

ABC's of DRG's: Basic glossary. RN 48:55–58, Jun 1985

Adams R, Duchene P: Computerization of patient acuity and nursing care planning. J Nurs Admin 5:11–17, Apr 1985

Dickey FG: The future of allied health education. J Allied Health 9:5–13, Feb 1980

Fosbinder D: Nursing cost/DRG: A patient classification system and comparative study. J Nurs Admin 16:18–23, Nov 1986

Friedman E: The dilemma of allied health professions credentialing. Hospitals 55:47–51, Feb 1981

Galloway JD: Duties and responsibilities of trustees. Health Management Forum 2:22–28, Spring 1981

Griffith H: Who will become the preferred providers? Am J Nurs 85:538–542, May 1985

McKibbin RC et al: Nursing costs and DRG payments. Am J Nurs 85:1353–1356, Dec 1985

Mowry MM et al: Do DRG reimbursement rates reflect nursing costs? J Nurs Admin 15:29–35, Jul/Aug 1985

Occupational health groups seek licensure in 26 states. Am Nurse 17:1, 20, May 1985

Saward EW et al: Health maintenance organizations. Sci Am 243:47–53, Oct 1980

Snook I: Hospitals: What They Are and How They Work. Rockville, Md, Aspen System Corp, 1981

Spitzer RB et al: Cost containment: Impact on nursing services and nursing education. In The Impact of Changing Resources on Health Policy, vol. 65, p. 87. A.N.A. Pub. No G 149. American Academy of Nursing, 1981

Taylor MB: The effect of DRG's on home health care. Nurs Outlook 33:290–291, Nov/Dec 1985

Thompson JD, Diers D: DRG's and nursing intensity. Nurs and Health Care 6(8):434–439, Oct 1985

9 | *Collective Bargaining*

Objectives

After completing this chapter, you should be able to

1. *Define the term* **negotiate.**
2. *Discuss the effect of federal labor legislation on collective bargaining for nurses.*
3. *Use the terms related to collective bargaining appropriately.*
4. *Identify at least two aspects of arbitration.*
5. *Explain the role of the* **Board of Inquiry.**
6. *List three items that should be considered in a contract for professional nurses.*
7. *Identify the problems related to the role of the nursing supervisor in collective bargaining.*
8. *Present concerns of nurses about joining a bargaining group.*
9. *Identify three advantages of having the state nurses' association serve as the bargaining agent for the state's nurses.*
10. *State points both for and against strikes by nurses.*
11. *Discuss changes seen in the 1980s in collective bargaining practices of nurses.*
12. *Discuss the* **grievance process.**

In 1974 amendments to the National Labor Relations act (NLRA) made it possible for employees of nonprofit health care institutions to bargain collectively. Before this time nurses, as well as several other professional groups, were excluded by law from organizing and negotiating collectively for salaries, working conditions, and benefits. Health care, which has come to be regarded as a fundamental right, was seen as an essential service — one that could not be disrupted. Initially, the right to bargain collectively was a controversial issue among nurses and other members of the health care team. Nursing had evolved as a profession that was characterized as one of dedication, service to humanity, and altruism. For nurses to work toward changes in their economic status would have been viewed as incongruous with these values.

But nursing has come of age. Today nurses are vitally concerned about such issues as nursing's image, autonomy, comparable worth, advancement of the profession, and economic welfare. They believe that people who choose nursing as a career should have the opportunity to have some voice in working conditions, length of working week, fringe benefits, and wages without losing face with the public at large, members of the medical profession, or other colleagues. This thinking was succinctly outlined in Muff's statement:

> We are not in this business out of charity, as altruists and nightingalists would have us believe. We are here to make money, to use our minds and our skills, to provide services to patients on our own terms. We need no longer apologize and feel guilty.[1]

As a new graduate you may enter the job market just as the contract negotiations reach a peak between health care institutions and nursing bargaining groups. It is likely that your educational preparation for nursing to date has provided little information about the process of collective bargaining, and you would therefore find yourself poorly prepared to make decisions that involve bargaining issues. If you are like many other nurses, you probably know little about the "rules of the game." Terminology may confuse you. If the negotiation process goes poorly, you might be faced with the decision of whether you want to join other nurses who have decided to strike, an ominous predicament for the new graduate who has just landed the first job.

In this section we provide some information that is basic to collective bargaining, in the hope that students reading it will have a better understanding on which to base decisions and actions.

Intelligent bargaining begins with an awareness of the process itself. The neophyte must understand that it is as the word *bargaining* implies: a set of procedures by which employee representatives and employer representatives negotiate to obtain a signed agreement (contract) that spells out wages, hours, and conditions of employment that are acceptable to both. A key word in this definition is negotiate. To *negotiate* means to bargain or confer with another party or parties to reach an agreement. Bargaining implies a discussion of the terms of the agreement and suggests that there will be give and take, that neither party will obtain all items asked for in the contract. The usual approach in negotiations is for representatives of the employees to ask for more than can be expected and for representatives of management to offer less. Some believe that if either party were to start from a realistic position, it would not allow room for bargaining and might be seen as a sign of weakness. Ideally, negotiations would proceed in a somewhat philosophical vein, moving toward reasonable compromises that could allow each side to win, but this does not always occur.

HISTORY OF COLLECTIVE BARGAINING

As early as the 1850s, Horace Greely, a reformer, publisher, and politician, was generating interest in and giving impetus to collective bargaining issues in his editorial columns of the *New York Tribune*. After the Great Depression that immobilized the United States in the late 1920s and early 1930s, several laws were enacted to help improve workers' conditions. Franklin D. Roosevelt was elected president in 1932, and his New Deal administration saw the passage of the National Industrial Recovery Act. Among the activities that resulted from this act was the creation of the National Recovery administration, whose purpose it was to administer codes of fair practice within given industries. The nation was called on to accept an interim blanket code that established for workers a 35- to 40-hour work week, minimum pay of 30 to 40 cents an hour, and prohibition of child labor.

On July 5, 1935, the NLRA became the national labor policy of the United States. Also known as the Wagner Act, the NLRA gave workers federal protection in their efforts to form unions and organize for better working conditions. It listed as unfair practices any actions on the part of employers that would interfere with this process. Wagner wanted management and labor to resolve their mutual problems through a system of self-government. This act also created the National Labor Relations Board (NLRB), a quasi-judicial body that was to ensure that the conditions of that legislation were properly enforced. Some of the duties of the NLRB include seeing that elections of union representatives are rightfully carried out, investigating charges of unfair labor practices on the part of either employer or employee, and judicially making decisions about violations of the NLRA and hearing appeals.

The original act used the term *labor organization,* which was defined in language that excluded nursing and several other professions, such as teaching and medicine, that were organized through professional organizations. Despite the fact that federal legislation had been written so as to exclude health care workers, nurses were not standing idly by and wringing their hands. During those early years of the 1900s nurses had fared no better than other workers — and perhaps worse. They worked long hours for little compensation under poor conditions.

By 1931 the American Nurses' Association (ANA) was publicly recognizing its obligation with regard to the general welfare of its members and developed, within their organization, a legislative policy speaking to this concern. In 1945 a committee was appointed by the ANA to study employment conditions. This study culminated in 1946 in the creation of an ANA Economic Security Program. This action was followed by the enactment of a resolution that would encourage state nurses' associations to act as exclusive bargaining agents for their respective memberships in the important fields of economic security and collective bargaining. The concept of professional collectivism, which emphasizes "that it is the responsibility of the professional to ensure high-quality care which, in turn, is dependent upon factors of interest to the profession — satisfactory working conditions and satisfaction with the work itself" grew out of this.[2] However, concern for the image of the nurse and nursing, prompted a no-strike policy to be officially adopted by the ANA in 1950, and it remained in effect until it was rescinded in 1968.

By 1947, with the impetus provided by the Economic Security Program of ANA collective bargaining between nurses and hospital administration had been implemented in several states and negotiated contracts were in effect.

In 1947 the original NLRA was amended through the Taft–Hartley Act (also known as the Labor Management Relations Act) and, because of heavy lobbying on the part of hospital management, it was written in such a way as to specifically exclude nonprofit hospitals from the legal obligation of bargaining with their employees. At the time, many hospital employers were developing contracts voluntarily with employees and were showing genuine concern about working conditions. Some states were mandating that state hospitals negotiate with all employees. But there was no federal requirement that this process would occur, and nursing suffered a serious setback.

Federal legislation passed in 1962 enabled employees of federal health care institutions to participate in collective bargaining. In 1967 investor-owned hospitals and nursing homes were also included, and the ANA was identified as the bargaining agent for the nurses of the Veterans' Administration hospitals. Legislation passed in 1970 saw the inclusion of nonprofit nursing homes in the collective bargaining process.

Finally, on August 25, 1974, Public Law 93–360 was put into effect; it amended the Taft–Hartley Act to provide economic security programs for those employed in nonprofit hospitals. Under Section 2-2 nonprofit hospitals had been excluded from the NLRA. When the act was amended, this section was repealed. Section 2-14 further defined health care institutions as "any hospital, convalescent hospital, health maintenance organization, health clinic, nursing home, extended care facility, or other institution devoted to the care of sick, infirm, or aged persons."[3]

These two changes brought health care facilities and their employees under the jurisdiction of the NLRB. Nurses finally were permitted to work through their professional association for better wages, hours, staffing conditions, patient–nurse ratios, and a voice in hospital governance in general.

In the health care industry, a strike or concerted work stoppage could have serious implications for the public. In an effort to ensure the least possible disruption of service, several significant amendments were attached to the NLRA passed in 1974. These changes include the following:

- Medical colleges are not afforded protection and coverage because they are not to be considered health care institutions.
- Hospital interns and residents are not afforded protection and coverage because they are not considered employees.
- Any union planning to picket, strike, or create a work stoppage against any health care facility must give a 10-day prior notice, in writing.
- Health care institutions that intend to terminate or modify a collective bargaining agreement must give a 90-day notice, rather than the 60-day notice applied to other industries.
- Parties in health care agreements who intend to modify or terminate a collective bargaining agreement must give a 60-day notice, rather than the 30-day notice applied to other industries, to the Federal Mediation and Conciliation Service (FMCS).

- Parties are required to participate in FMCS mediation.
- A Board of Inquiry may be convened if a strike or lock-out will "substantially interrupt the delivery of health care."[4]

UNDERSTANDING THE LANGUAGE

Union/Collective Action

Before continuing discussion of the bargaining process, some terms should be explained.

A *union* is an organized group of employees that negotiates and enforces labor agreements. Its major concern is the improvement of wages, hours, and working conditions of its members. When a branch or part of a professional association assumes this responsibility, as is done in nursing, the negotiating group may be known as a *collective action division*. It must work under the same legal constraints as unions. In nursing, the state association usually assumes this role because it is sufficiently large enough to possess needed financial resources and expertise, and at the same time is close enough to the members it represents to be sensitive to their needs. It provides legal counsel and representatives to assist with negotiations, may lobby on behalf of issues, or take part in other activities that would further the economic welfare of nurses.

National Labor Relations Board

The NLRB has the responsibility for administering the NLRA. It consists of a general council and staff and five members, each of whom has a staff. The NLRB has the responsibility to determine into which of the established groupings of hospital workers the various employees fall. Currently there are five groupings:

1. a unit of professional employees,
2. a separate unit for registered nurses,
3. a separate unit for office and clerical employees,
4. a separate unit of technical employees (including licensed practical nurses, x-ray technicians, and laboratory technicians), and
5. a unit of service and maintenance employees.[5]

In addition, the NLRB has two primary functions: (1) to conduct secret-ballot elections that will determine that the majority of employees of a unit desire the representation of a given union in collective bargaining procedures; and (2) to prevent and rectify unfair labor practices committed by employers or unions.

Issues in Labor Relations

An *unfair labor practice* is any action that interferes with the rights of employees or employers as described in the amended NLRA. It is not possible to discuss all of these in detail; however, some examples follow. An employer must not interfere with the employee's right to form a union or other organized bargaining group, join the group, or take part in the group's activities. The employer may not attempt to control a group, once organized, or to discriminate against its members in regard to hiring or tenure. Most important, the employer must bargain collectively and in good faith with representatives of the employees. Bargaining in good faith is a poorly understood term, but generally it means to require meeting at regular times to discuss, with the intent to resolve, any differences over wages, hours, and other employment conditions. It protects the employees if lawful strikes become necessary by giving them a right to be reinstated into their jobs.

Likewise, labor organizations have constraints placed on their activities. They, too, must bargain in good faith. They must not restrain or coerce employees in selecting a bargaining group to bargain collectively. They may not pressure an employer to discriminate against employees who do not belong to the labor organization.

One of the issues frequently brought up in negotiations that usually results in a dispute is that of *agency shop*. Agency shop is a contract arrangement between an employer and the union representing the majority of employees that requires those who do not want to be members to pay the union a fee instead of union dues. The obvious advantage of this requirement, from the workers' point of view, is encouraging membership in the union. Because the union is required to represent *all* employees, members or not, their desire to have a greater percentage of paying members is also obvious.

Setting Labor Disputes

When labor disputes arise, several actions can be taken to help resolve the differences. There may be *authoritative mandates*, by which a peaceful settlement will be encouraged by a president, secretary of labor, or other high-ranking or influential person. An *injunction* may be requested, which is a court order that requires the party or parties involved to take a specific action or, more commonly, to refrain from taking a specific action. This measure can forestall a strike. In some instances the institution or company may be subjected to *government seizure and operation*. Government employees are then used to run the plant, firm, or industry in question.

Arbitration

Mediators or *arbitrators* may be used. A mediator is a third person who may join the bargainers in early sessions to assist the parties to reconcile differences and arrive at a peaceful agreement. Mediation involves finding compromises, and the mediator is to assist with this. He or she must gain the respect of both parties and must remain neutral to the issues presented. An *arbitrator* is technically defined as a person chosen by agreement of both parties to decide a dispute between them. Thus the primary difference between a mediator and an arbitrator is that the mediator assists the parties in reaching their own decision, whereas the arbitrator has been given a mandate to actually make the decision for the parties if necessary. However, the terms mediator and arbitrator, and mediation and arbitration often are used interchangeably, and, in fact, a mediator may also serve as an arbitrator.

Arbitration may take several forms. It may be *mediation–arbitration*, in which an arbitrator joins the parties in the negotiation process before there are any serious disputes. The role of the arbitrator is to act as a mediator who will attempt to keep the parties talking, suggest compromises, and help establish priorities. If an agreement is not reached by a specified date, or if it appears that neither party is willing to compromise on an issue (called a *deadlock*), the mediator then assumes the role of an arbitrator and gives a decision based on the information gained in the role of mediator.

Another form of arbitration is called *binding arbitration*. This means that both parties are obligated to abide by the decision of the arbitrator. Some people see this as the least desirable alternative in settling disputes because it may result in a decision that is not satisfactory to either side but one by which both must abide. It has been suggested, in instances in which binding arbitration is to be used, that the parties spell out exactly which of the issues are to be decided by the arbitrator. Binding arbitration has the advantage of resolving deadlocked issues without a strike being called. It also encourages both parties, knowing that the arbitrator's decision may not please either side, to reach a compromise on their own.

The *final offer* approach is a type of binding arbitration. Employer and employee bargaining representatives reach agreement on as many issues as possible. The deadlocked issues and a final position from each

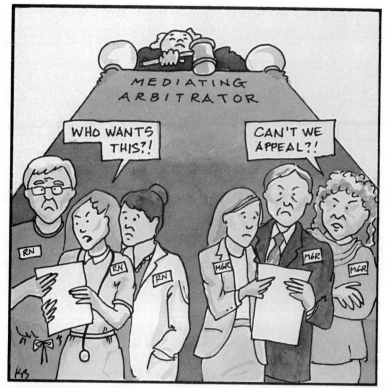

Figure 9–1. The arbitrator's decision may not really please either side.

side are then presented to the arbitrator, who is obligated to select only the most reasonable package. The arbitrator may not develop a third alternative, which would "split the difference." The final offer approach encourages both sides to come up with a fairly realistic package and serves to close the gap on issues.

One criticism of any type of arbitration is the expense involved. Arbitrators must be paid for their services. It is also criticized because it undermines voluntary collective bargaining and allows parties to avoid unpleasant confrontation with their own difficulties by shifting that responsibility to a public authority. However, this is useful to prevent the disruption of services.

Arbitration may also be defined as *interest* arbitration or as *rights* arbitration. When unresolved issues are submitted to an arbitrator for determination, it is known as *interest arbitration;* when there is a dispute over the application or interpretation of an existing agreement, it is known as *rights arbitration*. Arbitration is always considered the most formal of the types of third-party intervention.[6]

The Arbitration Process

Arbitration may be requested from the American Arbitration Association (AAA) or from available state mediation and conciliation services. The AAA is a nonprofit, nonpartisan organization that, for a nominal fee, will provide a list of qualified arbitrators. Other services, such as mediation and fact-finding, are also available through the AAA. The most frequent requests are directed to the *Federal Mediation and Conciliation Service* (FMCS), a government agency primarily involved in mediating disputes that arise out of contract negotiations. It can also furnish a list of competent arbitrators.

The FMCS was created by the Labor Management Relations Act of 1947 to conciliate and mediate disputes that could cause a disruption of interstate commerce. When the act was amended to include members of the health care field, this body was empowered with additional responsibilities that it was hoped would prevent or deter disruption of health care.

The FMCS becomes involved in the negotiation process when the regional office of the FMCS receives one of the notifications mentioned earlier, that is, the 90-day notice to modify or terminate an existing agreement, or the 60-day notice before the expiration date of the contract if the parties have not reached agreement by that time. A mediator will then be assigned to the negotiations.

The mediator will contact the spokesperson for both the bargaining agent and the employer and will try to arrange a mutually agreeable time and place for a meeting. He or she will try to assess the impact of work stoppage on the community, the status of the negotiation process and the relationship between the two parties, the critical issues that remain unresolved, and similar concerns. The mediator will also meet with each party separately to better understand the issues. After gathering all pertinent information from both parties, the mediator will submit the findings to the director of FMCS for evaluation. The director will decide whether to appoint an impartial *Board of Inquiry* (BOI) to engage in fact finding in cases in which a strike would seriously interrupt the delivery of health care of that area. If a BOI is appointed, both parties are notified of the Board's identity and the date of appointment.

The BOI may comprise one or more persons, but usually only one. Within 15 days after appointment the BOI must conduct hearings and issue a written report that includes the facts and recommendations for resolution of issues in the dispute. The parties may then accept or reject the recommendations, but it is hoped that the recommendations will assist the parties to reach a mutually agreeable settlement. Strikes or lockouts are prohibited until 15 days after presentation of the report.

The mediator may continue to work with the negotiating parties while the fact finding is being conducted and the report prepared, or may not enter negotiations until later. In either case the mediators have no authority to enforce any of their suggestions or recommendations. It is hoped that because of their neutrality, mediators can be a valuable resource and can create a constructive atmosphere for agreement.[7]

Strikes and Lockouts

When the negotiation process breaks down, lockouts and strikes are apt to occur. A *lockout* occurs when an employer closes a factory or other place of business to make employees agree to terms. One can readily see how undesirable this would be in the health care field, but it has occurred in some instances.

Strikes are of two kinds. An *economic strike* results from efforts on the part of employees to seek better economic benefits. *Unfair labor practice strikes* may be divided into two additional classifications: those caused or prolonged by the employer's unfair labor practice and those caused by the employees' unfair labor practice. If employees initiate an economic strike and during the strike the employer commits any of the actions that were described as unfair labor practices, the strike then becomes an unfair labor practice strike on the part of employers. *Sit-down strikes,* in which employees not only refuse to work but also refuse to leave the employer's property, are an example of unfair practices on the part of employees. Sit-down strikes have been uncommon in the health care industry. Employees who engage in unlawful activities during a strike or whose activities cause a strike to become unlawful are not entitled to reinstatement privileges.

Reinstatement Privilege

A *reinstatement privilege* is a guarantee offered to striking employees that they will be rehired after the strike, provided that they have not engaged in any unfair labor practices during the strike and provided that the strike itself is lawful. The hospital may replace a striking nurse during the strike. If strikers agree *unconditionally* to return to work, the employer is not required to replace the striking nurse at that time. However, recall lists are developed, and if the nurse cannot find regular

and equivalent employment, he or she is privileged to recall and preference on jobs before new employees may be given employment.

As stated earlier, nurses may lose their reinstatement privileges
because of misconduct during a lawful strike. For example, strikers may
not physically block other nurses and personnel from entering or leaving a struck hospital. Strikers may not threaten nonstriking employees
and may not attack management representatives. These types of activities usually do not occur in strikes conducted by nurses but are not
outside the realm of possibility.

Summary

In this section we have given an overview of collective bargaining
and an exposure to some of the language involved in the process. Those
who want to gain more information will be interested in an NLRB
publication titled *A Guide to Basic Law and Procedures under the National
Labor Relations Act,* which explains union shops, strikes, elections, and
other issues related to negotiations. It may be obtained by writing to the
NLRB office at 1717 Pennsylvania Avenue NW, Washington, DC
20570.

WHAT TO LOOK FOR IN A CONTRACT

So far we have discussed the negotiation process and its language.
We have talked broadly about negotiating wages, hours, and working
conditions. In this section we spell out in more detail specific provisions
that might be included in a contract.

A contract must meet certain specified criteria to be legally binding.
It must result from mutually agreed-on items arrived at through a
"meeting of minds." Something of value must be given for a reciprocal
promise, that is, professional duties for an agreed-on sum. Contracts can
be enforceable whether written or oral, but it is easier to work with
those that are written.[8]

Although each agreement will differ, most contracts have a fairly
general format that will include the following:

- A preamble stating the objectives of each party
- A statement recognizing the official bargaining group
- A section dealing with financial remuneration, including wages
  and salaries, overtime rates, holiday pay, and shift differentials
- A section dealing with nonfinancial rewards, in other words,
  fringe benefits such as retirement programs, types of insurance

available, free parking, and other services provided by the employer

- A section dealing with seniority in respect to promotion, transfer, work schedules, and layoffs
- A section establishing guidelines for disciplinary problems
- A section describing how grievance procedures will be resolved
- A section that may explicitly state codes of conduct or professional standards.

The contract may also include many other mutually agreed-on items, such as no-strike agreements and an arrangement for using an arbitrator to settle issues that become deadlocked.[9] Several other areas that are negotiable are important and should be mentioned. These may be in-

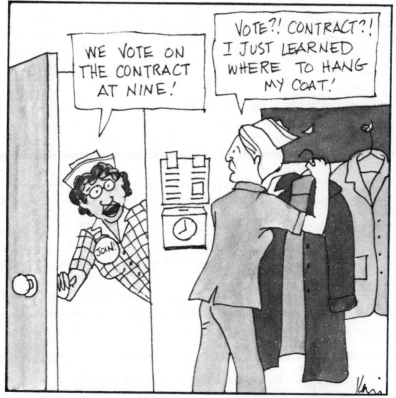

Figure 9–2. As a new graduate, you may find yourself poorly prepared to make decisions that are involved in bargaining issues.

cluded in the section dealing with professional standards or nursing care.

Cleland outlines the following items that should be considered in a contract that involves professional nurses. First of all, the contract should provide for shared governance; that is, that professional policy decisions should be developed by professional staff and administration who work jointly on the policy. This often takes the form of a nursing practice council or a professional performance committee. Second, the contract should provide for individual professional accountability. This would ensure peer evaluation of a practitioner's competence. Third, the contract should define the collective professional role. This spells out the responsibility of registered nurses as professional practitioners and describes their part in the planning of patient care. The purpose of this is to strengthen nurses' influence on the quality of care.[10]

It is important that, as a new graduate, you know whether there is a contract in effect in the institution from which you seek employment or in the community in which you plan to work. You should also be knowledgeable about the terms of that contract, if it exists, so that you might best fulfill your obligations and recognize and benefit from the provisions to which you are entitled. State nurses' associations can be contacted for this information and usually can provide a copy of any contracts that have been negotiated within that particular state.

ISSUES RELATED TO COLLECTIVE BARGAINING AND NURSING

The issues of collective bargaining that relate to the nursing profession can be divided into five major points of discussion:

1. The role of the supervisor in collective bargaining
2. The argument of professionalism versus unionism
3. The decision facing nurses about whether they want to join a bargaining group
4. Which bargaining group nurses should choose to represent them
5. Whether the individual nurse will decide to strike if negotiations break down and a strike is called

The Supervisor and Collective Bargaining

Historically, nursing has paid little attention to how the term supervisor has been used in the health care system. An employee observing another employee carrying out a procedure for the first time might be said to be "supervising" the activity. Likewise, charge nurses, head nurses, and possibly team leaders perform a different type of supervisory activity, that of supervising the care of patients and the actions of personnel. When the Taft–Hartley Act was amended to require non-profit hospitals to bargain collectively with their employees, problems arose regarding the definition of supervisor as written in the amendment. A *supervisor* was defined as

> any individual having authority, in the interest of the employer, to hire, transfer, suspend, lay off, recall, promote, discharge, assign, reward, or discipline other employees, or responsibly to direct them, or to adjust their grievances, or effectively to recommend such action, if in connection with the foregoing the exercise of such authority is not of a merely routine or clerical nature, but requires the use of independent judgment.[11]

In this sense, supervisors were not viewed as employees, but as agents of the employer, carrying out "supervisory acts for, on behalf of, and in place of the employer."[12] Therefore, if the person hired as supervisor were to become involved in the collective bargaining group and its workings, it could be ruled an unfair labor practice. The supervisor's participation could be viewed as "dominance" on the part of the employer.

Thus any person functioning within the health care system in any manner that met the above definition was excluded from the appropriate bargaining unit. Head nurses and supervisors were considered part of hospital management. With the Division of Economic and General Welfare of the ANA assuming a heavy role in the negotiation process, nurses found themselves in a dilemma. Those people who, for years, had assumed leadership positions among their peers could not do so when it came to determining working conditions. Membership in the association was not prohibited by law, but supervisors could not take part in the association's collective bargaining. In past years it often was the head nurses, supervisors, or perhaps the director of nursing services that pushed the staff nurses toward membership in the professional association and toward becoming involved in the activities of the organization. If the professional association assumed bargaining responsibilities, the supervisory personnel were restricted from applying this push, especially if they solicited membership or authorization cards.

In several instances in which the state nurses' association won elections to represent nurses at the bargaining table, hospital administration has objected that the state nurses' association was not a proper "labor organization" because it had supervisors as members and directors. When this challenge was raised in Alabama in 1968, the NLRB overruled the objection by emphasizing that all activity related to collective bargaining was carried out by members of the unit. There was no supervisor involvement with the collective bargaining process.

In Maryland in 1975 a similar challenge occurred that has come to be known as the Anne Arundel General Hospital case. In this instance the hospital had its own negotiating committee elected by the general membership of the employees. Again it was ruled, when challenged, that inasmuch as that chapter admitted no supervisors to its membership and had no employee supervisors as its officers or directors, it met the requirements of a bona fide labor organization.[13]

These challenges have posed some problems for the ANA. First of all, the organization had to determine that no person with a supervisory role was involved in directing or advising the activities of the Economic and General Welfare Commission or its committees. In addition, an effort was made to place professional association dues and collective bargaining section dues in separate accounts to ensure that there would be no commingling of funds. This separation of funds tends to further emphasize that supervisors are in no way involved in the bargaining process, although their right to belong to the professional association is valid.

Directors of nursing service became concerned about their relationship with the association if that group were to represent nurses in the institution. In some instances hospital management discouraged directors from belonging to the association. Directors and assistant directors were becoming increasingly vulnerable, and sometimes they were discharged without notice and with no recourse. In other instances directors resented having part of their professional dues used to fund the Division of Economic and General Welfare of the association when that group could not represent them and, in fact, could make their job more hectic.

Probably the saddest aspect of the issue is the schism that results between supervisor and nursing staff within the hospital. It is the supervisors and director that usually serve on key committees within an institution, in which they support, define, and encourage greater professional recognition of the registered nurse in the care-giving role. In the negotiation process these leaders are placed on the opposite side of the bargaining table. As supervisors and staff, who, as a total group, have united for quality patient care, align themselves with one side or the other, the terms "we" and "they" begin to carry more meaning than either should. In a heated dispute some bad feelings inevitably result.

Many state nurses' associations are working to keep nurses united, whatever their role in health care delivery, and they are attempting to find methods to represent the welfare of all members.

Professionalism Versus Unionism

Among the issues related to collective bargaining, the pitting of professionalism against unionism has probably received more space in recent nursing literature than has any other.

The argument against unionism has its roots in the history of nursing itself. Nursing was perceived by many, including nurses, as a selfless, all-serving, altruistic calling. The act of caring for others, even if that meant subordination of the individual to the goals of that care, was to be compensation enough for the services rendered. The strong religious influence that pervaded the early development of nursing added to this concept of the profession. Early leaders in nursing espoused this dedication to its arts. In 1893 Lavinia Dock stated

> Absolute and unquestioning obedience must be the foundation of the nurse's work, and to this end complete subordination of the individual to the work as a whole is as necessary for her as for the soldier.[14]

Some nurses today speak out against unionizing. Campbell questioned the wisdom of organizing into unions but with a little different focus than that given by Dock. Campbell wrote:

> In a union, not only is the ability to speak out individually diminished, but the type of care and the needs of our patients may be jeopardized due to strikes and decisions that may or may not be pertinent in a given area of practice. Nurses should be implementing and auditing standards that pertain to nursing. These standards should not be subject to scrutiny of an arbitrator who may or may not be knowledgeable about quality patient care.[15]

Another factor that has hampered the strong development of unionization in nursing is the fact that nursing is primarily a women's profession. Although more men now enter nursing, statistics gathered by the Department of Health and Human Services indicate that the number of males in nursing has increased only 0.3% in a 4-year period between 1980 and 1984, from 44,237 in 1980 to 57,199 in 1984.[16] This represents 3% of the registered nurses in the United States.

Early social beliefs that woman's role should be submissive, supportive, and obedient were extremely compatible with pervading concepts of the expectations that our society placed on nurses. The paternalism that has existed in the health care delivery system has also made the process of collective bargaining for nurses a slow one (see Chapter 1).

The combination of the role of women and the role of the nurse under earlier paternalistic practices had the nurse caring for the "hospital family," looking out for the needs of all, from patient to physician, and being responsible for keeping everyone happy.[17] The tendency to see the physician as the father figure in the health care system, and the nurse as the corresponding mother figure, has done little to promote the autonomy of nursing as a profession. Campbell echoed the tenor of this thinking when she wrote in 1980, "If we are to keep unions out of the profession we, as nurses, must make every effort to build loyalty and a family feeling among our fellow nurses."[18]

Throughout this discussion we have used the term *unionism* without qualification. Certainly 5 years ago it would not have been acceptable, and to some it is still not acceptable today. Unionism to some means gaining coercive powers and with that developing a nurses' public image that would have a detrimental effect on the profession. Some have feared that their white collars might turn "blue," recalling the traditional association of unionism with blue-collar workers.[19] However, most of the literature of today has stopped quibbling over the word *unionism*. When Barbara Nichols was president of the ANA, she wrote: "Too much time has been squandered on discussions of whether we are a union or a professional association. The American Nurses' Association is both."[20] Other authors go so far as to say that "if collective bargaining did destroy 'professionalism' it would be a blessing. This concept is a false god, a silver cross held up to ward off the evil spirits of fair play, decent conditions, and your rights under the law."[21]

Some believe that the collective action of nurses provides one of the best avenues for achieving professional goals and exercising control over nursing practice. As nurses are called on to assume greater and greater responsibility for complicated decisions, collective bargaining through a professional organization may provide the means to implement the concept of collective professional responsibility.[22]

Another reason given by nurses for not organizing is the impact that striking would have on the health care delivery system. Many believe that withdrawal of services would cause innocent people to suffer. (We will discuss the strike later in this chapter.)

Certainly the way that collective bargaining will be perceived by the nurse and by the public that is served will be primarily determined by the manner in which the bargaining is conducted. Nurses as a group need to develop the skills that are necessary to communicate to the public the importance of their role in health care delivery. They must be able to handle conflict situations and work toward resolution while maintaining integrity and dignity. Nurses need to become enlightened and informed, and they need more than a superficial understanding of the process of collective bargaining.

Finally, many think that nurses need to broaden their perceptions. Many nurses dichotomize issues into categories such as good/bad, right/wrong, best/worst. There is a need to endeavor to understand and make accommodations for differing points of view and to acknowledge that areas of compromise can exist.

To Join or Not to Join

Once the individual nurse has gained an understanding of collective bargaining and has developed a personal philosophy about the professional role, he or she will be ready to make a decision in regard to membership in the bargaining unit.

In working with students who are soon to embark on professional careers, we find that it is easier for them to decide whether to bargain collectively than it is to decide to part with the monies that are required for membership. Many nurses want better working conditions and higher salaries but are all too willing to let someone else fund these endeavors and work to achieve them.

Those who argue against an agency shop—largely the administration—contend that it begins to erode management's basic right to decide who will be employed.[23] It also takes away some of the freedom of the individual by eliminating the option of each nurse to decide whether he or she wants to belong to an organized group in order to work in a given hospital. This may serve as either an asset or a deterrent to recruitment, depending on the applicant's viewpoint.

Representation of Nurses

Of far greater controversy than whether nurses should unionize is the issue of which organization should represent nurses at the bargaining table. As mentioned earlier, this is determined by elections that are supervised by the NLRB. To become the certified collective bargaining representative of a group of employees, the organization in question must receive 50% of the votes cast, plus one.

When nurses first began to organize, the ANA, through the state nurses' associations, was the bargaining representative. This group still represents more nurses than all the other organizations put together. However, there has been a strong movement on the part of other organizations to vie for the representative position. A study conducted by Richard U. Miller in 1980 indicated that more than 30 labor organizations represent health care workers.[24] In addition to the ANA, which has been representing nurses since 1946, the major unions organizing nurses include The Federation of Nurses and Health Professionals/ American Federation of Teachers, which began organizing nurses in 1978; District 1199 National Union of Hospital and Health Care Employees, representing nurses since 1977; Service Employees International Union; and the United Food and Commercial Workers. The Teamsters Union also has been chosen by some nurses as their representative.

Nurses face another difficult decision when trying to decide which group can represent them best. Those who have strong allegiance to the ANA contend that only RNs should bargain for RNs. One of the reasons given for this position is that in collective bargaining, nurses face different issues than do other workers. In addition to concerns about salary, benefits, working conditions, and the like, nurses want also to negotiate questions pertaining to staffing, patient care concerns, and participation on joint hospital committees. Many believe that only nurses can effectively negotiate such items. These people contend that hospital administrations, fearing the power of labor unions, will bargain more constructively and positively with nurses themselves. They also believe that the ANA will be a stronger, more united organization if it serves as both the professional association and the bargaining agent.

Some believe that nurses compromise their collective bargaining powers when the recognized union is a group other than the state nurses' association. They think that when nurses do not bargain for themselves, the "organization shrivels and their influence on health care weakens."[25]

Others believe that another organization can represent nurses better. Chief among the arguments of this group is the issue of supervisor membership in the professional association (discussed earlier in this chapter). These same people would also contend that it is not realistic for one group (*i.e.,* the ANA) to work with the professionalism aspect of nursing as well as with the issues of wages, benefits, and working conditions.

Some would argue for two organizations, one to represent issues related to professionalism and another to negotiate salaries. If nurses choose to have one group involved in professional concerns (*e.g.,* codes of ethics, standards of care, and updating skills required in the practice of the profession) and a second group representing them at the bargaining table, there are some obvious drawbacks. First and foremost is the matter of cost because both organizations would be collecting dues. Many perceive the cost of belonging to the ANA and the state associations as very high, with dues of approximately $200 per year. Additional membership dues in another organization might be prohibitive. Second, there are those who believe that the union would become the dominant force between the two groups because money and working environment issues both speak strongly. There are no easy answers to this question, and it will certainly be one of the biggest issues facing nurses in the future.

To Strike or Not to Strike

Nurses, employers, and the public are served best when negotiations are truly in good faith and continue until resolution occurs. In some areas in which a strike has occurred, it took nurses months, and perhaps years, to regain lost salaries. The level of care to the community may have been placed in jeopardy during the time of the strike, and the public image of nursing may have been damaged. These are not desirable outcomes.

The negotiation process does not always move smoothly. The last alternative for the employer in pushing an issue is the lockout or layoff. For the nursing bargaining unit, the last alternative in forcing an issue is the strike. When negotiations reach this point, serious problems can occur. To some nurses the actual withholding of services to a public that needs them is abhorrent and is incompatible with personal definitions of professionalism. These people would favor no-strike clauses in contracts, coupled with binding arbitration. This eliminates the need to consider the strike as an alternative.

Other nurses believe that strikes are a necessary and justified means of achieving desired ends. In the early 1980s, when organized activities of nurses were embryonic, negotiations that reached the strike stage received fairly wide publicity. Today strikes have occurred frequently enough among nurses' bargaining groups to be no longer treated in a sensational fashion.

It is not always possible to anticipate how the general public will interpret a strike by professionals, especially if professional standards are an issue. Someone needing health care may be aware only that care is not available and may be angered by any disruption that could occur in the usual pattern of health care delivery. On the other hand, if the public perceives hospital management as being unreasonable and causing the change in services, the public sentiment may be supportive of nurses on strike.

One approach that nurses sometimes use to soften the impact of the strike on health care consumers is an agreement to continue to deliver services to critical care areas. Through this mechanism nurses continue

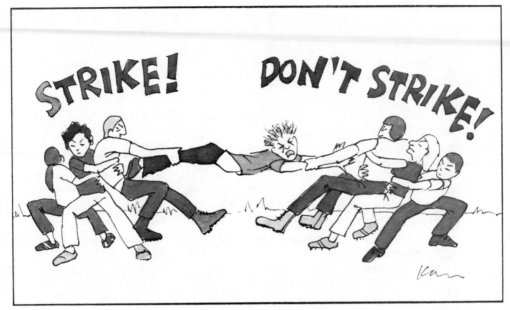

Figure 9–3. There are no easy answers to the strike issue.

to staff those areas of the hospital in which care is of an emergency nature. This often includes coronary and intensive care units, labor and delivery suites, emergency rooms, and emergency surgery units.

When a strike is voted by a majority of members of a bargaining organization, the individual nurse who was opposed to striking will have to decide whether he or she will abide by the vote of the majority, or whether he or she will go against the majority and cross picket lines to continue in the care-giving role. To strike may be contrary to personal beliefs, but to return to work while colleagues are striking may also be in conflict with values.

Changing Attitudes Today

At one time economic concerns and working conditions may have been the principal motivators for collective action. However, by the mid-1980s subtle, and at times not so subtle, changes were occurring throughout the United States with regard to collective bargaining, unionism, and labor–management relations. Some working in the area of contract management would report a shift from the adversarial relationship that had historically existed between the employee and the employer, which focused on salaries, work hours, and the like, to one that placed greater emphasis on the quality of work life. *Concession bargaining,* in which there is an explicit exchange in labor costs for improvements in job security, was seen to occur with increasing frequency. These changes have been seen in industry more than in nursing, although the strike of more than 6,000 Minnesota nurses was triggered by hospital practices related to the layoff of staff and the involuntary reduction of hours.[26]

A current trend often seen in health care institutions is an effort toward *union busting.* Although technically illegal when referring to methods used to get rid of an existing union, the term union busting has been expanded to include a wide range of legal activities that slow down collective bargaining. Pressured by rapidly escalating health care costs and influenced by the changing attitudes toward work, hospital administrators have hired consultants and law firms to assist and advise in discouraging and impeding organizational activities. This is also a counteraction to the courting by unions of the expanding groups of previously unorganized professional groups, such as physicians and nurses, as union membership among trade unions dropped. Anti-union organizing campaigns are usually aimed at strategies that will delay, and thus drag down the momentum of, organizing efforts. This could include challenging unit membership, attempting to decertify elections, and failing to bargain in good faith, thus drawing out the negotiating process.[27]

Organized nurses in some states have recently focused their bargaining energies on issues of pay equity. For example, nurses employed by the state of Pennsylvania lodged a complaint with the U.S. Equal Opportunity Employment Commission, charging discrimination against female employees, who earn an average of $3,000 less per year than the state's male employees in similar positions.[28] Nurses in Florida, Michigan, Washington, Alaska, California, and Illinois are also among those who have waged battles related to comparable worth.[29,30,31,32,33]

The Grievance Process

Although the grievance process is a somewhat different subject than collective bargaining, it is usually one part of a negotiated contract and therefore deserves some mention here.

The *grievance process* represents an established method to be used in the adjustment of grievances between parties. A *grievance* is "an allegation by any party functioning under a collective bargaining agreement that a violation of the contract has occurred."[34] Although grievances can be filed by either the management or the employee, most cases are filed by the employee.

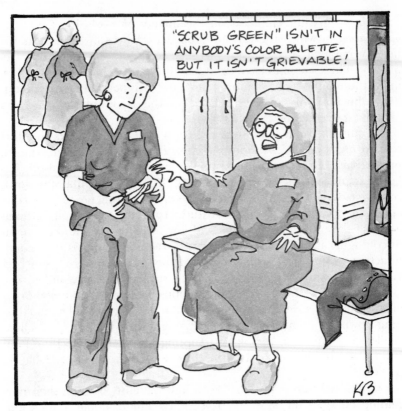

Figure 9–4. It is important to discriminate between complaints and grievances.

It is important to discriminate between complaints and grievances. Employees may have complaints that are not violations of the contract. For example, Nurse No. 1 may object that she was required to float from the postpartum unit to the nursery. She had been oriented to the nursery but preferred to work in the postpartum unit. Nurse No. 2 was required to float from a medical unit to a surgical unit to which she had not been oriented. If the contract in this hospital stipulated that no one would be floated to a unit to which they had not been oriented, Nurse No. 1 had a complaint, whereas Nurse No. 2 had a grievance.

The grievance process spells out in writing in the contract a series of steps to be taken to resolve the area of dissension. The usual steps are as follows:

1. The employee and the immediate supervisor talk informally about the disagreement. If not satisfied, the employee asks the bargaining representative from the institution (sometimes called a *steward*) to intercede.

2. The supervisor and the steward talk informally. If no agreement is reached, the grievance is put into writing and filed with the supervisor. Usually the contract specifies a given number of days in which this must occur. The supervisor will also respond in writing.

3. If the grievance is pursued, it moves to the next level of management. At this point, the original decision may be either upheld or overturned.

4. If the decision is not reversed and the employee still wants to pursue it, the problem goes to a committee. This committee usually is composed of union and management representatives. After reviewing the case, the original decision is either upheld or denied.

5. If the decision is still unsatisfactory to the employee, it is finally reviewed by the top administrator and the union president. If the decision is still unacceptable to the employee, the issue is presented to an arbitrator. The decision of the arbitrator is binding.

The procedure may sound like many steps that may take a great deal of time, and indeed this is true. Although most grievances are settled short of arbitration, they are still time and energy consuming. Grievances can be best avoided if everyone has a good understanding of the terms of the contract, and if sound personnel policies are developed and applied consistently and equitably.

CONCLUSION

We have attempted to present a comprehensive, although not detailed, explanation of the collective bargaining process and the issues that surround it. Each of you will need to examine these issues and resolve them according to your personal value system and your philosophy. To do so you will need to consider the issues at stake, the ramifications that any action will have on the health care of a given area, and the dictates of your own conscience. We hope that this chapter has provided information to assist you in any decisions related to collective bargaining that you may be required to make.

REFERENCES

1. Muff J: Altruism, socialism, and nightingalism: The compassion traps. In Muff J (ed) Socialization, Sexism, and Stereotyping, p 245. St. Louis, CV Mosby, 1982
2. Rutsohn PD, Grimes RM: Collective Bargaining: "Quo Vadis" for the Allied Health Professional. Allied Health 53, Fall 1977
3. Bryant YN: Labor relations in health care institutions: An analysis of Public Law 93–360. J Nurs Admin 8:28, Mar 1978
4. Douglas JM: Issues in Collective Bargaining for Nurses. National League for Nursing Publication Number 32–1874, pp 10–11. New York, National League for Nursing, 1981
5. Hemelt MD, Mackert ME: Dynamics of Law in Nursing and Health Care. 2nd ed, pp 70–71. Reston, VA, Reston Publishing, 1982
6. Castrey BG, Castrey RT: Mediation: What it is, what it does. J Nurs Admin 10:24, Nov 1980
7. Castrey BG, Castrey RT: Mediation: What it is, what it does. J Nurs Admin 10:24, Nov 1980
8. Rothman DA, Rothman NL: The Professional Nurse and the Law, pp 109–110. Boston, Little, Brown, 1977
9. Werther WB Jr, Lockhart CA: Labor Relations in the Health Professions: The Basis of Power — The Means of Change, pp 108–111. Boston, Little, Brown, 1976
10. Cleland V: Taft–Hartley amended: Implications for nursing — the professional model. J Nurs Admin 11:18, Jul 1981
11. Public Law 93–360, Section 2, 1974
12. Hemelt DM, Mackert ME: Dynamics of Law in Nursing and Health Care. 2nd ed, pp 70–71. Reston VA, Reston Publishing, 1982
13. Douglas JM: Issues in Collective Bargaining for Nurses. National League for Nursing Publication No. 32–1874, pp 10–11. New York, National League for Nursing, 1981
14. Dock LL: Nurses should be obedient. In Bullough V Bullough B (eds): Issues in Nursing: Readings Selected From Books and Periodicals to Form a Basis for Discussion of Problems in Nursing Today, p 96. New York, Springer–Verlag, 1966
15. Campbell GJ: In Opinions: Is bargaining unprofessional for nurses? AORN J 31:1289, Jun 1980
16. R.N. Ranks Grow to Nearly 2 million, says HHS: New Survey Shows 20-percent employment rise. Am J Nurs 86:603, May 1986
17. Ashley JA: Hospitals, Paternalism and the Role of the Nurse. New York, Teachers' College Press, 1976
18. Campbell GJ: In Opinions: Is bargaining unprofessional for nurses? AORN J 31:1289, Jun 1980
19. Stern EM: Collective bargaining: A means of conflict or resolution. Nurs Adm Q 6:18, Winter 1982

20. Nichols B: An open letter to the nurses of America. Am J Nurs 80:61, Jan 1980

21. Gideon J: Unions: Choice and mandate. AORN J 31:1205, Jun 1980

22. McClelland JQ: Professionalism and collective bargaining: A new reality for nurses and management. J Nurs Admin 13:36–38, Nov 1983

23. Cannon P: Agency shop and the nurse administrator. Nurs Adm Q 6:56, Winter 1982

24. Miller RU: Collective bargaining: A nursing dilemma. AORN J 31:1197, Jun 1980

25. Mallison MB: Weathering the economic climate. Am J Nurs 85:943, Sep 1985

26. 6,000 Minnesota RNs Strike Back at Layoff Trend. Am J Nurs 84:941, 948, Jul 1984

27. Ballman CS: Union busters. Am J Nurs 85:963–966, Sep 1985

28. Pennsylvania nurses call for pay-equity probe. Am J Nurs 85:924, Aug 1985

29. Comparable worth debate intensifies nationwide. Am J Nurs 85:924, Aug 1985

30. Michigan nurses fight to reform the civil service salary system. Am J Nurs 85:316, 317, 333, Mar 1985

31. Washington RNs ask lawmakers to fund salary hike for women. Am J Nurs 85:318, 333, Mar 1985

32. Resolute Contra Costa RNs show how to win a comp/worth base. Am J Nurs 85:317, Mar 1985

33. Judge slows down Alaska PHNs' search for comparable worth. Am J Nurs 85:332, Mar 1985

34. Werther WB, Lockhart CA: Labor Relations in the Health Care Professions: The Basis of Power—The Means of Change, pp 108–111, Boston, Little, Brown, 1976

FURTHER READINGS

Beletz E. Meng MT: The grievance process. Am J Nurs 77:256–260, Feb 1977

Cannon P: Adminstering the contract. J Nurs Adm 10:13–19, Oct 1980

Cappelli P: Plant-Level Concession Bargaining. Industrial and Labor Relations Review 39:90–104, Oct 1985

Delaney JT. Lewin D, Sockel D: The NLRA at Fifty: A Research Appraisal and Agenda. Industrial and Labor Relations Review 39:46–75, Oct 1985

Despres LM: A lawyer explains what the national labor relations act really says. Am J Nurs 76:790–794, May 1976

Eldridge I, Levi M: Collective bargaining as a power resource for professional goals. Nurs Adm Q:29–40, Winter 1982

Emanuel WB: Nurse unionization is dominant theme. Hospitals 55:121–128, Apr 1981

Emerson WL: Appropriate bargaining units for professional employees. J Nurs Adm 8:10–15, Sep 1978

Epstein RL, Stickler KB: The nurse as a professional and as a unionist. Hospitals 50:44–48, Jan 16, 1976

Flanagan L: Braving New Frontiers: ANA's Economic and General Welfare Program, 1946–1986 ANA PUBL 1986 #EC–144:1–30

Godfrey M: Most nurses deserve more pay. Nurs 77:10–11, Jul 1977

Godfrey M: Nurses salaries today: Where you can earn the most and the least. Nurs 77:81–97, Jun 1977

Godfrey M: Someone should represent nurses. Nurs 76:73–85, Jun 1976

Gross JA: Conflicting Statutory Purposes: Another Look at Fifty Years of NLRB Law Making. Industrial and Labor Relations Review 39:7–18, Oct 1985

Jordan CH: Collective bargaining and the road to self-determination. Nurs Adm Q 8:59–62, Winter 1982

Lunn S: Unions and continuing education. AORN J 31:1212–1216, Jun 1980

Luttman P: Collective bargaining and professionalism: Incompatible ideologies? Nurs Adm Q:21–28, Winter 1982

McEvoy P: Unionization or professionalization: What way for nurses? Nurs Mirror 141:70–72, Nov 20, 1975

Pettengill MM: Multilateral Collective Bargaining and the Health Care Industry: Implications for Nursing. J Prof Nurs 5:275–282 Sept–Oct 1985

Roberts RM, Cox JL, Baldwin LE, Baldwin LS: What Causes Hospital Nurses to Unionize? Nurs Forum XXII 22–30 Jan 1985

Smith GR: Unionization for Nurses: an Issue for the 1980's. J Prof Nurs 4:192–201, Jul/Aug 1985

So You're Interested in Economic and General Welfare for Nurses, Publication No. EC–124. Kansas City, American Nurses' Association, 1977

Stearns PM: Making a decision on organizing. AORN J 31:1208–1211, Jun 1980

Taft–Hartley amended. Series. Am J Nurs 75:284–295, Feb 1975

Tomlins CL: The New Deal, Collective Bargaining and the Triumph of Industrial Pluralism. Industrial and Labor Relations Review 39:19–34, Oct 1985

Yeagers J: Why I had to strike. Am J Nurs 77:874–875, May 1977

10 | The Political Process and Health Care

Objectives

After completing this chapter, you should be able to

1. State reasons why the political process is relevant to nursing.
2. Identify seven ways a person might affect the political process.
3. Discuss the significance of the Nurse Training Act.
4. Explain the major provisions of the Medicare and Medicaid acts that relate to health care.
6. Identify the major purposes of four additional federal legislative acts.
7. Discuss the various proposals related to a national health care system.
8. List common state-level legislative concerns.
9. Discuss common local political concerns.

Politics often is thought of as the way in which the government functions; in reality it is far more than that. Politics is the way in which people in a democratic society try to influence decision making and the allocation of resources. Resources include money, time, and personnel. Because resources are always limited, choices must always be made as to how they will be used. There is no perfect process for making optimum choices because in every instance some task, some program, or some product is left out. You will recognize that politics is a part of every organization, as well as part of government at every level.

RELEVANCE OF THE POLITICAL PROCESS FOR NURSES

Health care is very costly, and public dollars can be and are spent in many ways to provide health care. What part of the federal budget should be allocated to health care? Of the money allocated, what part should be used for preventive health programs, what part for research, what part for care and treatment, and what part for education? These questions are answered by legislation and by administrative decisions made by governmental agencies. If you have opinions on what is appropriate, or think that priorities as they are set currently are incorrect, or if you have ever been blocked in your attempt to provide health care to a client and family by learning that the one needing care did not have the necessary funds and that no public support was available for the care needed, the political process is relevant to you.

Your practice as a nurse is controlled by a wide variety of governmental decisions. One of the most basic is the nurse practice act of your state. In that document nursing is defined legally, and the scope of nursing practice is outlined. This document affects what you do each day that you practice. All of the philosophical discussions about the role of the nurse must return to the reality of what is the nurse's legal role. Do you care what that role is now, or what changes are made in it? Does it make any difference to you what education is required in that law or if that law requires continuing education? Answering yes to any of these questions underlines the relevance of the political process for you.

Many decisions are made within the various nurses' organizations (discussed in Chapter 12). These organizations speak for nurses in a variety of settings. Are you happy with the way they are spending funds paid in dues? Do you agree with all of the public statements they make? Do you support their mechanisms for decision making? Are you happy with the view the public receives of nurses and nursing from these organizations? Do you care what these organizations do with their resources? The political process is an important part of their functioning too.

AFFECTING THE POLITICAL PROCESS

Once you have decided that decision making affects you and your practice as a nurse in many crucial ways, your next concern is how to influence the process by which those decisions are made. Can you as an individual have an effect on such things as what legislation is submitted, what is passed, and the content of that legislation? The answer is yes you can, but not without effort and concern on your part. Each person must make a decision as to the level of personal involvement, but there is, in the broad realm of the political process, a place for everyone to function in a way that is comfortable. Some of the ways are outlined here.

Keeping Informed

To keep informed about legislation and health care, it is necessary to become familiar with the sources of information. Your daily newspaper can be an excellent source regarding significant legislation being proposed. This source is not complete, however, and you often learn of legislation after it has already been passed.

Television and radio news reports are valuable but may give only an overview of a particular piece of legislation being introduced. This overview may be helpful in alerting you to something that you want to study more intensively. Some television programs do discuss issues in depth. These programs usually make an attempt to present both sides of any issue to meet the Federal Communications Commission rules regarding equal time.

Professional journals usually devote some space to current legislative issues. This is done in the "News" section of the *American Journal of Nursing* and in the section entitled "Capital Commentary" in *American Nurse*. When major issues are being discussed, other nursing periodicals frequently contain articles of interest.

Nursing organizations or other health-related organizations may hold open meetings to present and discuss legislative issues. Often knowledgeable speakers are present who can help you to understand what is being proposed and the various potential effects.

Newsletters or journals of organizations that have a political focus provide information on what they see as current issues. These include consumer groups such as Common Cause, political groups such as Young Democrats and Young Republicans, and nonpartisan groups such as the League of Women Voters.

Copies of legislation are usually available through your congressional representatives (for federal matters) or your state representatives (for state matters). Along with copies of the legislation you may receive other informational material from a legislator. Government agencies affected by proposed legislation may also provide information about its potential effect.

Each source of information is valuable to you but should be weighed in terms of its known biases. Even the most objective-sounding report may be as greatly shaded with meaning by what is not reported as by what is reported. Considering what groups support and what groups oppose a particular viewpoint may help in identifying bias. Speculate whether the group and its members would tend personally to gain or lose by the passage of proposed legislation. Are there special interest groups voicing an opinion? When biases are very evident, be sure to also obtain information from those with divergent points of view. Decision making needs to rest on a firm factual basis.

Once you are informed about the current issues in legislation, you are better prepared to form a personal opinion about them and to try to influence the outcome of the political process. There are many ways you can affect that process.

Voting

Your individual vote on a ballot issue is significant. One of the unfortunate statistics in the United States is the low percentage of those eligible who are registered and vote. Although you cannot vote directly on most legislative issues, you can vote for candidates whose position you support.

It is a common practice to disparage the importance of the individual vote in any election. Recent major elections in this country have demonstrated again how important those votes can be. Recounts were necessary in several elections because the margin between the two candidates was only a few hundred votes out of the thousands cast. Absentee ballots are always available for those who cannot be present at their polling place on the day of the election. These must be requested well in advance of the election, however. Even one-sided votes with overwhelming support for or against one candidate or issue may strongly emphasize the position of the voting public, and thereby affect subsequent legislative and governmental decisions.

Shaping Public Opinion

Public opinion does influence the actions of legislators and regulatory bodies. You may help to shape that public opinion. As a registered nurse, your opinion about matters that affect health care will be significant as others make their own decisions. Share the knowledge you have gained while you research an issue. Don't be afraid to state your own opinion, although you must be prepared with evidence to support that opinion to be seen as a thoughtful health care professional. This does not mean that you must become an orator on every social occasion, but that you should use opportunities that arise to present your concerns to others.

Communicating with Legislators and Officials

Legislators are affected by the views of their constituents. Letters received usually are reviewed by the legislator's staff; views are tabu-

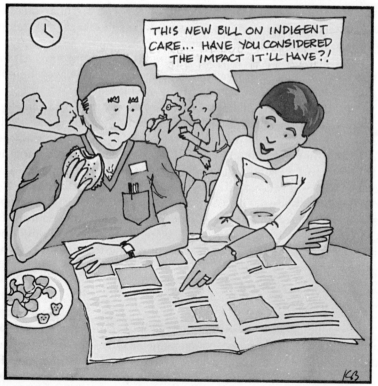

Figure 10–1. Sharing your opinions is one avenue of political involvement.

lated, and letters with significant opinions or information are directed to the legislator for individual consideration. Form letters and post-cards receive the least attention from a legislator. A carefully written personal letter that reflects thoughtful and informed opinion on an issue that that person is competent to evaluate receives the most attention. As a registered nurse you have expertise in an aspect of health care that can provide a valuable viewpoint. Legislators often appreciate personal anecdotes from your practice (with identities concealed, of course) that underscore your point.

Concern regarding rules and regulations of a specific department of government can be addressed to officials of that department. It is possible for officials to become insulated from the effects of their decision making. Communication from concerned citizens is important to them as well as to legislators. Letters to officials should reflect the same careful professional view as letters to legislators do to be most effective in influencing regulations (see Figs. 10–2 and Fig 10–3).

Telephone calls cannot usually be made directly to a legislator, but can be made to the legislator's office. Staff keep a record of all calls and the positions of callers. In some states a toll-free number is maintained for calls to legislators during the legislative session.

Telegrams are delivered by telephone within 5 hours of being sent. A mailgram is a less expensive type of telegram that is delivered in the regular mail on the next business day after you send it.

Visits to congressional or state representatives may also be an effective means of expressing your concerns. Appointments should always be made well in advance, or the person may not have time to speak with you. If your time is circumscribed (such as a limited visit to Washington, D.C.), you may have to modify your expectations and meet with a staff member who will relay your concerns. Plan carefully for a visit. It is often helpful to write out concerns and questions. Be sure to leave time for answers to the questions that you pose. Even when you disagree with the position taken by your legislator, be polite and present your concerns calmly. Rudeness will result in an unwillingness to listen to what you have to say.

Group Action

The political process within the nursing profession takes many forms. On one level it is the involvement of nurses in legislative and ballot issues. Nurses can be involved as individuals, but they have far more effectiveness when they work in groups. As the largest single

(Text continues on p. 316)

HOW TO WRITE YOUR CONGRESSMAN

How to learn their names . . .

Call your public library, local newspaper, or chapter of the League of Women Voters to learn the names and addresses of your U. S. senators, your representative to congress, your state senator(s), and your state representative(s), (called assemblyman in California, New Jersey, New York, and Wisconsin; delegate in Virginia and West Virginia).

How to obtain a copy of a bill

For a Senate bill, write or visit (no telephone requests filled) the Senate Documents Office, Washington, DC 20510; for a House bill, write or visit the Doorkeeper of the House, U. S. Capitol, Washington, DC 20515.

Ask for the bill by number and enclose a self-addressed and gummed label for fastest service. There is no charge.

Requests are normally filled the day received, unless the bill is out of print, and sent via first class mail. There is a limit of six items per day per person, and of three copies of one bill per person (or of one copy per bill if the bill is 60 pages or longer).

Request a copy of a state bill from the appropriate state legislator.

Copies of hearing record can be requested from the committee conducting the hearing, although they usually are not ready for distribution until several weeks after the hearing.

An alternate to the above procedures, for federal bills and hearing records, is to request a copy from your appropriate senator or representative.

(Reprinted by permission of the N.A.A.C.O.G.)

Fundamentals:

1. Address your letter properly: "Hon. _____, House Office Building, Washington, DC 20515", or "Senator _____, Senate Office Building, Washington, DC 20510".
2. Identify the bill or issue. Try to give the bill number or describe it by popular title.
3. Watch your timing. Inform your congressman while there is still time to take effective action.

Write to the right persons:

Concentrate on your own delegation. The representative of your district and the senators of your state cast your votes in the Congress and want to know your views.

Be brief:

Be reasonably brief. Your views and arguments stand a better chance of being read if they are stated as concisely as the subject matter will permit. It is not necessary that letters be typed — only that they be legible — and the form, phraseology, and grammar are not important.

Do:

1. Write your own views — not someone else's. A personal letter is far better than a form letter or signature on a petition. Form letters often receive form replies.
2. Give your reasons for taking a stand. The effects of a bill on a certain constituency will be far more helpful.
3. Be constructive. If a bill deals with a problem, but you believe the bill is the wrong approach, outline the correct approach. If you have expert knowledge, share it with your congressman.
4. Say 'well done' when it is deserved. Congressmen appreciate this from people who believe they have done the right thing.

Do not:

1. Don't make threats or promises.
2. Don't berate your congressman. If you disagree with him, give reasons for your disagreement.
3. Don't become a 'pen pal'. Quality is more important than quantity.
4. Don't demand a commitment before the facts are in. A bill rarely becomes law in the same form as introduced, it is possible for a writer to change his or her position once a bill reaches a floor.

The above material, excerpted from *Congressional Record, Nov. 2, 1977.* by Morris K. Udall, was prepared by the Washington office of The American College of Obstetricians and Gynecologists.

Figure 10-2.

HOUSE

HOUSE	CONSTITUENT	SENATE
Representative introduces bill. Clerk of the House refers it to appropriate committee.	Start with your letter writing campaign urging representatives and senators to cosponsor the legislation.	Senator introduces bill. Clerk of the Senate refers it to appropriate committee.
Committee chair refers bill to a subcommittee which holds hearings to examine arguments for or against the bill.	Write to each subcommittee member. Place special emphasis on members from your state.	Committee chair refers it to a subcommittee which holds hearings to examine arguments for or against the bill.
Subcommittee holds a 'mark-up' session to discuss and vote on the bill. A majority vote in favor moves the bill to full committee.	Request that your local paper print an article you've written. Meet with the paper's editorial board to urge its support.	Subcommittee holds a 'mark-up' session to discuss and vote on the bill. A majority vote in favor moves the bill to full committee.
Full committee reviews subcommittee hearing record and may hold additional hearings. A mark-up session is held and if the bill is approved it is reported to the full House.	Meet with your representative and senators in their home district offices. Send a copy of your paper's editorial to every member of the full committee.	Full committee reviews subcommittee record and may hold additional hearings. A mark-up session is held and if the bill is approved it is reported to the full Senate.

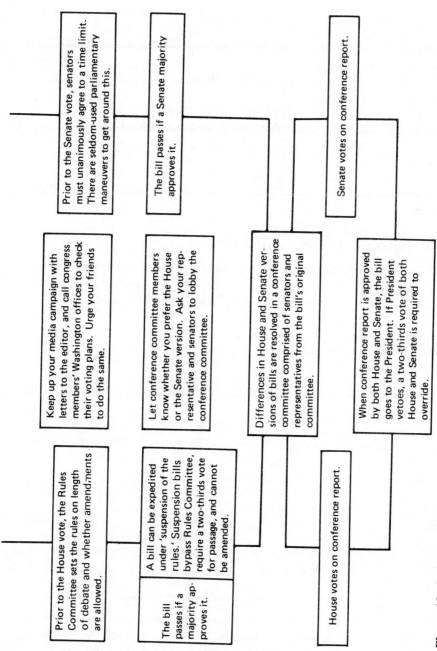

Figure 10–3. How a bill becomes a law.

Prior to the Senate vote, senators must unanimously agree to a time limit. There are seldom-used parliamentary maneuvers to get around this.

The bill passes if a Senate majority approves it.

Senate votes on conference report.

Keep up your media campaign with letters to the editor, and call congress members' Washington offices to check their voting plans. Urge your friends to do the same.

Let conference committee members know whether you prefer the House or the Senate version. Ask your representative and senators to lobby the conference committee.

Differences in House and Senate versions of bills are resolved in a conference committee comprised of senators and representatives from the bill's original committee.

When conference report is approved by both House and Senate, the bill goes to the President. If President vetoes, a two-thirds vote of both House and Senate is required to override.

Prior to the House vote, the Rules Committee sets the rules on length of debate and whether amendments are allowed.

A bill can be expedited under 'suspension of the rules.' Suspension bills bypass Rules Committee, require a two-thirds vote for passage, and cannot be amended.

The bill passes if a majority approves it.

House votes on conference report.

health care occupation, nurses have many votes, which is important to elected officials. In addition, although nurses do not have high incomes, when gathered together their financial contributions can be significant to a candidate or issue.

Most traditional nursing organizations are nonprofit groups, and therefore are limited in their political activity. The major role of these groups in politics is testifying as to facts and concerns within the health care area. The American Nurses' Association (ANA) has an office in the nation's capitol and tries to keep the nursing profession informed about legislative matters of importance to health care. The ANA also provides experts in the field of nursing to testify about proposed legislation. Most state and district nurses' associations have legislative committees that serve this function in their area.

Political Action Committees

To take a more active role in seeking passage of desired legislation and defeat of undesired measures, nurses have formed organizations called *political action committees*. These organizations are registered as political action groups, and thus have more freedom in the political arena. The American Nurses' Association Political Action Committee (ANA-PAC) is a political action organization. It actually lobbies for the passage or defeat of bills and can support candidates for public office. Since the 1976 general elections, ANA-PAC has raised funds that were used to support candidates for the Senate and the House of Representatives. Candidates were chosen for support based on their expressed and demonstrated stands on key health issues, such as national health insurance, funding for biomedical research, extension and funding of the Nurse Training Act, and third-party reimbursement for nurses. Not all endorsed candidates were supported financially owing to the limitations of the funds available. In 1984, 90% of the candidates endorsed by ANA-PAC were elected (*American Nurse,* January 1987).[1] The candidates' successes were attributable to many factors in addition to the support of ANA-PAC, but the effect of nursing support has been demonstrated.

The Nurses' Coalition for Legislative Action is an organization of 28 specialty nursing organizations that works on behalf of those organizations at the federal level. The Tri-Council is a coalition of the ANA, the National League for Nursing, and the American Association of Colleges of Nursing that also functions at the federal level. Both of these organizations provide expert testimony for committees and commissions that are considering health related legislation.

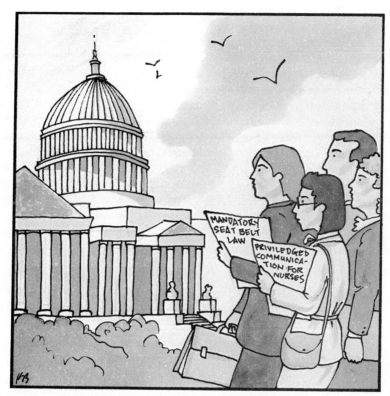

Figure 10–4. Nurses may lobby to get desired legislation passed by visiting legislators, by presenting information and arguments about the bill, and by writing letters.

Many states have political action organizations composed of nurses. In addition to these specific nursing groups for lobbying, there are more general lobbying groups with this focus, such as Common Cause (a consumer lobbying group), the League of Women Voters, and even church organizations. You may support these groups by simply donating money for their needs or by active involvement in the activities and the work of the group.

Although growth in size of these political action groups has not been rapid, it has been steady. In addition, nurses are gaining more sophistication in the political process. Both of these factors result in nurses' gaining increased power. There is still a long way to go before nurses have the same kind of power as that wielded by such groups as labor, education, and medicine, but change is occurring.

Testifying for Decision-Making Bodies

Many decisions relative to health care in general and to nursing are made by committees and commissions of the various levels of government. They frequently have hearings to gather information before decisions are made. As a nurse your testimony may have particular value when certain areas of health care are being considered. A nurse may testify as either an official representative of an organization or an independent individual. If you have an opportunity to testify, be sure to make your position clear so the decision makers know whether you speak for yourself or for a larger group. Prepare your testimony ahead of time, but try not to just read a statement. A less formal presentation is usually more interesting for the listener. Be prepared with sources for any facts and figures you present, and explain any technical terms you use. Most committees will accept written testimony if you cannot be there in person, but the personal presentation is usually more effective.

Individual Support for Legislation and Candidates

As an individual you may choose to support a specific piece of legislation by contributing money for publicity and campaigning or by personally working on a committee that is striving for passage of the proposal. Funds are needed for printing and distributing literature, newspaper ads, and television and radio announcements. Workers may be needed for secretarial tasks, to contact people in a door-to-door campaign, and to speak on behalf of the issue.

Supporting a candidate for public office is done in the same way. In our political system the reality is that those who have actively supported a candidate during an election campaign are listened to more closely when decisions are made. Working for a candidate is one way to make your view known.

Limitations on Your Political Activity

If you are an employee of any governmental agency, such as a public health department or the Veteran's Administration, there are restrictions on your political activity that do not apply to the general public. For the federal government, these restrictions are defined in the Hatch Act. The main focus of prohibited activities are those that have to do with supporting a particular political party by being an officer or party spokesperson. The Hatch Act also prohibits any activities on behalf of a party or in support of legislation that could be construed as providing support from the agency that employs you. This act does not interfere with your rights as a private citizen to support parties and candidates financially, to join political parties, to work for or against measures that will appear on a ballot, or to participate in nonpartisan (*i.e.,* not connected with a political party) elections as a candidate. Each state has its own version of the Hatch Act. If you are employed by a governmental agency of any kind, you should investigate the limitations that it may place on your political activity.

The Federal Government's Role in Health Care

The federal government operates in the health care field in a complex way. There are literally dozens of agencies, some with similar titles, and sometimes identifying which agency is responsible in which area is difficult. The following overview may help you to place some agencies in context.

Department of Health and Human Services

The Department of Health and Human Services (DHHS) is a cabinet-level administrative unit of the federal government. It was originally created in 1953 as the Department of Health, Education, and Welfare. The date of its origin points out how recent has been the view that the federal government should have a major responsibility in health care, and that this area was the equal of such aspects as defense. In 1980 a separate department was created for education and the remaining functions were retitled Health and Human Services. There are four major service divisions of DHHS (Table 10–1).

Office of Human Development Services. The Office of Human Development Services is responsible for four sections. The activities of these sections are primarily in the health prevention and welfare field.

Public Health Service. The Public Health Service encompasses all the activities relating to illness, disease states, and treatment. The sections of this division are much more obviously related to nursing concerns. The *Centers for Disease Control* maintain all statistics relevant to the epidemiology of various disease processes. Research is supported and recommendations are made for the control of communicable diseases both in the institution and in the community.

The *Food and Drug Administration* (FDA) regulates the use of medications and devices for both prevention and treatment of disease. It also sets standards for food labeling and for what may be added to foods.

Table 10 – 1. **Major Service Divisions of the Department of Health and Human Services**

Office of Human Development Services	*Social Security Administration*
Administration on Aging	Systems
Administration for Children, Youth, and Families	Governmental Affairs
	Family Assistance
Administration for Native Americans	Hearings and Appeals
Administration for Public Service	Operational Policy and Procedure Assessment

Public Health Service	*Health Care Financing*
Centers for Disease Control	Health Standards and Quality Bureau
Food and Drug Administration	Bureau of Quality Control
Health Resources Administration	Bureau of Program Operations
Health Services Administration	Bureau of Program Policy
National Institutes of Health	Bureau of Support Services
Alcohol, Drug Abuse, and Mental Health Administration	Office of Child Support Enforcement

The FDA also sets standards for allowable radiation and establishes rules regarding milk and shellfish sanitation, restaurant operation, and interstate travel facilities.

The *Health Resources Administration* is concerned with planning for the agencies and personnel to provide health care in the community. One aspect of this planning is planning for nursing, which is done through a Division of Nursing. Because the responsibility for all research endeavors has been transferred to the Center for Nursing Research in the National Institutes of Health, the Division of Nursing has a much more restricted budget. Recent legislation has eliminated many of the other programs that the Division used to administer, such as construction grants for schools of nursing and individual assistance for students at all levels of nursing education. There is concern in some circles of nursing that the Division of Nursing will lose much of the influence it has had.

The *Health Services Administration* provides leadership to communities in providing health care and provides direct health care to specific groups (*e.g.*, native Americans, migrants, mothers and children). The

Health Services Administration is an area that has received drastic cuts in funding as the federal government strives to transfer responsibility to local and state governments.

The *National Institutes of Health* (NIH) are agencies established for research and treatment of specific health problems. There are institutes for heart, lung, and blood problems, arthritis, metabolism and digestive disorders, allergy and infectious disease, neurological and communicative disorders and stroke, and many other areas of concern. It is within this agency that the National Library of Medicine operates as an agency to provide support for research activities.

The role of the *Alcohol, Drug Abuse, and Mental Health Administration* is to provide research and treatment for these problems. Public education is an important part of its function.

Health Care Financing. The Health Care Financing division administers the Medicare and Medicaid programs. As part of this responsibility it establishes policies and procedures for care providers and recipients. This division is charged with the responsibility of researching health care costs and methods of containing those costs. The Health Care Financing division also provides assistance to the states in their programs to provide health care to the needy.

Social Security Administration. The Social Security Administration oversees all of the funds that are dispensed under the Social Security Act. It provides a mechanism for establishing eligibility and dispensing funds, and furnishes an appeal system.

Center for Nursing Research

In the fall of 1985, against great administrative opposition, including a presidential veto by President Reagan, legislative supporters of nursing succeeded in establishing a Center for Nursing Research within the NIH. All research support was to be transferred from the Division of Nursing to this new center, and additional funds were authorized for start-up, organization, and research grants. Although the budget for nursing research is still just a fraction of the budgets of the other institutes within the NIH, a great many nurses think that this is a significant move toward putting nursing in the mainstream of research.[2] Some nursing leaders have expressed concern that nursing will lose autonomy and control in this new environment that is dominated by other disciplines.[3] There is no disagreement that nursing needs increased support of its research activities as it strives to establish a broader knowledge base for nursing practice.

LEGISLATION OF SIGNIFICANCE

In recent years many pieces of legislation have been passed that have critically affected nursing. These legislative acts are not static, however. They are constantly being changed and revised in light of current concerns. A few significant ones are presented here.

For each of these legislative acts the money actually received from the federal government depends on two separate legislative actions. The first is the authorization act. This outlines the rules under which funds can be expended and sets a ceiling on the amount of money that can be provided. The second action is the appropriations process. In this process the federal budget is determined and specific amounts of money are appropriated for actual spending. The amount appropriated cannot be more than the amount authorized, but it can be, and frequently is, less. Sometimes this is confusing because two monetary amounts may be reported in regard to the same act. Historically, a third factor has affected the amount of money available under a specific legislative act. The executive branch makes decisions about how and when funds that are available will be spent. If money that has been authorized and appropriated has not been spent by the end of the budget period, the funds must be reauthorized and reappropriated.

Nurse Training Act

The Nurse Training Act of 1964 (Title VII of the Public Health Service Act) was a significant factor in the growth of nursing education. It provided for financial assistance to schools of nursing and to students in those schools for 2 years and was renewed in 1966 for 2 additional years. In 1968 financial assistance to schools and students was continued under Title II of the Health Manpower Act. In 1971 federal aid to nursing education was again expanded. Moneys for constructing schools of nursing and for aiding the educational program were provided. Many of you have been educated in buildings or practice laboratories whose construction was funded under this act. Individual financial aid to students was also provided. A large number of your instructors may have had their graduate education made possible by this funding.

Although nurses think that the moneys were well used in a responsible manner, continued funding was not automatic. In 1973 and 1974 the Nixon administration made a concerted effort to curtail money spent on nursing education as well as on other health-related endeavors. Later both the Ford and the Carter administrations proposed drastic cuts in nurse training money. Nursing organizations fought long and hard through testimony and through providing public information to achieve passage of the new Nurse Training Act legislation. This was finally accomplished, although there were many compromises over what nurses had originally wanted to see passed. Many of you may have received individual financial assistance from money provided through this act. Schools have continued to receive financial support for programs.

A new version of the Nurse Training Act was passed in 1979 as Public Law 96 – 97. In addition to support for nursing students, nursing schools, and nursing research, this bill provided for an independent study of nursing personnel needs. The total amount of money appropriated was less than previous acts had provided. These funds are discussed more completely in Chapter 3.

Funds currently appropriated through the Nurse Training Act are limited. They provide for some advanced educational support and support for a few specific programs. Each year nurses have supported legislation to reinstitute the Nurse Training Act. Although there has been consistent support from some legislators, it has not been enough to alter the situation. Table 10 – 2 shows an overview of the Nurse Training Act and its provisions.

Medicare and Medicaid

In 1965, after years of effort and testimony by many health-related groups, (including the ANA) and with widespread public support, an amendment of the Social Security Act was passed. Title XVIII of the act, which has termed Medicare, provided for payment for hospitalization and for the purchase of insurance for meeting physicians' fees for people over age 65. Title IX of the act, which was termed Medicaid, provided funds for health care for the dependent population. Medicare and Medicaid have supplied an important health care resource but have not been without problems. Costs have been much larger and have risen faster than anticipated. There has been a great deal of publicity over instances of abuse and even fraud that have occurred in connection with these two programs.

The bill contained many provisions that have been significant for nursing. A definition of skilled nursing care in the original bill was

Table 10–2. **Federal Funding for Nursing Education Through The Nurse Education Act (in millions of dollars)**

Year	Authorization	Appropriation
1965	17.1	16.4
1966	42.9	37.5
1967	68.8	61.5
1968	80.3	61.9
1969	88.9	40.1
1970	95.0	49.0
1971	115.0	64.0
1972	201.5	122.8
1973	227.0	122.7
1974	254.5	150.3
1975	254.5	116.7
1976	161.0	127.5
1977	186.0	118.0
1978	206.0	119.5
1979	105.5	100.3
1980	103.0	100.3
1981	103.0	74.3
1982	103.0	46.4
1983	103.0	42.8
1984	70.8	42.3
1985	70.8	50.3
1986	54.1	—
1987	55.35	—
1988	56.6	—

Authorization figures: 1965–1981 from Kalish and Kalish, 1982.[4]
1982–1985 from Soloman, 1985b.[5]
1986–1988 from Nurses' Coalition for Legislative Action, Correspondence, 1985.[6]
Appropriation figures: 1965–1983 from Crosby, Facteau, and Donley, 1983.[7]
1984   from FY 1984, Dec. 1983.[6]
1985   from Solomon, 1984b.[8]

narrow and excluded many of the elderly who needed care in nursing homes. According to the bill, skilled nursing care was defined as requiring continuous, 24-hour care, including procedures administered by a person who has received skilled training and has a license to perform the care required. The care had to be diagnostic, curative, stabilizing, or rehabilitative. It could not be maintenance or terminal care, which are considered custodial and outside the scope of the covered situations. Nurses have felt that this definition eliminated from coverage many people who needed skilled care in maintenance, custodial, or terminal situations.

Through later efforts and testimony, the ANA was instrumental in getting the legislators to recognize that the definition of skilled nursing was a critical matter, and through a Senate subcommittee the ANA was asked to study skilled nursing care to provide background data for the Senate. Amendments to the Medicare – Medicaid Act of 1972 encouraged increased study of alternative ways of providing health care to contain costs. These alternatives included innovation in the use of nurses in expanded roles as well as the use of health maintenance organizations.

Amendments to this act were also responsible for mandating review and evaluation of health care. This was done in the interests of cost

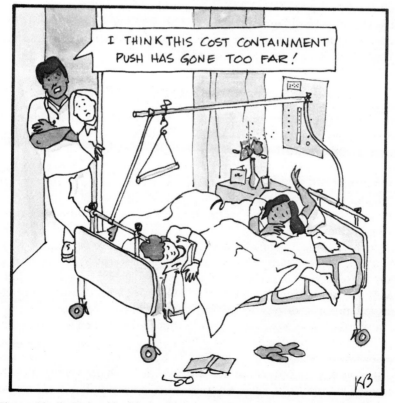

Figure 10–5. Federal legislation is encouraging hospitals to stop the rapid rise of health care costs.

containment. Within institutions, records of Medicare–Medicaid patients must be reviewed and compared with specific criteria for care.

In 1982 Medicare was revised by the 97th Congress to prevent the predicted bankruptcy of the system owing to rapidly escalating costs. The premium for Part B of Medicare (the optional portion that provides for out-of-hospital care) and the deductible that the individual must pay for covered service were increased. The system of payment was changed to prospective payment based on diagnosis-related groups. Many items that were previously funded separately were now included in the one prospective rate. A mechanism for reimbursing hospice care was included. There is still separate support for medical education and nursing education programs that are under the control of the hospital in which they occur, and this is meant to compensate for additional costs related to the teaching responsibilities of and the services rendered by those in such programs. Although the largest share of this fund is for residency programs for physicians, significant support has been available for nursing diploma programs. This funding source for nursing education programs in hospitals is in jeopardy, as increased efforts are being made to cut Medicare costs even further.

Evaluation of Health Services: Peer Review

The first provision for the systematic evaluation of health care services provided to the consumer was established through the Professional Standards Review Organization and utilization review set up by Medicare and Medicaid. As part of the 1982 revisions of Medicare, the evaluation process was altered. Hospitals are now required to contract with an external medical review organization, called a Utilization and Quality Control Peer Review Organization (abbreviated PRO). These organizations are established through contracts awarded by the secretary of health and human services through competitive bidding. Most of the PROs are statewide in scope and are required to have a substantial number of physicians represented in the organization in order to effectively set standards and review care. Evaluation may consist of preadmission, preprocedure, concurrent, or retrospective reviews. The purpose of the reviews is to determine whether the care given was necessary and whether it was given in the appropriate manner. For example, the reviews have resulted in an increase in the number of surgeries performed as day procedures on outpatients rather than as inpatient surgeries. This results in a significant economic saving. The PRO is also required to evaluate outcomes of care to assure that the changes that are made do not jeopardize clients.

Maternal Child Health Act, Title V

The Maternal Child Health Act was planned to improve health in the nation through benefits such as nutritional support, health supervision, and well-child care to mothers and children. Part of the money appropriated was earmarked for nursing research projects and nursing research training. Nurses who provide care are directly affected in their practice because the provisions of the act outline what care is funded and to whom that care can be provided.

Occupational Safety and Health Act

There has been a great deal of controversy over the provisions of Occupational Safety and Health Act (OSHA), which is designed to improve the safety of the working environment. The act specifies safety devices that must be present, such as goggles, showers, and eye washes, in areas where caustic chemicals are used. Other examples of safety regulations that have been developed under OSHA are safety switches required on machinery to prevent accidental engagement of gears during repair, and standards set for air purity and availability of masks and respirators in the working area. Many people think that the rules and regulations created by this act are too extensive and cumbersome. For example, the rules regarding ladder safety are extremely detailed and cover several pages. When one considers the enormous number of different pieces of equipment and envisions the quantity of regulations that exist to cover all these items, it is apparent that it would be almost impossible for any one person to know all the applicable regulations.

Nevertheless, the concern for the safety of the working person is of real importance to nurses. Occupational injuries are a major health problem in the adult population. They are costly not only in terms of health and personal loss, but also in terms of lost productivity for the employer. Nurses are affected by the provisions of this act in their work environments. They, too, are subject to injury and accident on the job.

A major concern in nursing is the high incidence of back injuries suffered by direct care personnel. Another, more recent concern is the potential hazard of the many toxic drugs, such as chemotherapeutic agents, that health care personnel may handle. Hospitals are being required to set up procedures for handling and disposing of such agents in a way that will protect staff at all levels.

Nurses in occupational health nursing are involved in another way. They may be part of the program for educating workers about job safety. In some situations safety precautions are time-consuming and uncomfortable, and workers may be tempted to ignore them. Nurses may be able to help workers understand the importance of following health and safety regulations. Occupational health nurses also work with management in planning to make the environment safer and in establishing appropriate procedures of caring for injuries.

Health Planning and Resources Development Act

In an attempt to provide coordinated community planning that would prevent duplication of costly services and the absence of necessary but unprofitable services, the Comprehensive Health Planning and Resources Development Act of 1974 was passed. Through a variety of organizations and agencies and supported by federal funds, communitywide and statewide planning occurred. Since that time the federal funds have not been appropriated to support these planning activities. In some states planning has continued with state and local support. Thus the federal legislation provided the initial direction and support for a needed service. In other areas planning has come to a standstill. Although some people oppose planning and would rather rely on the marketplace to control the availability of services, others would prefer a planning approach but find it impossible to fund such an approach in the current economic climate.

Other Significant Legislation

You may want to investigate other federal legislation and evaluate its impact on health care in general and nursing in particular. The Health Maintenance Organization Act of 1973 was passed to promote the development of prepaid health plans with a focus on health maintenance as well as illness care. Although health maintenance organizations have been in existence in the United States for many years, their growth was slow in many areas of the country owing to organizational and funding difficulties and, in some instances, state laws that hampered their growth. It was hoped that this would support the growth of the kind of comprehensive health care that is the focus of health maintenance organizations.

The Emergency Medical Services Systems Act of 1973 was funded to assist communities with the development of more effective systems to handle medical emergencies.

In 1983 an "orphan drug" bill was passed and signed into law. The purpose of this bill was to support and encourage the production of drugs that would be of benefit to only a limited number of people and therefore might not be financially feasible without some kind of outside support.

PROSPECTIVE LEGISLATION THAT WILL AFFECT NURSING

Each year many issues that affect nursing come before the House and the Senate. There are more issues that have never been resolved, and others are attempts to continue (or discontinue) previous provisions related to health care.

National Health Insurance

The United States is the only major industrialized country that does not have some type of government-sponsored health care for all citizens. Opinions are sharply divided over whether or not this is desirable. Public opinion appears to be moving toward support of some type of nationwide health care plan. Costs of hospital and medical care have risen much more rapidly than the general rate of inflation. Part of this rise is due to advances in treatment that require expensive equipment, laboratory work, and intensive care. People are also beginning to look at health care as a right rather than as a privilege available only to those who can afford it.

Through Medicare and Medicaid and the widespread effects of the military, public health, and Indian health systems, the federal government is already deeply involved in the provision of health care. How much greater that involvement should be is the subject of serious debate.

One factor that is creating more support for some type of statewide or national health plan is the increasing amount of uncompensated care being provided by some of the nation's health care facilities. When people are unemployed or underemployed they often do not have health insurance. These same people are often not eligible for public assistance for health care. When they have major health care needs, bills simply remain unpaid. Hospitals historically have absorbed these costs through spreading them out to those who do pay their bills. As insurance companies and the government become more stringent about reimbursement, this is becoming increasingly difficult and some hospitals will be in serious financial trouble if some method of assisting with this problem is not found soon.

A bill passed by the House of Representatives provides coverage of catastrophic medical costs for those on Medicare.[9] This coverage would begin after more conventional insurance runs out, to care for those whose care runs into the hundreds of thousands of dollars and bankrupts even middle-class families. This bill, however, still does not speak to the needs of those who are not covered by Medicare and who are unable to purchase conventional health insurance coverage. Even with only Medicare coverage, this bill still has many obstacles to pass before its provisions become reality.

Because the federal government has not acted, many states are beginning to look at the problem from a state perspective. Some questions that are being raised are, Is there a right to health care? If there is a right, what level of health care does this cover, *i.e.*, routine preventive services, surgery and hospitalization for all conditions, or only for serious life-threatening conditions, catastrophic conditions only, transplants and experimental treatments? These are difficult philosophical and ethical questions and there are no simple answers.

Reimbursement of Nursing Services

One key concern of nurses is whether nursing care will be directly reimbursed. This has been of special concern to primary health care nurses. The availability of funding for the care to be provided by nurses will, to a great extent, determine whether the public is able to use such services. Physicians (through the American Medical Association) have consistently supported provisions that would result in direct payment only to physicians or for care ordered by physicians. Other organizations of direct-care providers, social workers, nurses, psychologists, and so forth are seeking greater breadth in reimbursement possibilities. Third-party payment funds a large percentage of the health care in the United States, and if this avenue of funding is closed to nurses and other direct-care providers, then their ability to provide services is severely curtailed. Physicians believe that controlling access to third-party payment will control costs of health care. This limitation also preserves for the physician a unique position of power in the health care setting.

Labor Law Reform

Many nurses supported a bill to modify the National Labor Relations Act (see Chapter 9). This act would change procedures of the National Labor Relations Board (NLRB) and add measures that may be taken if either side in a labor negotiation violates the law. This law would provide that labor representatives be given equal time to talk with employees on the employer's premises if the employer has used work time to address employees in regard to issues. The bill also contains provisions that would help to lessen the delay between appeal to the NLRB and the time the case is heard.

Opponents of the legislation believed that it unfairly required the employer to support the efforts of the labor organization. They also believed that it changed the balance of power in favor of labor organizations, to the detriment of employers. Proponents feel that these changes are needed to effectively achieve a balance of power and to prevent violations of the labor laws. Whatever the outcome, labor laws are of significance to nurses as they become increasingly involved in the negotiation process.

Equal Rights Amendment

The Equal Rights Amendment (ERA) has provoked some of the most heated debates of any issue in recent years. The proposed amendment simply states that "rights provided under the Constitution shall not be abridged on account of sex." A further statement enables the legislature to enact laws as necessary to support this. Because the vast majority of nurses are women, this amendment would seem to have special significance in the field of nursing. The ANA and the National League for Nursing have strongly supported its passage.

Individual nurses do have varying viewpoints. Some see the ERA as crucial to professional recognition and advancement. They cite the historically low salaries of nurses and other women in the health care field and the lack of power that the nursing profession has had in health care as reflections of the status of women in our society. They believe that legal recognition of the rights of women will support efforts within nursing to achieve acknowledgement as a profession and will assist nurses in righting such historical wrongs as the relative salary gap. Concern also is expressed for the mental health of women. Strong arguments have pointed out that the position of women in society creates problems in mental health and in the way women are treated as clients in the health care system.

Other nurses oppose the passage of the ERA for a variety of reasons that seem to center on what they believe will be negative consequences for society if it is passed. Some think that passage of the ERA will further disrupt family life, which will be detrimental to the health and well-being of children as well as of women.

Most polls indicate that an actual majority of people in the United States favored the ERA. The system of ratification gives equal status to states with lesser populations and provides for ratification through state legislatures rather than by popular vote. This is designed to make the passage of a constitutional amendment a difficult process and made the ERA fail despite popular support. Although ratification of the ERA failed, the idea of having a constitutional amendment to guarantee equal rights has not been abandoned. Supporters have changed their strategy and attempts have been made to legislate equality in ways other than through a constitutional amendment.

STATE-LEVEL LEGISLATIVE CONCERNS

Many issues that vitally affect the health care area are decided at the state level. Because issues in each state differ, we will outline some general areas of concern.

State Institutions' Budget and Planning

Types of state institutions range from those for the care of the mentally retarded and the mentally ill to penal systems and institutions of higher education. Health care is often a consideration in all of these settings. When budgets are planned, such diverse concerns as immunization and contraception may be included or omitted from the planning. Nurses often can be a voice for those who are unable to speak for themselves in regard to their own health care needs. Sometimes nurses who work in these settings are unable to deliver quality care because of severe budgetary deficiencies. All nurses can support efforts to provide quality health care in such settings.

Nurse Practice Acts

Nurse practice acts are being discussed and revised in many states. The process is long and difficult, and requires intense effort on the part of nurses. Once a bill that has been carefully developed has been submitted to the legislative body, nurses must remain alert to changes and amendments that may substantially alter the intent of the original proposal. The bill must be followed through the legislative process until its passage.

LOCAL POLITICAL CONCERNS

The budgetary process always seems to be at the base of any political or legislative concern. Because there is a limited amount of money available, budgets are always developed with a series of compromises. To gain one objective it is sometimes necessary to recognize that there will be no funds for another. In most communities budgets for public health departments, school nurses, and so forth are developed over a period of several months. Hearings are often held, at which members of the public may ask questions and address the issues. Nurses have often found that involvement at this planning stage is most rewarding. Determining priorities for health is essential, and nurses often can speak with authority on these matters. Nurses actually employed in the department under consideration may be much more limited in making their views known because of regulations governing their action in the political sphere. For this reason it is significant that other nurses recognize the importance of community health. It is not only the practice of the public health nurse that is affected by the priorities of the agency. For example, the nurse who is employed in the hospital may wish to refer a discharged patient to a public health nurse for follow-up, only to find that, owing to changes in the ordering of priorities, home visits for the identified purpose are no longer being made.

In many communities, decisions about the allocation of federal money are made at the local level. Support for alternative health care centers, blood pressure screening, and senior citizen centers may depend on whether those who are knowledgeable about the benefits of these services are willing to voice their advocacy.

THE POLITICAL PROCESS WITHIN THE NURSING PROFESSION

Any large group of people that is organized into a body has a political process. All of the earlier discussion about the traditional political process is equally applicable to the politics of the profession.

On an individual level one is seldom able to influence such an organization meaningfully unless one is a member. This may create some conflict within the individual. If you do not agree with all that an organization is doing, the usual course of action is to withhold or withdraw your membership. When you are a member of a profession, you may find that this course of action presents more difficulties. The organization may continue to speak for the profession. If you are outside of the organization, you may find yourself without a voice on significant issues affecting your professional life. By joining a professional organization and actively involving yourself in it, you may be able to make your concerns and viewpoints heard.

If you decide to join a professional organization, you have an obligation to be an informed and concerned member. Your vote on candidates for local, state, and national office is important. Your activity on a committee or as an officer is necessary for the organization to function effectively. You have an obligation to be informed on issues that are before the organization and make your viewpoint known. The concerned involvement of many individual members will make an organization an effective voice for a profession. Chapter 12 describes many organizations related to nursing.

CONCLUSION

Political and legislative issues are an important aspect of planning for health care in our society. The informed and concerned nurse can make a significant contribution to society's health by actions in this arena of life.

REFERENCES

1. ANA-PAC achieves 90% success rate in 1986 elections. Nurse 19:1, 20, Jan 1987
2. Jacox AK: Science and politics: The background and issues surrounding the controversial proposal for a National Institute of Nursing. Nurs Outlook 33:78–84, Mar/Apr, 1985
3. Dumas RG, Felton KG: Should there be a national institute for nursing? Nurs Outlook 32:16–22, Jan/Feb, 1984
4. Kalisch BJ, Kalisch PA: The Politics of Nursing. Philadelphia, JB Lippincott, 1982
5. Solomon S: Nursing's legislative agenda, round one. Nurs Health Care 6:296–298, Jun 1985
6. FY 85 health appropriations. Testimony of the American Nurses' Association to the Labor, Health and Human Services Subcommittee of the House Appropriations Committee. #34–323. Washington, DC U.S. Government Printing Office
7. Crosby L, Facteau L, Donley R: Priorities for nurse training act legislation: A national survey of nursing deans. Image 15:107–110, Fall 1983
8. Solomon S: Update: Nursing education funds, NIN, DRGs and education. Nurs Health Care 5:302–303, Jun 1984
9. Morrissey KL: Congress turns attention to nursing agenda. Nurs and Health Care 8(7):378–379, Sep 1987

FURTHER READINGS

Althouse HL: How O.S.H.A. affects hospitals and nursing homes. Am J Nurs 75:450–453, Mar 1975

The American Nurse. American Nurses Association, monthly newspaper

Archer H: From bill to law: The legislative process. Imprint 23:26, Dec 1976

Archer S, Goehner P: Nurses: A Political Force. Belmont, CA, Wadsworth Health Sciences Division, 1982

Archer S, Goehner P: Speaking Out: The Views of Nurse Leaders. New York, National League for Nursing Publication No. 15–1847, 1981

Brown B, Gebbie K, Moore JF: Affecting nursing goals in health care. Nurs Adm Q 2(3):17–31, 1978

Capitol Commentary. Am Nurse (regular column)

Diers D: A different kind of energy: Nurse power. Nurs Outlook 26:51–55, 1978

Dumas RG, Felton G: Should there be a national institute for nursing? Nurs Outlook 32:16–22, Jan/Feb 1984

Hughes E: Learning about politics. Am J Nurs 79:494–495, Mar 1979

Humphrey C et al: The Emergence of Nursing as a Political Force, pp 1–90. New York, National League for Nursing Publication No. 41–1760, 1979

Humphrie S: Legislation. AORN J (regular column)

Jacox AK: Science and politics: The background and issues surrounding the controversial proposal for a National Institute of Nursing. Nurs Outlook 33:78–84, Mar/Apr 1985

Johnson R: Legislative Commentary. Imprint (regular column)

Kalisch B, Kalisch P: Politics of Nursing. Philadelphia, JB Lippincott, 1982

Maraldo P: Politics: A very human matter. Am J Nurs 82:1106–1111, Jul 1982

Also see the official publication of your state nurses' association.

Unit IV
Career Opportunities and Professional Growth

11 | Employment in Health Care

Objectives

After completing this chapter, you should be able to

1. *Discuss societal and educational factors that have caused changes in the abilities of the new graduate.*
2. *Define* **competency** *as it applies to nursing.*
3. *List major areas of competence that are of concern to employers.*
4. *List six consistent expectations of employers of new graduates.*
5. *Identify two areas in which expectations differ widely.*
6. *Discuss ways of coping with expectations.*
7. *Set personal career goals.*
8. *Write a letter of application and a résumé.*
9. *Prepare for an employment interview.*
10. *Discuss the concept of burnout and its relationship to stress.*
11. *Discuss how "comparable worth" relates to nursing compensation.*

After completing an educational program, you, as a new graduate, will want to get out into the real world and practice your nursing skills. In the past such a goal was rather simple and straightforward. Early in the 20th century almost all graduate nurses performed private-duty nursing. The nurse was hired by a patient or family to provide care during a particular episode of illness or disability. Some nurses specialized in maternity cases, in which they cared for new mothers and infants; others specialized in caring for persons with long-term illnesses, such as strokes. The nurse was expected to live at the patient's residence and assume 24-hour responsibility for the patient's care. This might even include preparing special foods for the convalescing patient. Nurses hired as graduate nurses in hospitals usually were head nurses, supervisors, or directors.

CHANGES IN NURSING

By the 1930s the employment situation began to change. More graduate nurses were hired to provide patient care. Employment practices became modernized, and nurses were no longer expected to be on duty for 24 hours a day when engaged in private-duty nursing. Regular work schedules were established in hospitals. Nurses still worked split shifts — morning and evening of the same day with a period in the afternoon off — and there were few employee benefits (paid holidays, vacations, and so forth), but the beginnings of change were there. Most nurses now worked in a hospital or an institution.

World War II had a major impact on nursing. Because women were essential to the war effort, it became acceptable for married women to continue working. Women nurses were valued members of the armed forces and attained elevated status by becoming officers in the military. Nurses in the Army had to learn to be assertive in managing their responsibilities, and many brought this quality back to the hospital. Wanting to be of service to a country at war, women who might never have considered nursing because of its previous status now entered the field.

The expansion of the hospital or institutional job market for nurses was also influenced by population growth; advances in medicine, with more surgeries being performed and special care required that was available only in a hospital; and the dramatic increase in the number of hospitals.

The noninstitutional job market also grew. Since the early 1900s, when Lillian Wald established a visiting nurse service, community health nursing has continued to develop. Nurses were pioneers in bringing health care to people's homes and in focusing on prevention of illness through consumer education.

Other areas of nursing in the community began to widen as well. More nurses were working in industry. Conditions for workers improved and action regarding their health became part of law, custom, or contract. Nurses also worked in school districts, and the field of school nursing started to expand.

Nurses began to provide primary health care. *Primary care* is that segment of health care that furnishes both the initial contact with the health care system and the longitudinal supervision of health care needs. Perhaps the first primary health care was provided by the nurse midwives of the Frontier Nursing Service in Kentucky in the 1920s. These midwives assumed overall responsibility for the care of childbearing women during pregnancy, delivery, and the postpartum period. Nurses who give primary care have been considered to function in an expanded role that requires additional specialized education.

Another early group that expanded practice were the nurse anesthetists who organized the Association of Registered Nurse Anesthetists in 1931 and assumed responsibility for accrediting programs to prepare nurses in this specialty field. Nurses outside of institutions were still a minority.

After World War II, nursing grew geometrically, extending to many areas at once, and the nation experienced a shortage of nurses. Because of this shortage, many other categories of health care workers were created, but roles and relationships were not carefully planned.

PATTERNS OF CARE DELIVERY

The *case method* was the first system used for the delivery of nursing care in the United States. A nurse worked with only one patient and was expected to meet all of that patient's nursing needs. Often the nurse lived in the patient's home as well as "specialing" that patient in the hospital. This one-to-one relationship had many advantages as far as care was concerned, but the nurses worked long hours and were poorly paid. Advancing technology and changes in cost made this kind of care impractical.

The *functional method* of care delivery emerged during the Depression. This method allowed for the care of increased numbers of patients in hospitals and for advancing technology. Hospitals were primarily staffed by nurses and student nurses, with only a few nursing assistants.

Specific tasks were assigned according to the level of skill required for performance. The system was economical and efficient, but it had the disadvantage of fragmenting care. Communication among the different persons who cared for the patient was difficult, and often the patient had no idea who was in charge of his or her care.

The concept of *team nursing* was introduced in the early 1950s. This approach to patient care is based on having a group of people of different levels of skill assigned to a group of patients. The team works together, with each member performing those tasks for which he or she is best prepared. In the original concept the team was led by a registered nurse, and a central aspect of its function was the *team conference,* in which the team members planned patient care together. The potential for high-quality care is present in team nursing, but the time required for team conferences and the necessity for constant communication can interfere with achieving the ideal. There remains the concern that the patient feels as if no *one* person is concerned for his or her care. Nurses may also feel some frustration at the lack of autonomy. Without team planning, team nursing may become functional nursing in reality.

Many hospitals have returned to a *total patient care* type of assignment, in which a registered nurse (RN) or licensed practical nurse (LPN), depending on the needs of the patient, is assigned for all care needs. This nurse cares for a group of four to six patients, depending on how acutely ill each patient is. This returns a greater sense of autonomy to the nurse and makes him or her feel like a whole person and not a collection of tasks to the patient. By maintaining a broad range of skills, the nurse can enjoy the satisfaction that comes from seeing the whole picture.

The newest approach to the delivery of nursing services, *primary nursing,* is an extension of the total patient care concept. A registered nurse is designated primary nurse and is assigned 24-hour responsibility for a patient's care. The primary nurse does the initial assessment and plans the patient's care. When the primary nurse is on duty, he or she cares for the patient. During other shifts or on the primary nurse's day off, another nurse, called an *associate nurse,* cares for the patient. It is the responsibility of the associate nurse to carry out the plans made by the primary nurse.

Many nurses find greater job satisfaction in primary nursing. Patients express satisfaction in knowing who is responsible for their care and in having one person with whom to discuss their concerns and problems. Although far more nurses are required for this method of care delivery, studies show that, because of the many factors involved, it is no more expensive than other methods.

One problem with primary nursing is the role of the primary nurse. In most facilities every nurse serves as the primary nurse for a few patients and as the associate nurse for the patients of primary nurses on other shifts. Sometimes the nurse finds it difficult to follow plans made by another if there is disagreement. Another concern is the level of expertise and commitment required of all nurses. Because there is no team leader to help pull things together, patient care will suffer if a nurse is not fully competent to perform all the required tasks.

EMPLOYMENT OPPORTUNITIES

The economic position of the nurse in the hospital has improved rapidly because of the extension of laws governing fair labor practices to nonprofit institutions and because of the advent of collective bargaining. The number of positions for registered nurses in hospitals has risen as care has become more complex.

The number of men in nursing, which remained relatively small for many years, is beginning to increase as society reassesses its attitude toward labeling jobs as woman's or man's work. Men have been attracted by the improving economic picture of nursing and in turn have not been reluctant to advance it still further.

The growth of autonomy for the registered nurse is even more marked outside the hospital setting. Community health nurses have always operated much more independently. The focus on health care is shifting from illness to health. With the growth of community health and the many other roles that nurses begin to fulfill in community mental health centers, women's health care delivery systems, maternal–infant care programs, and outpatient and primary care, the percentage of nurses employed in nonhospital settings is constantly rising. Because most of these positions require a baccalaureate degree and specialized educational programs, the new graduate is still most often employed in the hospital or long-term care institution.

The hospital environment today is affected by all that has gone before. In some settings, there are remnants of the paternalistic attitudes that were prevalent in the years when women were expected to accept the hospital as the family surrogate during training and employment. This attitude may coexist with one that expects today's nurse to be an independent decision-maker. Emphasis is placed on the nurse's need for breadth and depth of theory to cope with the complexities of caring for the acutely ill. At the same time pangs of nostalgia may be expressed for the days when nurses "really knew how to work" and did not worry about so much "booklearning."

Unlike graduates of the hospital programs of the past, you may be unfamiliar with the hospital as an employer. Your contact with the institution may have been brief as you focused your time on learning. You may have questions regarding employer expectations and your own role as an employee in an institution.

All of these factors bring you, as a new graduate, into a world of uncertainty but one also filled with opportunity and promise.

COMPETENCIES OF THE NEW GRADUATE

Considerable controversy exists within the nursing profession concerning which skills the new graduate should possess and to what level of proficiency. In diploma programs, which graduated most nurses of the past, students spent enough hours in direct care that, on graduation, they were prepared to accept almost any nursing position in the hospital where they received training and perform with skill all the procedures commonly used in that institution.

Both nursing education and the nature of the hospital have changed. The hospital population now comprises a much higher percentage of acutely ill patients with complex problems. Extended-care facilities now look after many of the more convalescent patients. Complexity of care has increased as more new procedures and techniques have been introduced. Nurses are expected to make knowledgeable decisions about the moment-by-moment care of the patient, day-to-day concerns, and discharge planning. In order to do this competently, nurses need a greater base in theory.

Changes in nursing education that were caused by a variety of social and economic factors have resulted in students spending less time directly caring for patients (see Chapter 2). The time that is spent is carefully planned and structured for optimal use, making the students' learning experiences as productive as possible. However, the chance of every student being able to practice every skill is slim. Nursing educators have tried to bridge this gap by using practice laboratories and teaching general principles.

Another factor affecting beginning competency is the mobility of the nursing population. Students no longer can expect to work as graduate nurses in the same hospital where they learned their skills. As a result, many nurses begin their careers far from the location of their education where equipment, policies, and procedures may differ.

Nursing administrators believe that because of these factors, new graduates need considerable supervision and direction before they are ready to assume full responsibility. This lengthy time of teaching and orientation places a heavy cost burden on the first employer, and thus on the patient.

The variance between the needs of the employment setting and the ability of the new graduate to perform has created considerable tension between nursing administration and nursing education. In some cases this has led to increasing distance between the two sectors and a lack of cooperative action, each one blaming the other for the continued existence of the problem. Nursing administrators believe that educators need to do more to increase the competence of new graduates; nursing educators think that the expectations of employers are unrealistic and should be adjusted to the reality of today's beginning practitioner. They further claim that today's new graduates have many capabilities and can quickly acquire greater skill competence. Fortunately, in some areas the tension has provoked mutual dialogue and constructive attempts to solve the problems.

The National League for Nursing (NLN) has been studying the whole area of competencies of the graduate nurse (see Chapter 2). Differentiating the competencies of the graduates of the various types of educational programs has been a major part of the task.

In April 1978 the Council of Associate Degree Programs of the NLN developed and approved a statement of the competencies of the associate degree graduate. Members of the council were also asked to plan for implementation of the statement. Competency was defined as

> a combination of demonstrated cognitive, affective, and/or psychomotor capabilities derived from the activities of the associate degree nurse in the various roles in the practice setting. Stated in broad terms, a competency is the integration of more specific behaviors.[1]

The statement is quite extensive and speaks of competencies in assessing, planning, implementing, and evaluating care. The descriptions must be somewhat general because they are intended for all graduates of associate degree programs from around the country. Below are two examples.

Assessing

    1. Collects and contributes to the data base (physiological, emotional, sociological, cultural, economic, and spiritual needs) from available resources (*e.g.*, patient, family, medical records, and other health team members).

Implementing

    3. Maintains and promotes adequate respiratory function

through the implementation of nursing protocols and oxygen therapy (*e.g.*, positioning, IPPB, etc.).[2]

The Council of Baccalaureate and Higher Degree Programs of the NLN has published a statement of the "Characteristics of Baccalaureate Education in Nursing." Part of this statement lists the competencies expected of the baccalaureate graduate. Most of the descriptions are related to cognitive abilities, such as using nursing theory and synthesizing theoretical and empirical knowledge. Attributes such as accepting responsibility and accountability and collaborating with others are included. The descriptions are broad and do not speak to any specific competencies as they have been defined by other groups.[3]

The most comprehensive statement on competencies issued by the NLN is "Competencies of Graduates of Nursing Programs," which was accepted by the Board of Directors of the NLN in April 1979. A task force examined all four levels of nursing education (practical nursing, diploma, associate degree, and baccalaureate) and were assigned to

1. identify the common core that runs through all levels of preparation;
2. identify differences in programs in terms of competencies;
3. identify areas of omission or emerging areas for which competencies need to be specified and to which attention must be given at the appropriate program level; and
4. present a working paper to the board of directors by April 1979.[4]

The result was a paper that defined many key words in nursing education, reviewed the literature relevant to the topics being considered, and presented the conclusions of the task force. The knowledge base, the practice role, and the competencies of each level were outlined. The task force concluded that there was still some ambiguity and lack of discrimination in the statements with regard to minimal expectations of new graduates of the various programs. The task force has recommended continued study of this topic and discussion among all the groups representing the numerous programs involved so that the differences in breadth and depth can be more clearly identified. In 1982 the NLN published the results of the task force's study.[5]

Many other groups have also worked on statements to describe competencies of new graduates. The deans and directors of associate degree programs in Florida have formulated a statement of competencies that was published by the Florida State Board of Education. The statement comprises four assumptions about the practice of the associate degree graduate, and each assumption has a list of competencies relating to it. Approximately 68 competencies are listed. The statement defines *competency* as "the basic understanding of and ability to perform a nursing activity."[6] The expected level of skill at the activity is satisfactory performance and evaluation by an instructor in the educational program. This performance and evaluation may take place in either a patient care situation or a practice laboratory.

Because the statement is used to describe a more limited group (one state's associate degree graduates), it is more specific than that developed by the NLN. One major section deals with the use of the nursing process, and another discusses technical skills in detail. For example, under "Hygienic Care," such things as "administering and/or supervising oral care, skin care, and care of hair, hands and feet" are explicitly stated.[7] Under the section on "Elimination," competencies such as "inserts, irrigates, and removes tubes (*e.g.*, rectal, urinary, levine)" and "performs ostomy care" are listed. The statement includes descriptions of workload competency of care for four to six patients and team leading two or three others in the care of eight to ten patients.[8]

The New Mexico System for a Nursing Articulation Program developed a statement of the "Minimum Behavioral Expectation of New Graduates from New Mexico Schools of Nursing." This statement outlines competencies for graduates of practical, associate degree, and baccalaureate degree nursing programs. Broad categories such as nursing process, communication, change, and management were described in relationship to each level of practice. A detailed list of tasks appropriate to each degree was also included.[9]

Throughout the nation other groups are wrestling with statements that delineate the competencies of new nursing graduates. Similarities and patterns are emerging. The outline of theoretical knowledge and functioning in regard to the nursing process seems to be the most consistent. The most divergent opinions seem to be in the area of skill or task competency. Some groups provide exhaustive lists, and others offer more general guidelines. Even with the statements, employers are often asking for further clarification of skills. Have these graduates only the necessary theoretical knowledge to perform the skill? Have they actually performed the skill? If so, was it in a practice laboratory only, or was it in a patient care situation? Does competence mean that the new graduate can function independently, or will some supervision still be needed?

In addition to theoretical knowledge, use of nursing process, and skill competency, speed of performance is a concern of new employers. As a student, your patient care load may be limited to two or three patients and might not encompass a full shift. This schedule allows you to focus your time on maximum learning, but it may not give you the opportunity to work within the realistic time and workload constraints of the employment situation.

Further complicating the picture is the confusion surrounding competencies of the graduates of the three types of nursing education programs. Although statements have distinguished between levels of functioning, many employers do not differentiate expectations. Some employers state that new graduates have not clearly demonstrated differences in competencies. This has created confusion in the minds of nurses, employers, and the public over the role of the registered nurse prepared in each type of educational program.

THE EMPLOYER'S GENERAL EXPECTATIONS OF THE NEW GRADUATE

What is expected of the new graduate varies in different facilities and in different geographical areas. Expectations are affected by various factors in the community.

A hospital that serves as a learning environment for nursing students may be accustomed to hiring people who have experience in that facility and are familiar with its physical plant and its policies and procedures. Such hospitals may expect a more rapid transition to the role of the registered nurse than hospitals that do not have students and are used to hiring people who have no prior experience with the facility.

Large hospitals may have a staff development program and a well-developed orientation program. Newly hired nurses are not expected to function on a unit until they have completed the orientation program. In small hospitals all orientation may be more informal. This may be beneficial for the person who sees such orientation as an individualized program. However a small hospital may not have the resources to allow the same amount of time for orientation as that allowed by a larger hospital.

Urban facilities may be accustomed to the different backgrounds of nurses from other parts of the country, or even from foreign countries. Facilities in rural areas may have experience only with those who have similar backgrounds and may build expectations based on a narrower view of what competencies students should have had.

Most facilities that employ newly graduated registered nurses expect them to demonstrate the following competencies:

    1. Possess the *necessary theoretical background* for basic patient care and for decision making. Many employers believe that new graduates of today are *very* competent in this area. For instance, the new graduate should understand the signs and symptoms of an insulin reaction, recognize it when it occurs, and know what nursing actions should be taken. When assigned an immobilized patient, the new graduate is expected to be aware of the potential problems related to immobility and what independent nursing measures should be initiated to prevent the development of complications.

2. Be able to use the nursing process in a systematic way. This includes assessment, planning, intervention, and evaluation. New graduates should be able to write and use nursing care plans. Depth and comprehensiveness may be expected to be related to educational preparation (associate degree, bachelor of science degree, or diploma). Some employers ask that a nursing care plan be written as part of employment screening.

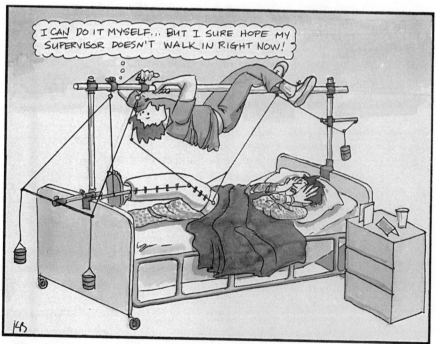

Figure 11–1. New graduates are expected to know both their own abilities and when to seek appropriate help.

3. Recognize their own abilities and limitations. Employers may be able to assist if nurses ask for help and direction but cannot accept the risk to patients created by nurses who do not know their own limitations.

4. Understand the record-keeping function. However, employers recognize that the ability to do this independently in patient care is not possible until the new graduate is given time to learn the charting system used in the facility. The new graduate is expected to recognize the need for recording certain data but might need to ask questions about where and how to chart. It is anticipated that the nurse would keep accurate, grammatical, and legible records.

5. Understand and have a commitment to a work ethic. This means that the employee takes the responsibility of the job seriously and will be on time, takes only the allowed coffee and lunch breaks, and will not sign off ill unless truly ill. It also means that the new graduate recognizes that nurses are needed 24 hours a day, 365 days a year, and that this may require sacrifices of personal convenience, such as working evening shifts or on holidays.

6. Possess skill proficiency in the basic nursing care procedures that often are carried out by nursing assistants. This includes such things as giving baths and performing general hygienic measures. In some settings nurses will be carrying out these tasks, whereas in different settings they will be directing others who do them. In either case, proficiency is essential.

The tasks that are generally reserved for the registered nurse represent the area of widest diversity. These include passing medications to an entire unit of patients, caring for intravenous infusions, performing sterile procedures such as catheterization, and assisting a physician with such complex procedures as a spinal tap or thoracentesis.

Some facilities provide extensive orientation programs in which every skill is checked before the new graduate is allowed to proceed independently. Other employers expect the new graduate to perform the skill if able or to ask for help if unable. Often employers are flexible in their expectations, so that it may be acceptable if a given person seems to have proficiency in a reasonable percentage of skills. Other employers have a list of skills in which proficiency is mandatory, although speed may

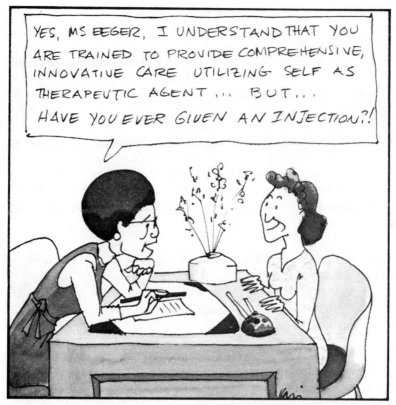

Figure 11–2. Employers are often concerned about an applicant's specific technical skills.

not be expected. Also, there may be a difference between what the employer would wish and what the employer will accept.

7. Functioning with acceptable speed. This is another area in which expectations vary greatly. Most employers state that they accept that the new graduate will be slower; however, they may vary in how much slowness is acceptable and how soon they feel that slowness should be overcome. Generally, an orientation period is planned. An acceptable speed of function is reflected by ability to carry out a usual registered nurse assignment within the shift. Thus, if the usual patient assignment for a registered nurse is the care of six moderately ill patients, the new graduate is expected to accomplish this by the end of the orientation period.

PROBLEMS OF TRANSITION FROM STUDENT TO PROFESSIONAL

With all of this controversy, the new graduate often feels caught in the middle. As a student, you may feel that you are expected to learn a tremendous amount in an alarmingly short time. The expectations may seem high and in some ways unrealistic. Then, as a new graduate suddenly thrust into the real world, you may feel insecure and think that your educational program did not adequately prepare you for what is expected of you. On one hand you are expected to function like a nurse who has had 10 years of experience, but on the other hand your new ideas may not be considered because you have so little experience. You may become frustrated because you do not have time to deal with a patient's psychosocial problems or teaching needs.

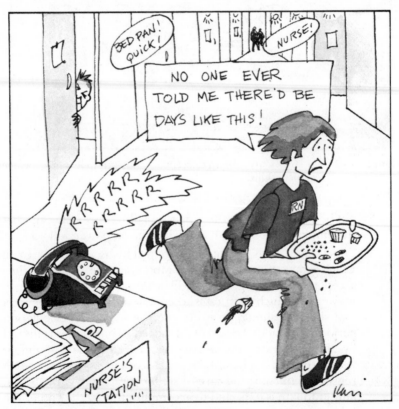

Figure 11-3. Some new graduates are disillusioned by the working conditions that they find on their first job.

As a student, you are taught that the "good nurse" never gives a medication without understanding its actions and side-effects and that evaluating the effectiveness of the drug is essential. As a staff nurse, you may find that the priority is getting the medications passed correctly and on time and that there is little or no time to look up 15 new drugs. As for evaluation, that becomes a dream. How can one evaluate the subtle effects of a medication in the 2 minutes spent to pass the medication to a patient one does not know? The individually and meticulously planned care that was so important to you as a student may become a luxury when you are a graduate. Often the focus is on accomplishing the required tasks in the time allotted, and it is efficiency in tasks that may earn praise from a supervisor.

It may seem impossible to deliver quality care within the constraints of the system as it exists. New graduates may feel powerless to effect any changes and may be depressed over their lack of effectiveness in the situation. Marlene Kramer has called the feelings that result from such a situation *reality shock.*[10] She states that the new graduate may experience considerable psychological stress, and that this may contribute to the problem. The person undergoing such stress is less able to perceive the entire situation and to solve problems effectively.

At this point some nurses become disillusioned and leave nursing altogether. Others begin to "job hop" or return to school, searching for the perfect place to practice perfect nursing as it was learned. Some push themselves to the limit, trying to provide ideal care and criticizing the system. They may end up being labeled nonconformists and troublemakers. Still others give up their values and standards for care and reject ideals as impossibly unrealistic expectations that cannot be sought in the real world. These persons simply mesh with the current framework and become part of the system.

There is an alternative to these nonproductive coping methods. It is possible to create a role for yourself that blends the ideal with the possible, one in which you do not give up ideals, but see them as goals toward which you will move, however slowly. In order to do this you need to be realistically prepared for the demands of the real world.

Coping with Expectations

One way of meeting the challenge is to assess yourself as you approach the end of your educational program. Consider what your competencies are. Think about the seven areas of expectation: (1) theoretical knowledge, (2) use of the nursing process, (3) self-awareness, (4) record keeping, (5) work ethic, (6) skill proficiency, and (7) speed of functioning.

Second, gain information about what the employers in your community expect from new graduates. This can be done by talking with practicing nurses, requesting interviews with nursing administrators, meeting with the faculty, and contacting recent graduates who are currently employed. Try to get specific information.

After you have gathered this information, try to correlate it with a realistic appraisal of your own ability to function in accordance with the employer's expectations. If you identify any shortcomings, the time to try to remedy them is before graduation. For example, if the registered nurse is expected to pass medications for an entire unit while meeting time criteria, then new graduates know that they must soon meet this standard. You might consult with your clinical instructor to arrange for experiences that would help you to perform this task with greater ease.

If you recognize that you consistently have difficulty functioning within a time frame, you might obtain employment as a nursing assistant while still in school; this will give you more experience in organizing work within the time limits that the employer sees as reasonable. If you identify a lack in certain skills, you might register for extra time in the nursing practice laboratory to increase your proficiency. You could even time yourself and work to increase speed as well as skill.

If you have formed a habit of frequently being late for class, you can change. Perhaps part of your problem is your personal physiology. You might find that you work more effectively on the evening or night shift.

As you plan for your first job, you can examine the psychological challenges to be met. Understanding that you are not alone in your feelings of frustrations is often helpful. It may be useful to form a support group of other new graduates who meet regularly to discuss problems and concerns and seek solutions jointly. You can also gain valuable reinforcement from other nurses in your work setting. Many have successfully dealt with the problems you face and are able to provide support and help. This "preceptor" relationship has often been lacking in nursing and needs to be cultivated.

When confronted with areas of practice that you would like to see changed, weigh the importance of the issue. Use your energies wisely. The "politics of the possible" is important to you. Learn the ways of the system in which you work and how to use that system for effective change. You, as a person, are important to nursing, so it is important that you neither burn yourself out nor abandon the quest for higher-quality nursing care; you should be able to continue to work toward improving nursing and bringing it closer to its ideals.

Many hospitals are attempting to help new graduates deal with reality shock. Some are doing it by making orientation programs more comprehensive and by providing an experienced nurse to work as a preceptor to the new graduate. Nurse internships have been created to provide a planned and organized transition time during which the new graduate participates in a formal program, including classes, seminars, and rotations to various units of the hospital. An *externship*, which is a program for student nurses during the summer before the last year of the basic program, has been used in some areas as a mechanism to ease the transition from student to new graduate. In this program the student nurse is employed as a nursing assistant but participates in a planned program that introduces the role of the registered nurse. You may wish to inquire whether hospitals in your area have developed any of these or other programs to assist you when you are a new graduate.

PERSONAL CAREER GOALS

In caring for patients, you are involved in the process of goal setting. Many nurses recognize the value of this in patient care but never transfer the concept to their personal lives. Nursing is such a broad field with so many possible directions that, without carefully setting goals, you might drift for years.

Focusing Your Goals

You may want to focus on a broad area of clinical competency, such as pediatric nursing, or on a more restricted area, such as neonatal care. Clinical areas available for concentrated effort become more varied as health care becomes more complex. Emergency care, coronary care, neurologic and neurosurgical nursing, and specialties in the care of persons with ear, nose, and throat disorders are just a few of the clinical possibilities. Nurses specialize in aerospace nursing, enterostomal therapy, and respiratory care as well as operating room nursing and postanesthesia care. Opportunities for additional education and for practice in most clinical specialties are now available for any registered nurse, regardless of his or her initial educational background.

Some specialty areas are in the primary care field, such as the woman's health care specialist, the family nurse practitioner, and the pediatric nurse practitioner. Increasing numbers of these programs require a baccalaureate degree for entry, but some admit any registered nurse with experience in the field.

Another approach may be to focus your goals on the setting in which care is delivered, such as acute care, long-term care, or community care. As health care needs expand, these separate realms of care delivery are all demanding more specialized knowledge. Even within the individual area of focus there are differences. For example, within the community there are ambulatory-care settings, public health nursing agencies, occupational health nursing departments, and day-care facilities.

Yet another way of focusing your goals is according to functional categories. Although nurses are initially thought of as direct-care providers, they are needed in many other positions. For example, there is need for those who would move into supervisory and administrative capacities, those who teach, and those who conduct nursing research. Nursing also lends itself to writing, to community service, and even to political involvement.

You may decide to set your goals in relation to all three types of foci. That is, you might identify a clinical area, a care setting, and a functional category.

Setting Your Goals

The first step in setting personal career goals is a thorough self-assessment. Determine how your abilities and competencies correspond to your own expectations as well as to those of the employers. Other factors to explore are your likes and dislikes, the situations or types of work you particularly enjoyed as a student. Also, it is important to recognize the area in which you were most comfortable. Were there areas in which you or your instructor felt that you were an above-average student? Consider your health and personal characteristics in relationship to types of work. Do you have physical restrictions? Do you prefer working independently, or with others? How do you respond to close supervision or to relative freedom in the job setting? Do you work well with long-term goals and a few immediate reinforcements, or do you need to see results quickly? Another factor to consider is your own geographic mobility; would you be willing to move or travel as part of a job? Both your personal responsibilities and preferences operate in this arena.

As you plan ahead you need to examine the entire field of nursing. What types of jobs and opportunities are open to you? What education and personal abilities are needed in these areas? Are you interested? Does the education you have meet the educational requirement? Are avenues for additional education available to you? All of these considerations are important as you plan for the future.

Career goals need to be both short and long term. They will help you to plan your future constructively. This does not mean that goals are static. Just as patient goals must be realistic, personal, and flexible, so must your own goals.

Short-term goals will encompass what you want to accomplish this month and this year. What do you want to do and what do you want to be? One recent graduate stated that her short-term goal was to have 2 years of solid experience in a busy metropolitan hospital.

Long-term goals represent where you want to be in your profession 5 to 10 years from now. The long-term goal of the graduate referred to above was to work in a small, remote community in which she would have the opportunity to function autonomously.

Although both long- and short-term goals will be revised as your life evolves, they will guide you in making day-to-day decisions more effectively.

MAKING GOALS REALITY

Philosophical questions regarding goals must be resolved by practical approaches. As a new graduate, your first goal simply may be to get a job in nursing (especially if you live in one of the areas of the country that has more limited opportunities for registered nurses).

Whatever the situation, you are more likely to realize your goals if you are prepared to present yourself in the best possible way to a prospective employer. Many of you have held different jobs in the community as students and as adults. You may be familiar with and competent in the "job-search" process. Others of you have never applied for the kind of job that truly could be considered the beginning of a career. Different expectations are held by both employers and prospective employees in such a situation.

Letter of Application

Writing a letter requesting an interview is an excellent way to approach many prospective employers. A letter may be dealt with at the recipient's convenience, whereas a telephone call may interrupt a busy schedule. There are fewer chances for misunderstanding if your request is in written form and if you receive a written reply.

Your letter of application should be written in standard business form (see Sample Letter of Application). Make it brief and clear. Introduce yourself and your purpose for writing in the first paragraph so that the reader immediately has an understanding of the subject. You may then want to briefly state your reasons for applying for a position with this particular employer. The more specific the reasons, the better the impression you are likely to make. When asking for an appointment, indicate the times you might be available and how and where you can be contacted. Thank the person for considering your application, and close. You should be able to include this information on one page. Remember, the employer is a busy person and will thank you for facilitating his or her job. Another point to remember is that the letter represents *you*. You will be judged on spelling, grammar, clarity, and neatness as well as on the letter's content. Ask a friend or family member to double-check your first draft if you have any questions about its correctness. A written résumé should accompany your letter.

The Résumé

The appearance of your résumé is important, since it presents your image to the employer. It should be neatly typed on standard-sized

---

SAMPLE LETTER OF APPLICATION

432 N.W. 85th St.
Seattle, WA 98117
Nov. 15, 1987

Ms. Jane Jackson, RN, MN
Director of Nursing Services
Evergreen General Hospital
Kirkland, WA 98002

Dear Ms. Jackson:

I am interested in a position as a registered nurse in your medical unit. I graduated in June of this year and took my state board examination in July. In September I was notified that I had passed and I now have my license.

In addition to my clinical experience at Shoreline Community College, I have had extensive volunteer experience and extra educational experiences related to gerontology and care of the elderly. This information is included in my attached résumé. I would like an appointment to discuss employment possibilities. I am currently working evenings as a health care assistant and therefore I can be reached by telephone (363-8320) during the mornings from 8:00 a.m. to noon or by letter at the above address. I will call your office next week to ask for a specific appointment.

Sincerely,

Lisa Sanger

white paper so that it is easy to handle, file, and read. A résumé that is individually typed (or reproduced well enough so that it appears to be) usually will be more positively received than a carbon copy or a poor-quality photocopy. To achieve legibility use wide margins, spacing, indentation, and numbering to separate different sections and topics. You might want to underline important items in red or highlight them with an asterisk to draw swift attention. When an employer is reviewing many résumés, anything that facilitates the job and makes you stand out is an advantage.

The content of your résumé is critical. Organize it into groups of information. Include personal information, work experience, educational background, volunteer or community work, awards and honors, and references. In each group list the most recent items first.

Under personal information give your name, age, address, and telephone number. If you will be moving, indicate the date the move will be effective, and provide an alternate method of contacting you after that date. A permanently settled relative or friend who would be willing to forward your mail would be appropriate. Indicate the date your license will be effective and whether you have a temporary permit to work as a nurse (if that is required in your state). Employers are not permitted to ask about marital status and dependents. However, you may choose to add this information.

Work experience should give a complete employment history with no unexplained gaps in time. For example, if you spent 15 years as a homemaker since your last employment, include those dates and state "homemaker" after them. For each job you held include address, dates employed, position, and duties. The prospective employer would be especially interested in a previous nursing assistant position or any other position that demonstrates your knowledge of or experience in some area of health care or the assumption or responsibility. If you have had only one or two part-time jobs during your educational program, it would be appropriate to include them in detail. However, if during your educational program you held 15 part-time jobs, it is appropriate to list significant ones that offered valuable experience. In one line write, "Various part-time jobs to finance schooling: clerk and waitress. Individual names provided on request." Include the overall dates for this period.

Educational background should cover your nursing education and any specialized courses or postgraduate work you have done. It is appropriate to note any college-level work. Do not include high school information because graduating from a nursing program is the significant education. If you attended any special workshops, include those as a separate section.

Choose the items you list under volunteer and community work carefully. If you are 40 years old, the fact that you were student-body president in high school would probably be considered irrelevant. However, if you went from high school directly to nursing education, this information could be important in demonstrating your leadership ability. Your participation in any community organizations such as the Parent-Teacher Association and service in any leadership roles that would be significant to an employer should be noted, with descriptions. In some instances you may want to list briefly the skills or abilities gained from a particular activity. For example, if you worked as a volunteer for a Planned Parenthood Clinic, you might specify that your duties included individual client counseling in relation to family planning methods. Simply stating that you were a volunteer might not communicate the level of responsibility you assumed.

List awards and honors that would demonstrate your competence or leadership ability. Items that deal with your position in a social organization usually would not be included. You may omit this section if you feel that you have nothing pertinent to enter.

Be selective in choosing the persons you will list as references. Consider the people who know you and would be able to present you in a positive way to a future employer, and who would have credibility with the employer. Seek the person's permission before giving him or her as a reference. Most commonly you should provide as one reference someone who has known you personally for a relatively long time and who could attest to your ability to relate with others and to such attributes as personal integrity. A second reference may be an instructor or supervisor from your basic educational program. This person would be able to affirm your ability in the nursing field. A third reference should be someone who has employed you and who can describe your work habits and effectiveness as an employee. Include full names with title (if any), addresses, and telephone numbers so that the employer will be able to contact the references easily. When seeking permission to use someone as a personal reference, you might outline what particular emphasis you want that person to make, for example, "If you are contacted, I would particularly like you to provide information about my work habits and effectiveness as an employee." (See Sample Resumé of a Recent Graduate.)

The Interview

As you plan for an employment interview, you need to consider your appearance, your attitude and approach, and what the content of the interview will be.

SAMPLE RESUME OF A RECENT GRADUATE

Resume

Personal Data

Jill Smith
16002 Greenwood Avenue
Seattle, Washington 98133
Telephone: (206)546-4896

*Single
*Excellent health
*Age 26

Education

Shoreline Community College, Seattle, Wash. 1985 to 1987, A.D.N. (Overall G.P.A. 3.0 out of 4.0*)

University of Washington, Seattle, Wash. 1983 to 1985. General studies. (Overall G.P.A. 2.9 out of 4.0.*)

Conference: Pain Management. Sponsored by the State of Washington Associated Nursing Students. May 18–19, 1986.

Work Experience

June 1982 to present:
   Valley General Hospital
   400 S. 43 Street
   Renton, Washington 98005
   Title: Nursing assistant
   Duties: Worked in the obstetrical unit giving care to mothers and infants. Occasionally floated to give direct patient care on general surgery unit.

June 1984 to June 1986:
   The Boeing Company
   Seattle, Washington 98100
   Title: Clerk-typist
   Duties: Typed reports. Was responsible for making sure that clear, understandable language was used.

Volunteer Experience

Odessa Brown Mental Health Center, Seattle, Washington. Jan. 1987 to present. Volunteer counselor. Duties included assisting persons to use the community resources fully. Required ability to work with a wide variety of persons.

Community Activities

Member, Washington Cross-Country Ski Association, Seattle, Washington

References

Mrs. Celia Hartley, Director of Nursing   Phone: 546-4743
Shoreline Community College
Seattle, Washington 98133

Mrs. Elizabeth Nowlis, Supervisor   Phone: 386-9685
Valley General Hospital
Renton, Washington 98005

Mr. John Jefferson, President of the Mountaineers   Phone: 756-3427
9634 West Corliss Avenue
Seattle, Washington 98006

*Age, sex, marital status, ethnic origin, and religion are all optional. Employers may request a transcript of grades. Grades need not be included.

Your personal appearance is likely to evoke some type of response from the interviewer. Consider what you would like that response to be and dress appropriately. This would mean that what you wear when applying for one type of job might be inappropriate when applying for another type of job.

For example, if you were applying for a position at a hospital, you would wear businesslike clothing, such as dress pants and shirt or a suit or dress. Being neat and well groomed contributes to a businesslike atmosphere. If you were applying for a position in a walk-in health care clinic that offered services to persons who are uncomfortable in a traditional environment, it might be appropriate to wear the casual clothing worn by the workers at the clinic. You need to make a conscious decision about the impression you want to create. Although some may wish that appearances had no effect on the opinions of others, remember that, in reality, appearance often does make a significant difference.

When you go to the interview, take a copy of your résumé with you. This can help you to feel more confident if you have forms to fill out, or if questions about statements on your résumé arise during the interview.

When you arrive at an interview you will need to be sensitive to the problems and concerns of the interviewer. If it is apparent that untoward events are demanding his or her attention, you might state that you are aware of the difficulty, and you could ask for another appointment. Your sensitivity to the interviewer's cues are evidence of your sensitivity to patients' cues.

Your manner in the interview is also important. Although the employer expects you to be nervous, he or she will be interested in whether your nervousness makes you unable to respond appropriately. Remember, you are a guest and an applicant. Wait to be asked to sit down before you take a chair. Avoid any distracting mannerisms, such as chewing gum or fussing with your hair, face, or clothes. Be serious when appropriate, but do not forget to smile and be pleasant. The interviewer is also thinking of your impact on patients, visitors, and other staff members.

The interview should be a two-way conversation in which you will be gaining as well as giving information. Think through the situation before you go to the interview and outline information that you want to obtain and questions that you want answered. You may find it advantageous to write out your questions before going to the interview so that they are clearly stated and you do not forget the things that are important to you in the tense atmosphere that often exists in an interview situation.

During the interview you will discuss a variety of subjects. The interviewer may direct the flow of topics or may encourage you to bring up the ones that concern you. Applicants who focus initial attention on the nonprofessional issues of wages and benefits may be viewed as more concerned about themselves than about nursing. Therefore, if you are asked to present questions, you would be wise to ask professional questions first. You will be expected to be concerned about how nursing care is given and by whom, where responsibility and authority lie, the philosophy underlying care, the availability of continuing education, and where you would be expected to fit into their overall picture. Before you leave be sure to cover such topics as hours, schedules, pay scales, and benefits.

Time spent reflecting on your personal views will be valuable when you come to an interview. Remember that an interview is a chance for you to sell yourself to an employer, a chance to present yourself as a valuable addition to their nursing staff, and an opportunity to determine how you will fit into that work setting.

RESIGNATION

When you decide to leave a nursing position, it is important that you provide the employer with an appropriate amount of time to seek a replacement. The more responsible your position, the more time the employer will need. For a staff nursing position you should strive to provide 1 month's notice unless an urgent matter requires that less notice be given. Notice of resignation should be in a letter. The letter is directed to the head of your department, often the director of nursing. Carbon copies should be sent to other supervisory people, such as the head nurse and the supervisor.

The letter of resignation is important in concluding your relationship with the employer on a cordial and positive basis. The feelings that are left behind when you resign will influence letters or recommendation and future opportunities for employment with that agency. Give a reason for your resignation as well as the exact date when it will be effective. If you have accrued vacation or holiday time and want to take the time off or be paid for it, clearly state that. Comment about positive factors in the employment setting and acknowledge those who have provided special support or assistance in your growth.

If you are resigning because of problems in the work setting and want to note them, do so in a clear, factual, nonemotional way. Avoid attacking anyone in a personal way and do not make broad, sweeping

---

SAMPLE LETTER OF RESIGNATION

18520 Dayton Avenue
Seattle, Washington 98133
Nov. 20, 1987

Mrs. Jane Johnson, R.N.
Steven's Memorial Hospital
21600 75th Avenue W.
Edmonds, Washington 98020

Dear Mrs. Johnson:

I have just received notice of acceptance for a position in the Mission of Mercy Hospital in Calcutta, India. Therefore I wish to resign effective after December 31, 1987.

My time spent with Steven's Hospital has been valuable to me not only in terms of gaining self-confidence as a new graduate, but also in giving me many very special professional and personal relationships. All of the nursing staff have my thanks for their support and assistance as I grew in nursing. Although I look forward to my new position, I do leave with some regrets.

Sincerely,

Mary Taggart

cc: Marie Moore, R.N.
     Head Nurse ICU/CCU

---

negative comments. Try to make the letter a clear and reasonable statement of your position as a professional (see Sample Letter of Resignation).

MAINTAINING COMPETENCE

Regardless of whether a formal program of continuing education is required, the nurse has an obligation to society to maintain competence and continue practicing high-quality, safe care. Continuing education may occur through learning on the job, through reading of professional publications, or through attending classes. There are television courses, programmed instruction programs, and examinations related to journal articles. Any of these avenues may be appropriate, depending on the circumstances. Some nurses may want to advance through specialty or higher education.

Appendix B contains a list of nursing journals printed for national circulation in the United States. This list does not include any periodicals that are directed toward a wider health care audience or those focused around a specific disease problem unless it specifies a nursing audience. The length of this list gives you some idea of the volume of new information that is available in the field of nursing. No one can keep up with it all. You will need to decide what topics are important to your practice and to your growth as a professional. This brings you back to personal goal setting.

BURNOUT

Burnout is a form of chronic stress related to one's job. It can be identified by feelings of hopelessness and powerlessness, accompanied by decreased ability to function both on the job and in personal life. Burnout primarily occurs in nurses who work in particularly stressful areas of nursing, such as critical care, oncology, or burn units. It also occurs in other areas when staffing is inadequate or interpersonal relationships are strained.

Symptoms

Symptoms of burnout include both physical changes and psychological distress. Exhaustion and fatigue, frequent colds, headaches, backaches, and insomnia all may occur. There may be changes in disposition, such as being quick to anger or exhibiting all feelings excessively. As burnout progresses, ability to solve problems and make decisions decreases. This frequently results in an unwillingness to face change and a tendency to block new ideas. There may be feelings of guilt, anger, and depression because one cannot meet the expectations for doing a "perfect job."

In response to these feelings, some nurses quit their jobs and move on to other settings. These other settings may not even be in nursing. Others remain in their jobs but develop a personal shell that tends to separate them from real contact with clients and co-workers. The person may become cynical about the possibility of anyone doing a good job and may function at a minimal level.

Causes

Many causes of burnout have been discussed in the literature. Prominent among them is the conflict between ideals and reality. Just as this is a problem for the new graduate, it is also a problem for the experienced nurse. In trying to achieve the ideal, the nurse drives harder and harder and becomes critical of environment and of self. Nurses see themselves as being responsible for all things to all people and often take on more and more responsibility, thus increasing their own stress level.

Another cause of burnout is the high level of stress that results from practicing nursing in areas that have high mortality rates. Continually investing oneself in patients who die can take a tremendous toll on personal resources. In addition, the demand is constant for optimal functioning.

Institutions that are inadequately staffed may also place great stress on nurses. The patients are in need of care, the nurse has the skills to provide the care, and yet the patients do not receive good care. The nurse typically tries to do more and more, staying overtime, skipping breaks and lunch, and running throughout the shift. Despite this effort, there is little job satisfaction because the things that are left undone or that are not done well seem to be more apparent than all the good that was accomplished.

Preventive Actions

Burnout can best be prevented by mounting a stress-reduction effort involving the nursing staff, supervisory personnel, the hospital administration, and other health care workers. The most important aspect seems to be bringing burnout into the open and acknowledging the existence of the problems. This alone helps the individual nurse move away from the feelings of separation and alienation that often accompany burnout. Whatever the problems, they seem less frightening if they are defined as "normal" and if the individual nurse does not see himself or herself as the only person not performing as the "perfect nurse."

A second step is to provide for group discussions during which nurses can share feelings and specific concerns in an accepting atmosphere. This sharing may lead to concrete plans to reduce the stress created by the setting. For example, if one source of stress is conflicting orders between two sets of physicians involved in care, a plan might be developed whereby the nurses no longer take responsibility for the conflict, but refer the problem to some authority within the medical hierarchy. This type of resolution is possible only when the problem of burnout is being addressed by the whole health care team.

Giving nurses more control over their own practice often decreases stress. This action is limited by the constraints of the setting, but it may involve flexible scheduling, volunteering for specific assignments, and participation in committees that determine policies and procedures.

Rotating nurses out of high-stress areas before they become "burned-out" may allow them to rebuild resources and return to the job with enthusiasm. This can be done only if there is no stigma or blame attached to the need to rotate, and if other nurses are available for replacement. In patient care areas that are known to be stressful, it is helpful to have a counselor available for nurses. Consulting with this counselor should be viewed by the staff as a positive step and not as an admission of some lack or fault. The counselor needs to be someone who understands the setting and who has the skills to assist people in coping with stress.

As an individual nurse, you also can take actions to prevent burnout. These are the same general actions that are designed to control stress in any aspect of life. Paying attention to your own physical health is an important preventive measure. This includes maintaining a balanced program of rest, nutrition, and exercise. Another important point is not to subject yourself to excessive changes over short periods, since changes increase stress. You may decide, for example, not to move at the same time you change to a different shift. A period of "wind down" or "decompression" after work helps you to avoid carrying the stress of the workplace into your private life. This period may be physical exercise, reading, meditation, or any different activity. The activity you choose should not create more demands and increase stress. An important resource is someone who is willing to listen while you ventilate your feelings and talk about your problems. Sometimes this is a family member or personal friend, but it may be more appropriate for this to be a co-worker.

Burnout is a serious concern in the nursing profession, but there are strategies for managing it. If you are in a high-stress situation, you need to plan for prevention *before* you become burned-out.

SEX DISCRIMINATION IN NURSING

There are two major areas in which there is concern about sex discrimination in nursing: the issue of comparable worth and the discrimination against men in nursing.

Comparable Worth

Nursing has been, and still is, a field made up predominantly of women (see Chapter 1). Nursing has also been a poorly paid profession for most of its history. Although collective bargaining has resulted in increased nursing wages and benefits, there is still concern that compensation does not match the value of the job done by nurses. Many relate this to the fact that all women's occupations have historically been poorly paid.

Laws exist in many states that prohibit explicit sex discrimination in salary for a given job. For example, if both men and women are hired by an airline as flight attendants, they must be compensated on the same basis. This principle has been expanded to encompass jobs that are essentially the same work, although the titles may differ. The janitor

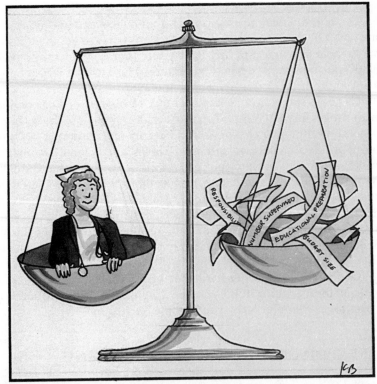

Figure 11–4. Jobs may be studied and assigned points of rank based on educational requirements, skills required, level of responsibility, and authority.

and the maid may have different titles, but if they have essentially the same tasks, then they must be paid on the same basis.

The next step that many women would like to see accepted is the principle of compensation based on comparable worth. Jobs may be studied and assigned points or rank based on educational requirements, skills required, level of responsibility, and authority. Those with the same points or rank are considered to be of *comparable worth*, although the actual substance of the work may differ. Alaska has a law barring discrimination in pay for work of comparable character.

Many women feel that differing jobs of comparable worth are not compensated equally because of sex discrimination. Most jobs that are found to score high in education, skill, responsibility, and so forth and that have low salaries are those jobs that have historically been held by women. Nursing is one example of such a field. Secretaries and teachers are other occupational groups that have traditionally had low wages relative to the level of responsibility required.

Groups of women have brought suit against employers, charging sex discrimination based on failure to provide equal pay for jobs of comparable worth. One such suit was filed by a group of public health nurses in Alaska.[11] They complained that their salaries were significantly lower than those of physicians' assistants, whose educational qualifications were not as high. Because the physicians' assistants were primarily men and the nurses were primarily women, the nurses claimed that they were being discriminated against because of their sex. Even though they were not successful in their suit, they have not given up their stand. A federal judge in Washington State ruled that the state must pay jobs of comparable worth comparable wages, and that state is moving ahead with plans to alter its compensation schedules. There is strong opposition to the concept of comparable worth throughout many segments of society. Therefore, any gains in this area will not be made without a great deal of effort. Continued action, both nationally and statewide, to obtain legal recognition of comparable worth as a basis for compensation can be expected.[12]

Discrimination Against Men

Men in nursing have also expressed concern about sex discrimination. Their concern is not monetary, but is related to being allowed to practice in all areas of nursing. In some facilities or areas men are not allowed to care for women patients, or if they are allowed to care for women, restrictions are placed on them in terms of obtaining consent for care from each patient.

Those who support the limitations on the practice of men in nursing state that it is a matter of providing for the modesty and privacy of the woman patient. This position was upheld by a court decision in favor of a hospital that refused to assign a man to a nursing position in labor and delivery.[13] The argument was made that the patient did not have free choice of a nurse, but rather was assigned a nurse for care, and therefore the restrictions were appropriate.

Those who oppose limitations on the practice of men in nursing state that as a professional, whether man or woman, the nurse should always consider the privacy and modesty of a patient of either gender. This can be done without excluding anyone from providing care in any area. By careful assessment the nurse can determine the true needs of the patient and plan for appropriate avenues to deliver that care. Furthermore, the point has been made that men as physicians have not been excluded from any branch of medicine and this has not created problems. Physicians are not always chosen by the patient either. House staff are assigned, referrals are made to specialty physicians, and many group plans designate a physician to provide care. Women nurses care for men patients in all situations. This has been accepted because women are seen in a nurturing, mothering role that the public associates with nursing.

The American Assembly for Men in Nursing (see Appendix B) provides a forum for the concerns of men in nursing and opposes any limitations on opportunities available to men.

Anti-male sexism in the United States was discussed by R.J. Kus.[14] He pointed out that society stereotypes men just as feminists have criticized that it stereotypes women. He makes a strong case for the importance of nurses examining the stereotypes they hold about men. Stereotypes narrow our thinking and interfere with people being able to develop to their fullest potential. It is appropriate for women in nursing to examine their own behavior and identify whether they have been guilty of perpetuating outmoded stereotypes of the nurse and supporting a type of discrimination toward men that they would fight to eliminate for women.

OCCUPATIONAL SAFETY AND HEALTH

Nurses have expressed concern regarding safety in the working environment for many years. A significant number of nurses are employed as occupational health nurses, and a specialty organization of such nurses has been active since 1942. However, nurses have often failed to look at their own workplaces in terms of optimal safety. There are many hazards in the hospital environment that can be a significant threat to nurses' long-term health.

Transmission of infection is a major concern when caring for infected patients. The presence of resistant organisms causes extra concern and makes treatment difficult. All hospitals have an infection-control officer, usually a registered nurse, who has the expertise to guide the staff in planning appropriate isolation procedures. The hidden danger for nurses lies in those patients who have not been diagnosed as having an infection and for whom infection-control measures have therefore not been instituted. AIDS (acquired immune deficiency syndrome) has created a reevaluation of all approaches to infection control and of health care workers' obligations to provide care for those with communicable disease. The individual nurse must assume responsibility for his or her own protection through conscientiously carrying out appropriate aseptic measures at all times. Employers must be held accountable for providing the supplies and environment to make this possible.

Nurses who have frequent contact with blood and blood products and those engaged in intravenous therapy have a special risk for exposure to hepatitis B. Although a vaccine exists to protect against this disease, the vaccine itself is not without hazards, and therefore a discussion with a physician regarding risks versus benefits is appropriate before undertaking immunization.

Anesthetic gases can increase the risk of fetal malformation and spontaneous abortion in pregnant women who are exposed on a regular basis. Standards exist for waste-gas retrieval systems and the allowable level of these gases in the air. Nurses working in operating rooms should seek information on the subject and expect that hospitals will provide a safe environment.

Chemotherapeutic agents used in the treatment of cancer are extremely toxic, and nurses who work in settings where such agents are prepared and administered should seek additional education regarding their administration, not only in relationship to the patient's safety, but also in relationship to personal safety.

Contact with many medications, especially antibiotics, during preparation and administration may cause the nurse to develop sensitivity. This may not only create transitory problems, such as a hand rash, but may also be a threat if treatment for a serious infection is compromised at some later date. Other medications are absorbed through the skin and may produce an undesirable effect.

Employees have a right to expect their employers to provide the safest working environment possible. Some hospitals employ an occupational health nurse to examine the working environment and employment practices in order to promote health and safety on the job. Nurses themselves, however, have often been lax in recognizing on-the-job hazards and acting for self-protection. This can be likened to the response of those who continue to smoke, regardless of their knowledge of the health hazards of smoking, or those who fail to wear seatbelts, although they know that the statistics show decreased fatalities in auto accidents when seatbelts are worn. Some people continue to do those things that they know are detrimental to their health and well-being. Unfortunately, nurses are no exception.

CONCLUSION

Many new graduates suffer from reality shock when they are confronted with their first position as a registered nurse. This is caused by the wide discrepancy they find between the ideal world of nursing as they learned it and the real world of nursing in which they attempt to practice. New graduates can ease their transition through this time by gaining an understanding of the world of employment, the forces that have helped to shape it, and some of the factors that exert pressure on that setting. The world of nursing practice is not without its problems for the practicing nurse either. Knowing what some of those problems are before you begin may help you to be more effective as you seek to make nursing all that it can be.

REFERENCES

1. Council of Associate Degree Programs. National League for Nursing: Statement on the Competencies of the Associate Degree Graduate, p 1. New York, National League for Nursing, 1978
2. Council of Associate Degree Programs, National League for Nursing: Statement on the Competencies of the Associate Degree Graduate, p 3. New York, National League for Nursing, 1978
3. Council of Baccalaureate Degree Programs, National League for Nursing: Characteristics of Baccalaureate Education in Nursing. New York, National League for Nursing, 1979
4. National League for Nursing: Working Paper of the N.L.N. Task Force on Competencies of Graduates of Nursing Programs. Pub. No. 14–1787. New York, National League for Nursing, 1979
5. Competencies of Graduates of Nursing Programs, Pub. No. 14–1905. New York, National League for Nursing, 1982.

6. Florida State Board of Education: Competencies of the Associate Degree Graduate, p 2. Tampa, State Board of Education, 1977
7. Florida State Board of Education: Competencies of the Associate Degree Graduate, p 5. Tampa, State Board of Education, 1977
8. Florida State Board of Education: Competencies of the Associate Degree Graduate, p 6. Tampa, State Board of Education, 1977
9. S.N.A.P. Project: Minimum Behavioral Expectations of New Graduates from New Mexico Schools of Nursing. Albuquerque S.N.A.P. Project, University of Albuquerque, Division of Nursing and Allied Health, 1977
10. Kramer M: Reality Shock. St. Louis, CV Mosby, 1979
11. PHN's win first round in equal pay case. Am J Nurs 82(7):1028, Jul 1982
12. House tackles pay equity issue: Kennedy to Introduce Legislation. Am J Nurs 83:7, Jan 1983
13. Arkansas judge rules male nurse out of labor/delivery. Am J Nurs 81:1253, Jul 1981
14. Kus RJ: Stages of coming out: An ethnographic approach. West J Nurs Res 7(2):177–194, May 1985

FURTHER READINGS

American Hospital Association: Statement on a Hospital Employer's Minimum Expectations of a Registered Nurse. Chicago, American Hospital Association, 1966

Bellocq JA: Comparable worth: Implications for nursing. Prof Nurs 1:3:131–137, May/Jun 1985

Buechler DK: Help for the burned-out nurse? Support groups. Nurs Outlook 33:4:181–182, Jul/Aug 1985

Career Guide: Nurs 79; Nurs 80 (monthly feature)

Career Planning Guide. New York, National Student Nurses Association (annual publication)

Dailey AL: The burnout test. Am J Nurs 85:3:270–272, Mar 1985

Godfrey M: The dollars and sense of nurses' salaries. Nursing's 1979 Survey, Part 1, 96, Sep 1979; Part 2, 97, Oct 1979

Heine CA: Burnout among nursing home personnel. J Gerontol Nurs 12:3:270–272, Mar 1986

Hicky JV: How to reduce stress and avoid burnout. Nurs 15:4:7–9, Apr 1985

Kramer M: Reality Shock. St. Louis, CV Mosby, 1974

Nelson LJ: The nurse as advocate: For whom? Am J Nurs 77:851, May 1977

Nursing Opportunities. RN (annual publication)

Protect Your Employment Rights, Publication No. L–04. Kansas City, American Nurses' Association, 1979

Schiponi CC: From the ideal to the real. Am J Nurs 78:1034–1035, Jun 1978

What Every Nurse Should Know About Signed Written Agreements. Publication No. L–03. Kansas City, American Nurses' Association, 1979

Wiley L: Job interviews: Oh boy! Are they important. Nurs 77:65–69, Aug 1977

Cuthbert BL: Please list three names. Am J Nurs 77:1596–1599, Oct 1977

Styles MM: The uphill battle for comparable worth: How it can be won; why it won't be easy. Nurs Outlook 33:3:128–132, May/Jun 1985

Vance C et al: An uneasy alliance: Nursing and the women's movement. Nurs Outlook 33:6:281–285, Nov/Dec, 1985

12 Organizations For and About Nursing

Objectives

After completing this chapter, you should be able to

1. *Identify various reasons for the number of nursing organizations in existence.*
2. *Identify the purposes of the major structural units of the American Nurses' Association (ANA).*
3. *Discuss the activities and programs of the ANA.*
4. *List some of the activities of the National Student Nurses' Association.*
5. *State the purpose of the National League for Nursing (NLN).*
6. *Identify those who are eligible for membership in the NLN and the ANA.*
7. *Discuss the major programs and services of the NLN.*
8. *Identify the purpose of accreditation.*
9. *Identify a major thrust of the specialty organizations.*
10. *Name one honorary nursing organization.*
11. *List two goals of the newest educationally oriented nurses' organization.*
12. *Identify some of the different groups of nursing organizations that exist.*

A student once said that it seems that every time nurses identify a problem, their first action is to form a new organization. This is an exaggeration but has some remnants of truth. To the person initially introduced to the great number of nursing and nursing-related organizations, it may all seem confusing.

A serious concern in the field of nursing is the overlapping of function and interrelationships between some of the various organizations. Unfortunately there has been a spirit of competition rather than one of cooperation in some situations in the past. Because nurses traditionally have had lower income, the decision of whether to join none, one, or several organizations has often been an economic as well as a philosophical issue.

Nursing organizations have recently put forth a concerted effort to

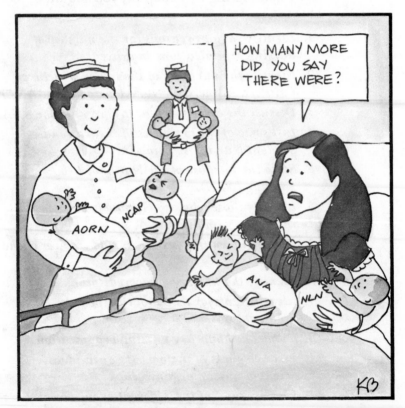

Figure 12–1. The large number of nursing organizations may seem overwhelming.

promote cooperation. Nurses, as a whole, seem to be better informed about the various organizations, and they generally receive better salaries than in the past. Unfortunately this has not resulted in significantly greater participation by professional nurses in their organizations. Some people specifically do not join because of philosophical differences, but many nurses seem to be apathetic and do not recognize the importance to the profession of nurses acting together. In an address to the 1978 American Nurses' Association (ANA) convention, Senator Daniel Inouye of Hawaii remarked that nurses are the single largest group of health care providers, and that as a result, they have potential for power in affecting change if they work together.

AMERICAN NURSES' ASSOCIATION

The ANA, the professional association for registered nurses, had its origins in a meeting of nursing leaders at the World's Fair in Chicago in 1890. Through their suggestions and efforts, the alumnae organizations of ten schools of nursing sent delegates in 1896 to a committee to organize a professional association. The resulting organization was called the National Associated Alumnae of the United States and Canada. The name was changed in 1899 to the Nurses' Associated Alumnae of the United States and Canada. In 1911 the organization split into Canadian and American groups because the state laws of New York (where the organization was incorporated) did not allow for representatives from two countries. The name *American Nurses' Association* was adopted in the United States.

Membership

In 1982 the ANA adopted a different organizational format, moving from a direct, individual membership to a modified federation structure. Figure 12–2 outlines this structure. The ANA membership is composed of state nurses' associations. The individual nurse belongs to the constituent state organization. Each state is free to establish its own membership plans; however, membership is limited to registered nurses. The only exception to this is the admission to membership of some new graduates who have not yet passed state board examinations. In addition to this change in membership, the Association has made significant changes in how the functions of the organization are to be carried out.

In 1984 there were more than 1.8 million registered nurses in the United States.[1] Of these, approximately 185,000 belong to the ANA.

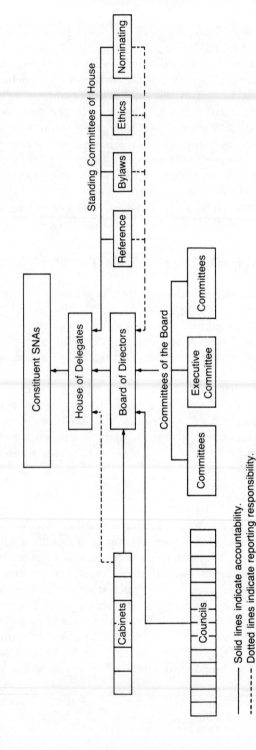

Figure 12–2. A.N.A. structure showing accountability and reporting relationships. (Am Nurs 10, Nov/Dec 1982)

— Solid lines indicate accountability.
------- Dotted lines indicate reporting responsibility.

From this you can readily see that most nurses do not participate in this organization. The figures are somewhat misleading, however, because it is safe to assume that many of the registered nurses who do not join the organization are not practicing, whereas those who are leaders in the profession usually do join. Nevertheless, although the association is the official voice for the profession, less than half of the registered nurses are members.

One reason for the low level of membership is its high cost. Dues to the national association and the state and district associations are paid together, and in most areas of the country they are more than $250.00 per year. Another reason given for not joining is lack of time to participate in activities. Many nurses have dual responsibilities of job and home, and they have no time for a professional organization. Other

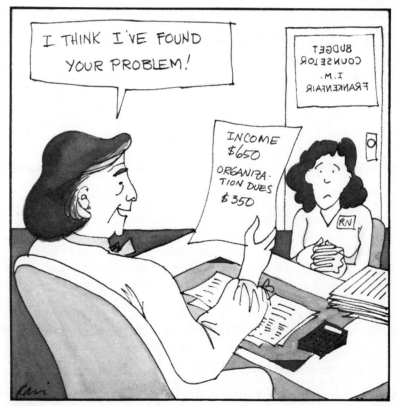

Figure 12-3. Deciding which organization to join may entail a financial as well as philosophical judgment.

nurses do not see how the benefits available through the association are personally valuable. Some explain that they are just not interested in the issues and concerns in which the organization is involved. Lastly, there are those who do not join because they do not agree with the position of the ANA on major issues.

Those who are active in the ANA believe that its work is severely hampered by the low level of membership. The organization is limited in funds because of the small number of members. Because some specific programs, such as those involved with collective bargaining, are costly to the association, there has been a strong move to require nurses to belong to the association if it serves as a bargaining agent. In some states the state association has set a specific percentage of staff that must be members before they will become the bargaining agent.

A current controversy involves differing views over what the purpose of the professional organization should be. Many people believe that the major concern should be what the organization can do for the individual nurse. Others believe that a truly professional view looks at what the individual may contribute to the profession through the organization. Some think that the organization should not be an advocate in the realm of economic security, whereas others see this as essential. Another point of controversy is the organization's stand on political issues.

Policy-Making

Every year at the ANA convention, members of the *House of Delegates*, who have been selected to represent each state nurses' association, meet. The power to set policy and direction for the organization rests with the House of Delegates. This body often takes an official stand on a controversial issue. In the time between conventions, it is the duty of the organization to carry out the directions of the House of Delegates.

The members of the House of Delegates also vote for candidates for all elective offices in the organization. A *board of directors* is elected to oversee the functioning of the association. The board makes policy decisions during the time between conventions, although it must stay within the framework of the decisions made by the House of Delegates. The officers of ANA (president, vice-president, secretary, and treasurer) are also elected and sit on the board.

The ANA has a large, professionally staffed office in Kansas City. Although the volunteers in the organization are essential, the many and varied tasks could not be accomplished without the full-time staff. The staff members range from professional business executives and research personnel to secretaries. The *executive director* is the chief administrator of the organization and is hired by the board. Throughout the history of the organization the executive director has always been a nurse with administrative expertise. The executive director works cooperatively and supportively with the president and the board.

The ANA supports committees that work on such policies as the ANA Social Policy Statement[4] and the Congress on Nursing Practice's suggested state legislation.[5] These activities are ongoing efforts to support the advancement of nursing as a profession.

The ANA also supports research on topics related to the profession itself, such as the historical patterns of licensure.[3]

Organizational Structure

There are many components of the ANA. The policymaking bodies have already been discussed. Other organizational units were developed to enable the organization to address particular needs.

Cabinets are groups organized to carry out specific responsibilities of the organization. There are six cabinets: Nursing Education, Nursing Practice, Nursing Research, Nursing Services, Economic and General Welfare, and Human Rights. Each cabinet is composed of five members elected by the House of Delegates and two members appointed by the Board of Directors. The Board determines the chairperson. These cabinets are charged with setting standards, recommending policies and actions, and responding to concerns of those within the organization.

Councils are related to areas of practice. There are currently 15 councils: Community Health, Gerontological, Maternal and Child Health, Medical–Surgical, Psychiatric and Mental Health, Continuing Education, High-Risk Perinatal, Intercultural, Nurse Researchers, Nursing Administration, Nursing Home Nurses, Primary Health Care Nurse Practitioners, Specialists in Psychiatric and Mental Health, and Clinical Nurse Specialist. Any member of a state nurses' association may join a council. The councils serve as a forum for discussing relevant concerns and planning for continuing education, and as a resource for recommending standards, positions, and policies. An executive committee for each council is elected at the annual meeting of the House of Delegates. It is through the Councils that certification is being conducted (see Chapter 4).

Standing committees deal with the business and organizational functions of the ANA. These committees are determined by the bylaws and are permanent. The bylaws, finance, and membership promotion committees are examples of standing committees.

Special committees and *task forces* are set up to deal with a particular problem at a particular time. For example, a special task force of the ANA was appointed to develop a statement on scope of practice. This task force reported back to the House of Delegates at the 1987 ANA convention.

The *Constituent Forum* comprises the presidents and executive directors of the state nurses' associations. This group meets to discuss concerns of common interest, to study issues, and to present a unified voice from the state nurses' associations on topics of national interest. For example, in 1986 the forum recommended that future membership in the Association include both professional and technical nurses. This recommendation was presented to the Board of Directors of ANA.[2]

Activities

The ANA has been referred to many times throughout this book. As a professional association, it has been involved in all the issues that nursing has confronted. The activities of ANA are carried out by committees, cabinets, councils, and other parts of the organization. There has not been universal support within the nursing community for all the activities that the ANA has championed or for the stands that it has taken. With any group as large as nursing, it is perhaps inevitable that there should be a wide range of viewpoints.

In addition to its activities, the ANA provides direct services to members. These include access to a group professional liability insurance plan and group insurance for health, disability, and accident coverage. From time to time the ANA also provides access to group travel arrangements and purchasing discounts.

Publications and Educational Materials

Through its educational services the ANA produces and distributes a wide variety of educational materials, such as films for nursing, as well as a biennial report entitled *Facts About Nursing*. This report provides basic statistical information used by many organizations and individuals. Reports of committees and commissions and special studies supported by the ANA are also published.

The American Nurse is the official organ of the Association; official announcements of Association business are published in this paper. The paper also contains current news of relevance to nursing and health care, editorials, letters, and classified advertisements. *The American Journal of Nursing* is the official journal of the organization. It is published monthly and contains some current news, but its major focus is professional articles. It is published by the American Journal of Nursing Company in New York City and retains autonomy over its own content. The American Journal of Nursing Company is wholly owned by the ANA.

The organization also publishes many pamphlets and informational resources that are of value to nurses. A complete list of publications is available from the organization.

ORGANIZATIONS RELATED TO THE ANA

As the official professional association, the ANA is related to three other organizations in a special way.

National Student Nurses' Association

The National Student Nurses' Association (NSNA) is the professional organization for students in schools of nursing and was started in 1952. Although it works with the ANA and the National League for Nursing (NLN) it is a fully independent organization.

A major project of the NSNA is "Breakthrough into Nursing," which is designed to recruit and maintain the enrollment of minorities in schools of nursing. The project has enlisted nursing students to speak to minority teenagers to interest them in nursing early in their scholastic careers, and to act as preceptors and tutors to increase the retention of minority students when they enroll in schools of nursing.

The NSNA frequently is asked to testify before congressional committees when issues relevant to nursing education are being considered. In this role the organization becomes the public voice for all student nurses.

Although the NSNA is an autonomous organization, it has close ties with the ANA. Members of the NSNA serve on selected committees within the ANA, speak to the House of Delegates at the ANA convention to provide a student viewpoint, and work together with the ANA in regard to current issues.

In 1975 the NSNA developed a Student Bill of Rights (Fig. 12–4). this document carefully balances the rights of students with the responsibilities of students. It supports the view of students as competent adults who are engaged in an educational program. The rights outlined relate to the educational program itself, to the rules and policies of the institution, and to freedom in personal life and decision making.

N.S.N.A. STUDENT BILL OF RIGHTS

The following Student Bill of Rights and Responsibilities was adopted by the NSNA House of Delegates in April 1975.

1. Students should be encouraged to develop the capacity for critical judgment and engage in a sustained and independent search for truth.

2. The freedom to teach and the freedom to learn are inseparable facets of academic freedom: students should exercise their freedom with responsibility.

3. Each institution has a duty to develop policies and procedures which provide and safeguard the students' freedom to learn.

4. Under no circumstances should a student be barred from admission to a particular institution on the basis of race, creed, sex, or marital status.

5. Students should be free to take reasoned exception to the data or views offered in any course of study and to reserve judgment about matters of opinion, but they are responsible for learning the content of any course of study for which they are enrolled.

6. Students should have protection through orderly procedures against prejudices or capricious academic evaluation, but they are responsible for maintaining standards of academic performance established for each course in which they are enrolled.

7. Information about student views, beliefs, and political associations which instructors acquire in the course of their work should be considered confidential and not released without the knowledge or consent of the student.

8. The student should have the right to have a responsible voice in the determination of his/her curriculum.

9. Institutions should have a carefully considered policy as to the information which should be a part of a student's permanent educational record and as to the conditions of its disclosure.

10. Students and student organizations should be free to examine and discuss all questions of interest to them, and to express opinions publicly and privately.

11. Students should be allowed to invite and to hear any person of their own choosing, thereby taking the responsibility of furthering their education.

12. The student body should have clearly defined means to participate in the formulation and application of institutional policy affecting academic and student affairs.

13. The institution has an obligation to clarify those standards of behavior which it considers essential to its educational mission and community life.

14. Disciplinary proceedings should be instituted only for violations of standards of conduct formulated with significant student participation and published in advance through such means as a student handbook or a generally available body of institutional regulations. It is the responsibility of the student to know these regulations. Grievance procedures should be available for every student.

15. As citizens and members of an academic community, students are subject to the obligations which accrue them by virtue of this membership and should enjoy the same freedom of citizenship.

16. Students have the right to belong or refuse to belong to any organization of their choice.

17. Students have the right to personal privacy in their living space to the extent that the welfare of others is respected.

18. Adequate safety precautions should be provided by schools of nursing, for example, to and from student dorms, adequate street lighting, locks, etc.

19. Dress code, if present in school, should be established by student government in conjunction with the school director and faculty, so the highest professional standards possible are maintained, but also taking into consideration points of comfort and practicality for the student.

20. Grading systems should be carefully reviewed periodically with students and faculty for clarification and better student–faculty understanding.

(Reprinted by permission of the National Student Nurses' Association, Inc © 1978)

Figure 12–4

Each state has a state student nurses' association that operates in the same relationship to the state professional organization as the NSNA does to the national organization. State conventions and workshops are held in many states. State issues are addressed by the state association in the same way that national issues are addressed by the NSNA. Local student nurses' organizations may or may not exist in individual schools of nursing. These local organizations may be closely tied to the state and national groups, or they may be independent. It is possible for an individual student to join the state and national student nurses' organizations even if no local counterpart exists.

In the past it was not uncommon for schools of nursing to require membership in the student nurse organization at local, state, and national levels. With increasing emphasis on student rights and freedom of choice, this practice is no longer followed and has led to recruitment problems for many of the student nurse organizations. Students are very busy, with full lives and limited funds. Some do not understand that the efforts of the organizations benefit them in larger ways that are not immediately visible. The activities of the student organization cannot occur without a wide membership base for funding and for credibility. Certainly the profession of nursing as a whole and the situation of the individual nursing student would be adversely affected if the NSNA did not remain a viable and active force.

International Council of Nursing

The International Council of Nursing (ICN) is the international organization for professional nursing, with membership composed of national nursing organizations. The ANA, as a constituent member of the ICN, sends delegates to its convention and participates in its activities. The ICN is interested in health care in general and nursing care in particular throughout the world. It works with the United Nations when appropriate and with other international health-related groups, such as the International Red Cross.

The ICN concerns itself with such issues as the social and economic welfare of nurses, the role of the nurse in health care, and the roles of the various national nursing organizations throughout the world and their relationships to their governing bodies. The primary governing body of the organization is the Council of National Representatives, which meets biennially.

The ICN has representatives of 98 national nurses' organizations. Every 4 years a quadrennial congress is held. This meeting is open to all nurses and to delegates from the national organizations. Activities of the organization are carried out by the officers, volunteer nurse members of constituent organizations, and employed staff. Headquarters of the ICN is in Geneva, Switzerland.

American Nurses' Foundation

The American Nurses' Foundation (ANF) was established by the ANA as a tax-exempt, nonprofit corporation for the purpose of supporting research related to nursing. The Board of Trustees of the ANF is composed of members of the Board of Directors of the ANA, other nurse members, and non-nurse members from other health-related fields and from the public. It is autonomous.

Since the establishment of the ANA Commission on Nursing Research in 1970, the focus of the ANF has changed. A three-pronged approach has been established in which the first objective is to conduct policy analyses to provide nursing leaders and public policymakers with the information they will need for decision making. The second objective is related to developing a group of "nurse scholars" who would engage in further study in such areas as journalism and public policy. Support is directed toward independent study, research, and doctoral and postdoctoral work. The third objective is to facilitate the research and educational activities of ANA. This includes providing consultation and funding for those groups within the ANA that wish to initiate projects.

To accomplish its varied objectives, the ANF solicits gifts and contributions from individuals and organizations. These gifts are tax-deductible. The $62,000 in research grants awarded in 1986 brought the total that the ANF has contributed to nursing research since 1955 to $1.5 million.[5]

American Academy of Nursing

The American Academy of Nursing (AAN) was established by the ANA as an honorary association within the ANA. The original members were chosen by the Board of Directors of the ANA. The AAN is now an independent organization, and new members are selected by those currently in the AAN. Those elected to the AAN are called Fellows and may use the title Fellow of the American Academy of Nursing (FAAN). The purpose of this organization is to recognize those nurses who have made significant contributions to the profession of nursing in general.

THE NATIONAL LEAGUE FOR NURSING

Another major nursing organization is the National League for Nursing (NLN), which was established in 1952. This organization fused seven organizations or committees into one. The groups were the National League of Nursing Education (1893), the National Organization for Public Health Nursing (1912), the Association of Collegiate Schools of Nursing (1933), the Joint Committee on Practical Nurses and Auxiliary Workers in Nursing Services (1945), the Joint Committee on Careers in Nursing (1948), the National Committee for the Improvement of Nursing Services (1949), and the National Nursing Accrediting Service (1949). Originally the National League of Nursing Education was organized under the title of the American Society of Superintendents of Training Schools for Nurses of the United States and Canada. Established in 1893, it represents the first nursing organization in the United States. The name was changed to the National League of Nursing Education in 1912.

A nonprofit coalition, the NLN extends membership to members of the health care team, interested laypersons, institutions concerned with nursing service and nursing education, as well as to registered nurses. Its prime purpose is to promote quality nursing care. The NLN works to assure that nurses optimize their own resources in the delivery of health care and strives for the continuous improvement of nursing education. The organization works in a complementary, rather than competitive, manner with the ANA. Whereas the ANA speaks as the official voice of nurses, the NLN seeks to unite the interests of nursing with those of the community. In the attempt to accomplish this, the NLN offers two major classifications of membership: that which is open to agencies that provide nursing services or nursing education and that which is open to any interested person. Each member has one vote on issues, and each agency has two votes that are designated to two individual members representing the agency at the conventions. Business sessions are held at biennial conventions, at which times issues are voted on and decisions are reached. Just as the ANA is sometimes criticized for championing causes unpopular with the nursing majority, so sometimes the NLN is criticized for its conservatism. Like any membership organization, the League takes positions and makes decisions according to the will of the majority. Because its membership encompasses lay consumer advocates, nursing educators from each kind of nursing education program, nursing service administrators, members of health-related disciplines, and registered nurses who want a voice in assuring quality education and service, divergent opinions are to be expected.

Organizational Structure and Membership

The NLN is organized at two levels, the national level and the constituent units. Throughout the United States there are 46 constituent units that may represent a state, several states, part of a state, or simply a large metropolitan area. The emphasis is on establishing constituent units according to the needs and interests of a given area. Individual members, totaling some 18,000, join the national organization through a constituent unit; however, if there is not an active unit in the area, the NLN may be joined directly at the national level. People may also join through one of the forums. Obtaining membership in a forum automatically enrolls one as an individual member in the national and constituent leagues. (NLN forums, which serve special interest groups, are discussed later in this section.) In 1988 the individual dues were $50 nationally, plus the amount assessed by the constituent unit. Forum dues are higher and vary with the forum. Nurse members receive reduced rates for professional liability insurance, and all members get a free subscription to the official journal, discounts on other publications and workshops, low-cost insurance rates, and several other optional membership benefits.

One of the recent changes in NLN membership structure has been the addition of several forums, which bring together persons with special interest. Until 1984 only one forum existed with NLN, the National

Forum for Administrators of Nursing Service, also referred to as the Executive Forum. As the name implies, membership in this forum is limited to nursing executives (directors of nursing) and to those who are next in line and carry titles such as associate or assistant, who are responsible for nursing services in hospitals, long-term care facilities, and community health agencies, as well as to faculty in graduate nursing programs who are responsible for the full-time instruction of content related to administration of nursing service.

In 1984 the National Forum on Computers in Health Care and Nursing was initiated. This forum was created for health care professionals who are interested or involved in computer technology.

The most recent forum, the Society for Research in Nursing Education Forum, became part of NLN in 1986, although the Society was founded in 1983. It is a membership group for educators and researchers who want to be in the vanguard of nursing education research. A major activity is the annual Conference on Research in Nursing Education. Each year a book of abstracts is published that serves as a comprehensive resource on current nursing education research. An interested person may join solely as a member of the forum and receive forum and League benefits, or join as a member of both the forum and the local NLN constituent league.

Another membership group represents agencies, and numbers approximately 1,800. This group comprises nursing education programs, home care and community health agencies, and nursing departments in hospitals and related facilities. Agency members are served by six program councils: Associate Degree Programs, Baccalaureate and Higher Degree Programs, Diploma Programs, Practical Nursing Programs, Community Health Services, and Nursing Service for Hospitals and Related Facilities. Individual members may elect to belong to one or more of the councils or the forum, in which they participate without vote in the concerns of those groups. Agency members of the education councils and the Council of Community Health Services determine accreditation criteria and elect members of the Board of Review and the appeal panel for accreditation of their respective groups. All council and forum members are kept aware of events through newsletters from the national office and through annual meetings.

The individual and agency members are responsible to the Board of Directors, which is composed of the five elected officers, the chairmen of the executive committee of the six councils and of the forums, twelve elected directors, two appointed directors, and four members of the executive committee of the Assembly of Constituent Leagues. All positions are open to non-nurse members and to nurse members, although only once has a non-nurse been elected president. Standing and special committees, which may be either elected or appointed, work through the Board of Directors.

The NLN provides four major services: accreditation, consultation services, continuing education, and evaluation and testing. In addition, the NLN assumes an active role in assuring that nursing has input into health policymaking. It provides information to the U.S. House of Representatives, the U.S. Senate, the Administration, and other policymakers and keeps the membership alert to key legislative issues.

Accreditation

Most students are aware of the accreditation services, especially if they are attending an NLN-accredited school. Accreditation, which is voluntary, is one of the oldest services provided. Initially this was done by the National Nursing Accrediting Service, which, as mentioned earlier, was merged with other groups to form the NLN. The goals of accreditation include providing the public with well-prepared nurses, guiding students in the selection of a program, assuring the public of the quality of the school and its faculty, and stimulating the continued improvement in schools. Designated by the U.S. Department of Education and by the Council on Postsecondary Accreditation as the accrediting body for all nursing programs the NLN currently accredits more than 1,400 educational programs. The NLN also sponsors an accreditation program for community health and home care programs, which assures consumers that an agency meets national standards for care. The NLN has been working with the U.S. Department of Health and Human Service to obtain "deemed status" for NLN's Accreditation Program for Home Care and Community Health. If deemed status is granted, NLN-accredited agencies would automatically be certified to participate in the Medicare home care program without going through the Medicare survey process.

The schools and agencies seeking accreditation request this service and pay for it. Working with published criteria and guidelines, each school or agency prepares a rather involved self-study. After completing the self-study the school or agency is visited by representatives of the NLN. These visitors are either educators from other NLN-accredited schools, or community health experts from accredited agencies, whichever is appropriate to the group seeking accreditation. These representatives have been specially selected and prepared to serve as voluntary visitors for the NLN. Their purpose in visiting the school or agency is to clarify, amplify, and verify the content of the self-study. The visitors

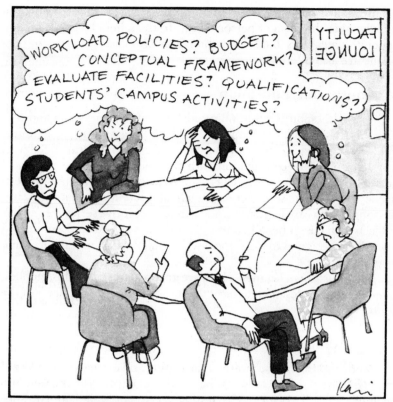

Figure 12–5. Preparation of a rather extensive self-study is part of the accreditation process.

prepare a report that, after being shared verbally with the school, is sent to the NLN. Accreditation is subsequently granted or withheld by a Board of Review, whose members are elected by each council. The Boards of Review meet twice each year for the purpose of reviewing programs. More and more schools and agencies are recognizing the value of NLN accreditation and are participating in the program.

A list of NLN-accredited programs is published each year in *Nursing and Health Care* and is available in pamphlets listing accredited schools and agencies.

Consultation

The NLN also offers consultation to schools that are seeking to improve their programs or that are initiating new programs, and to health agencies that are seeking to improve services. This consultation usually takes the form of personal visits to the school by paid staff and appointed members, but consultations at NLN headquarters or by telephone are also offered.

Continuing Education

The NLN sponsors continuing education (CE) workshops and conferences throughout the country, often repeating a workshop in different locations to spare nurses and others the expense of travel. Subjects are determined in consultation with the councils and are geared to current needs and interests. Curriculum, research, accreditation, testing, and evaluation, student recruitment and retention, political awareness and health care legislation, and a nurse executive series are regular subjects for CE. The NLN has recently developed and conducted workshops designed to assist the new graduate with the state licensing examination.

The constituent leagues, which are grouped by regional assemblies, offer workshops designed to meet the interest of particular areas of the country.

Evaluation and Testing

Students also may be aware of the testing and evaluation services of the NLN for it is the only testing service exclusive for nursing and health-related disciplines. The testing service provides pre-entrance testing to programs preparing practical and registered nurses, as well as to graduate nursing programs. It also prepares achievement tests that can be administered to students who are enrolled in practical and professional programs while in school, and proficiency examinations for nursing service personnel.

Research

When the U.S. government needs figures on nursing education, it cites data gathered by NLN's Division of Research. The division is a primary provider of statistics on nursing education, each year surveying all schools of nursing and of practical nursing for enrollments, admissions, and graduations. It also conducts a yearly survey of newly registered nurses for characteristics of employment. Every 2 years the nurse–faculty census is taken; every 3 years data are gathered on men and minorities in schools of nursing. These data are published in the annual *Nursing Data Book*. The division also publishes the yearly "blue books," which contain essential information on state-approved schools of nursing and of practical nursing.

Among special research projects in 1982, the division conducted studies on the source of income of nursing schools, the cost of nursing education, and the staffing patterns in hospitals (the last of which took into account the variable of patients' illnesses).

Other Services

The career information service answers the thousands of inquiries that come in every year about nursing education by mail and telephone. The NLN publishes annual lists of accredited schools of associate degree, baccalaureate, master's, diploma, and practical nursing programs, plus a list of doctoral programs and information on scholarships and loans. (Each of these booklets carries a minimal price.)

The Division of Public Policy and Research monitors the vital signs in Washington, D.C., and communicates its findings on legislation affecting nursing and nursing education through a monthly column in *Nursing & Health Care* and a quarterly newsletter, *Public Policy Bulletin*. Sometimes League spokespersons offer testimony on legislation or rulings significant to the organization. The Division of Public Policy and Research is not a lobbying group (NLN's tax status prohibits such activities), but it does work closely with the ANA's political action committee.

Throughout this book, and especially in Chapter 2, we have referred to the NLN publications. As a nursing student you are already aware of the monthly magazine *Nursing & Health Care*, the official organ of the NLN. This journal focuses on administrative and educational concepts, better methods of care delivery, expanding roles and practice, and material on nursing theory and research. It does not carry articles on direct patient care or specific clinical material. The NLN also has a publications unit, which brings out papers and monographs of selected workshops or topics, the various research and recruitment materials, and nursing studies.

The NLN consistently has pushed for better services for the consumer through improved education of nurses and improved delivery of services. In 1982 the NLN became concerned about the question of the nurses' public image and consequently appointed a Task Force on Nursing's Public Image.

Students who wish to learn more about the NLN and its functions are encouraged to obtain the pamphlet *This Is the National League for Nursing* (Publication No. 41 – 1532), available from the NLN in New York (see Appendix B for address).

At the 1987 Biennial Convention of the National League for Nursing, the membership was introduced to a new proposal for organizational structure. The name proposed for the new organization was the *National League for Health Care, Incorporated;* its work would be accomplished through subsidiaries. These subsidiaries would function independently; each would have its own board of governors, but would ultimately be responsible to the NLHC, Inc., Board of Trustees. The NLN membership body, as it is now known, would constitute one of the major subsidiaries. Others might be in home health care and in the publishing areas.[7] This proposal was also accompanied by a revision of the mission and goals statement, which was approved by the membership. The approved mission statement reads as follows: "The National League for Nursing advances the promotion of health and the provision of quality health care within a changing health care environment by promoting effective nursing education and practice through collaborative efforts of nursing leaders, representatives of relevant agencies, and the general public."[8]

You are encouraged to stay alert to future changes in the organizational structure of the NLN.

SPECIALIZED NURSING ORGANIZATIONS

In addition to the two major nursing organizations described, there are many other nursing organizations that have a special focus. These groups may have local organizations only in larger population centers; however, nurses may often join the national organization, regardless of whether there is a local chapter.

Clinically Related Organizations

Some of the earliest specialty organizations were related to specific clinical fields of nursing. A major focus of these organizations is continuing education related to the nursing specialty. Many of these groups also have some mechanisms, such as certification, for recognizing achievement in the field. Among them are groups that began as auxiliaries to specialty physicians' organizations. As more members joined and nurses became more active, the groups became autonomous. For educational purposes, many of the specialty organizations hold their annual or biennial national meetings at the same time and location as the specialty physicians groups (see Appendix C for a complete list).

One concern has been the overlapping of purpose and action between the Councils on Practice of the ANA and the corresponding specialty organization. One attempt to promote more cooperative effort was the creation of the Federation of Specialty Organizations and the ANA. This organization has held national meetings and has especially addressed concerns regarding credentialing. It appears to be serving as a much needed forum for dialogue.

Groups Related to Ethnic Origin

As the movement for self-determination and preservation of identity arose within ethnic groups in the United States, nurses within ethnic groups began to unite for a greater voice in health care. Some groups are nationally organized. Other ethnic groups may be organized on a more local level.

Honorary Organizations

The AAN, which is part of the ANA, is perhaps the most prestigious nursing honorary organization in existence today.

Sigma Theta Tau is a national organization established in collegiate schools of nursing to recognize those with superior ability, leadership potential, and contribution to nursing. Candidates may be asked to join during the senior year of a baccalaureate program or any time thereafter.

Alpha Tau Delta is a professional nursing fraternity. Students who are enrolled in baccalaureate nursing programs and demonstrate scholarship and personality characteristics in line with the organization's professional goals are eligible for membership.

Religiously Oriented Organizations

The National Council of Catholic Nurses and the Nurses' Christian Fellowship (primarily a nondenominational Protestant group) were organized to assist nurses to share concerns and integrate their work and their religious beliefs. These two organizations place special emphasis on meeting the patient's spiritual needs and on dealing with ethical issues.

Educationally Oriented Organizations

There has been a great deal of change and development since the 1960s as nursing education has moved more into the educational setting. During this time there has been an increasing emphasis on educational methods, curriculum development and research. Within several major geographical regions of the United States, an organization open to schools of nursing and often to members of the state boards of nursing was developed to promote interstate and interinstitutional cooperation in seeking pathways to improved nursing education. Membership in these organizations is not open to individuals, but to institutions (see Appendix B). These organizations are the Western Institute of Nursing (WIN), the Council on Collegiate Education for Nursing of the Southern Regional Education Board (CCEN/SREB), and the New England Board of Higher Education (NEBHE), the Midwest Alliance in Nursing (MAIN), and the MidAtlantic Regional Nursing Association (MARNA).

One of the newest national organizations is the National Organization for the Advancement of Associate Degree Nursing (NOAADN). Organized in 1986, this group was the outgrowth of the development of several state organizations. The first state to initiate an organization was Texas, where the first chapter was started in 1984.

The NOAADN has four purposes: to speak for associate degree nursing education and practice, to reinforce the value of associate degree nursing education and practice, to maintain endorsement of registered nurse licensure from state to state for the associate degree nurse, and to retain the registered nurse licensure examination for graduates of associate degree nursing programs. To fulfill these goals, seven objectives have been incorporated into the bylaws of the organization that relate to activities soliciting support for associate degree nursing, including legislative activity.

Membership is open to individuals, states, agencies, and organizations, with varying dues assessed each group. In 1987 *AD Nurse* became the official publication for this organization.

The American Association of Colleges of Nursing (AACN) was formed to assist collegiate schools of nursing to work cooperatively to improve higher education for professional nursing. Membership is restricted to deans and directors of programs that offer a baccalaureate degree in nursing with an upper-division nursing major and that are part of a regionally accredited college or university. Likewise, hospital schools of nursing have formed the National Association of Hospital Schools of Nursing, the aim of which is to support quality education in diploma programs.

The National Council of State Boards of Nursing, Inc. (NCSBN), was organized in 1978 to replace the Council of State Boards that had been part of the ANA. The purpose of this organization is to provide a forum for the state boards to act together regarding matters of common concern, especially the development of the licensing examination.

There is one delegate from each state board to this council. One reason given for establishing the independent organization was to avoid any potential conflict of interest between the legal licensing authority and the professional organization. Although delegates to the 1978 ANA convention expressed dismay over this change, the ANA did vote to develop a liaison with the new council. The actions of this council are particularly important because its membership represents the *legal* authority for control of nursing education and nursing practice. Although each state board must operate within its own laws, it does have authority to establish many specific rules and regulations. Working together, the state boards hope to promote uniform standards for the nursing profession.

The National Association for Practical Nurse Education and Service (NAPNES) informs the public about the role of the licensed practical nurse, promotes quality education for the practical nurse, develops guidelines and criteria for continuing education for practical nurses, and works with other groups that have similar or related interests. This organization has both institutional and individual memberships available. Institutional memberships are held by schools, practical nurse associations, health agencies, and others with concern for practical nursing education. Individual memberships are open. Many registered nurses who are employed in practical nursing education are members.

The North American Nursing Diagnosis Association (NANDA) is open to individuals as well as to group members. The purpose of this group is to work toward a uniform terminology for nursing diagnosis and to share ideas and information regarding this topic.

Political Action Organizations

There are specific rules and regulations governing the conduct of individuals and groups in the political realm. A nonprofit professional organization may provide expert testimony in regard to an issue but is prohibited from actively lobbying on the behalf of either legislation or a candidate. As nurses have become more politically active, one of the routes they have chosen has been for the formation of specific political groups. The financing of these groups must not be related to any nonprofit organization, and membership must be voluntary. Political action groups are free to undertake lobbying efforts as well as to work on behalf of candidates. Many individual states have political action organizations for nurses. The ANA political action committee is the national political action group (see Chapter 10).

Miscellaneous Organizations

The Gay Nurses' Alliance was an outgrowth of the movement of homosexuals to be accepted without having to disguise their sexual orientation. This group has primarily focused on the issue of gay rights.

The American Assembly for Men in Nursing was formed for men who feel that, as a minority in the profession, they need to speak on issues with a united voice.

Nurses House Inc. provides assistance for nurses in need. It originated from a bequest in 1922 from Emily Bourne, who donated $300,000 to establish a country place where nurses might find needed rest. As the need for a specific residence decreased, those who had become supporters of this endeavor sold the estate and invested the proceeds. Income from the investment and other funds donated by nurses and friends of nurses are used to provide guidance and counseling for nurses with emotional and chemical dependency problems, encouragement to homebound nurses, and temporary financial assistance to RNs who are ill, convalescing, or unemployed. Nurses House seeks members to continue these activities and donations to support them.

OTHER HEALTH-RELATED ORGANIZATIONS

There are a great many other health-related organizations in the United States. Some are open to nurses as members, and others have more restricted membership. Often the activities of these organizations affect the health care climate in which the nurse works. Knowledge of these organizations may help you to respond more effectively to their actions.

Health-Problem-Related Groups

Many organizations focus on a particular illness or group of illnesses, such as the American Heart Association. Public information and education are usually a major part of their efforts. In addition, many of these groups actively support research, professional education, and patient care. Nurses may join these groups as much as any member of the public might because of an interest in supporting the work. In addition, nurses may join such groups because they also make available special educational opportunities regarding patient care. Nurses may actively participate in these organizations, serving on committees and running for office. Some of these organizations hire nurses to serve various educational roles.

Organizations of Other Health Care Professionals

Most health care professionals have a professional association. It is rare, however, to find as large a number of organizations as there are for nurses. One exception is the number of professional organizations for physicians. In addition to the American Medical Association, there are many clinical specialty organizations. These groups focus on the recognition of competence and continuing medical education within their specialty area.

The National Federation of Licensed Practical Nurses (NFLPN) is one of the professional organizations for practical nurses. The NFLPN has worked with the ANA in regard to some of its activities, and actively supports the need for the practical nurse in health care.

Other professional groups, such as occupational therapists, physical therapists, medical record administrators, and dietitians have their own professional organizations.

The American Hospital Association (AHA) is an organization of accredited hospitals throughout the country. The AHA focuses on concerns common to institutional health care providers. The American Nursing Home Association serves the same function for nursing homes.

Accrediting Organizations

Many organizations are important to nurses because they exert their influence through the process of accrediting institutions. Although the state legally may license an institution or allow it to function with regulation, accrediting bodies commonly set standards that reflect sound, not minimal, standards. Thus, among hospitals, some are allowed to function by the state, although they do not meet the more rigid criteria set by the Joint Commission on the Accreditation of Health Care Organizations (JCAHCO), formerly the Joint Commission on the Accreditation of Hospitals (JCAH).

Often a great deal of power is wielded through the criteria set by the accrediting body. One way that nurses have worked to alter conditions for delivering nursing care is by persuading the accrediting body to alter their criteria.

Accreditation of educational institutions is another important concern. Although the NLN accredits nursing programs on a voluntary basis, those nursing programs that are part of colleges and universities are reviewed by the body that accredits the institution as a whole. Thus a single program may seek approval by the state board of nursing, by the NLN, and by the collegiate accrediting agency. This system may help to maintain quality in nursing education, but it may also create difficulties if the requirements of the various groups differ.

CONCLUSION

Any discussion of all the organizations related to nursing may seem confusing. It cannot be the most stimulating topic you have encountered; however, these organizations have far-reaching effects on the field of nursing and therefore will have a personal impact on you. We hope the information presented here will help you to be somewhat conversant with the many organizations and perhaps feel securer when others begin to sprinkle their conversations with the "alphabet soup" of nursing acronyms. A more comprehensive listing of nursing-related organizations is included in Appendix B. We wish you good fortune as you make your personal decisions about membership.

REFERENCES

1. RN ranks grow. Am J Nurs 86:603–604, May 1986
2. Forum considers nursing scope statement. Am Nurse 19:1, Jan 1987
3. Snyder ME, LaBar C: Issues in professional practice. I. Nursing: Legal authority for practice. Kansas City, American Nurses' Association, 1984
4. Nursing: A Social Policy Statement. Kansas City, American Nurses' Association, 1980
5. Congress for Nursing Practice: The nursing practice act: Suggested state legislation. Kansas City, American Nurses' Association, 1981
6. Foundation awards $62,000 in research grants. Am Nurse 18:18, Nov/Dec 1986
7. Proposed organizational structure for the National League for Health Care, Incorporated, and the National League for Nursing. Nursing & Health Care 8 (5):300–304, May 1987
8. Proposed mission and goals for 1987–1989 biennium. Nursing & Health Care 8 (5):298–299, May 1987

FURTHER READINGS

ADN educators organize new group to fight for RN license. Am J Nurs 86:862, Jul 1986

A.N.A. Bylaws, Publication No. G-77. Kansas City, American Nurses' Association, 1979

ANA honors nursing leaders. Am J Nurs 82:1142, Aug 1982

Christy T: The first fifty years. Am J Nurs 71:1778–1784, Sep 1971

Convention 1982: ANA votes federation. Am J Nurs 82:1246, Aug 1982

Ensor B: What the SNA's are doing. Am J Nurs 82:581–585, Apr 1982

Facts About Nursing, Publication No. 76–77. Kansas City, American Nurses' Association, 1983

Moses ML, Hardy M: It all happened on American Airline Flight 545. A.D. Nurse 2:6–7, Jan/Feb 1987

NSNA turns thirty. Am J Nurs 82:1024+, Jul 1982

Schmidt MS: Why a separate organization for state boards? Am J Nurs 80:725–726, Apr 1980

Appendix A:
State Boards of Nursing

State Boards of Nursing*

State/Address	Licensure Fees†	Temporary Permit	Continuing Education	Nurse Practitioners
Alabama				
Board of Nursing Suite 203 One/East Building 500 East Boulevard Montgomery, AL 36117	Examination: $45 Endorsement: $55 Renewal: $35/2 yr	Required to practice *Eligible:* New graduates awaiting exam results (3 mo for those awaiting endorsement)	None required	Permitted to practice Certification
Alaska				
Board of Nursing Licensing Dept. of Commerce Div. of Occupational Licensing Box D-LIC Juneau, AL 99811-0800	Examination: $50 Endorsement: $50 Renewal: $20/2 yr	Required to practice *Eligible:* New graduates from accredited programs awaiting exam results (3 mo for those awaiting endorsement)	None required	Permitted to practice Advanced Nurse Practitioner Authorization by board required
Arizona				
Board of Nursing Suite 103 5050 N. 19th St. Phoenix, AZ 85015	Examination: $45 Endorsement: $45 Renewal: $20/2 yr	Required to practice *Eligible:* Applicants for license who meet requirements (4 mo)	None required	Permitted to practice Certification as Registered Nurse Practitioner

State / Board	Fees	Interim permit	Continuing education	Notes
Arkansas State Board of Nursing Suite 800 University Tower Building W. 12th Street and University Avenue Little Rock, AR 72204	Examination: $41.50 Endorsement: $75.00 Renewal: $25/2 yr	Required to practice *Eligible:* New graduates awaiting exam results (3 mo for those awaiting endorsement)	None required	Licensed to practice Titled: Registered Nurse Practitioner (RNP)
California Board of Registered Nursing Suite 200 1030 13th St. Sacramento, CA 95814	Examination: $80 Endorsement: $30 Renewal: $40/2 yr	Required to practice *Eligible:* New graduates awaiting exam results (6 mo for those awaiting endorsement)	30 contact hours/2 yr	
Colorado Board of Nursing Room 132 1525 Sherman Street Denver, CO 80203	Examination: $36 Endorsement: $42 Renewal: $18/2 yr	Required to practice *Eligible:* New graduates awaiting exam results (4 mo for those awaiting for endorsement)	20 contact hours/2 yr	Permitted to practice No special license Function on RN license
Connecticut Board of Examiners for Nursing Dept. of Health Services 150 Washington St. Hartford, CT 06106	Examination: $30 Endorsement: $30 Renewal: $10/yr	Required for new graduates prior to results of first examination	None required if license remains current	Nurse practice act is written in broad terms. No special title given

(continued)

State Boards of Nursing* (continued)

State/Address	Licensure Fees†	Temporary Permit	Continuing Education	Nurse Practitioners
Delaware Board of Nursing O'Neil Building P.O. Box 1401 Dover, DE 19901	Examination: $30 Endorsement: $30 Renewal: $30/2 yr	Required for practice *Eligible:* New graduates awaiting exam results (60 days for those awaiting endorsement)	None required	Must be certified and graduate of an approved program
District of Columbia Nurses' Examining Board 5100 Wisconsin Ave. N.W. Suite 306 Washington, DC 20016	Examination: $20 Endorsement: $40 Renewal: $24/yr	No temporary permit available Cannot practice until licensed	None required	No law allowing or denying permission to practice
Florida Board of Nursing Suite 504 111 East Coastline Boulevard Jacksonville, FL 32202	Examination: $97 Endorsement: $62 Renewal: $22/yr	Required to practice *Eligible:* New graduates awaiting exam results (60 days for those awaiting endorsement)	24 contact hr/yr	Permitted under law Advanced Registered Nurse Practitioner in one of three categories: Nurse Anesthetist, Nurse Midwife, Advanced Nurse Practitioner

404

State / Board of Nursing	Fees	Temporary Permit		Advanced Practice
Georgia Board of Nursing 166 Pryor Street S.W. Atlanta, GA 30303	Examination: $60 Endorsement: $60 Renewal: $30/2 yr	Required to practice *Eligible:* First-time writers of NCLEX-RN and applicants for endorsement or reinstatement	None required	Permitted to practice Must apply for special designation as Nurse Practitioner
Hawaii Board of Nursing Box 3469 Honolulu, HA 96801	Examination: $50 Endorsement: $65 Renewal: $40/2 yr	Required to practice *Eligible:* New graduates awaiting results of first examination (those awaiting endorsement)	None required	Permitted to practice No special licensure required
Idaho Board of Nursing Room 203 413 West Idaho Street Boise, ID 83702	Examination: $60 Endorsement: $60 Renewal: $30/2 yr	Required to practice *Eligible:* New graduates until examination results received. Endorsement applicants for 90 days	Required for Nurse Practitioners and Nurse Anesthetists	Permitted to practice under special Nurse Practitioner Rules and Regulations that include passing a certification examination given by an organization recognized by the Board of Nursing

(continued)

405

State Boards of Nursing* (continued)

State/Address	Licensure Fees†	Temporary Permit	Continuing Education	Nurse Practitioners
Illinois				
Dept. of Registration and Education Third Floor 320 West Washington Street Springfield, IL 62786	Examination: $25 + exam costs Endorsement: $25 Renewal: $20/2 yr	Required to practice *Eligible:* Those who have applied and met requirements for license while awaiting permanent license for up to 12 months New graduates must practice under direct supervision of an RN	None required	Practice in accordance with definition of RN
Indiana				
Indiana State Board of Nursing One American Square Suite 1020, Box 82067 Indianapolis, IN 46282	Examination: $30 Endorsement: $30 Renewal: $20/2 yr	Temporary permit available, $10	None required	

Iowa				
Board of Nursing 1223 East Court Des Moines, IA 50319	Examination: $40 Endorsement: $56 Renewal: $36/3 yr	Required to practice *Eligible:* New graduates awaiting exam results (90 days for those awaiting endorsement)	4.5 continuing education units (45 contact hr) every 3 yr	Licensed under titled Advanced Registered Nurse Practitioner (ARNP)
Kansas				
Kansas State Board of Nursing Suite 551-S 900 S.W. Jackson Topeka, KS 66612-1256	Examination: $60 Endorsement: $60 Renewal: $25/2 yr	Required to practice *Eligible:* New graduates awaiting exam results	30 continuing education units (30 contact hr) every 2 yr	Graduate of approved program with clinician experience as Advanced Registered Nurse Practitioner and Certified Registered Nurse Anesthetist
Kentucky				
Kentucky Board of Nursing Suite 430 4010 Dupont Circle Louisville, KY 40207	Examination: $85 Endorsement: $50 Renewal: Active: $30/2 yr Inactive: $20/2 yr	Required to practice *Eligible:* New graduates awaiting exam results (4 mo for those awaiting endorsement)	30 contact hr/2 yr	Registered as an Advanced Registered Nurse Practitioner (ARNP) with specialty designation

State Boards of Nursing* (continued)

State/Address	Licensure Fees†	Temporary Permit	Continuing Education	Nurse Practitioners
Louisiana Louisiana State Board of Nursing 907 Père Marquette Building 150 Baronne Street New Orleans, LA 70112	Examination: $35 Endorsement: $30 Renewal: $15/yr	Required to practice *Eligible:* New graduates awaiting exam results (90 days for those awaiting endorsement)	None required	Permitted in the following categories: • Primary Nurse Associate (also known as nurse practitioner) • Certified Nurse Mid-wife • Certified Registered Nurse Anesthetist • Clinical Nurse Specialist
Maine Board of Nursing 295 Water Street Augusta, ME 04330	Examination: $40 Endorsement: $40 Renewal: $10/yr	Required to practice *Eligible:* New graduates awaiting exam results (90 days for those awaiting endorsement) Foreign nursing graduate awaiting exam results	None required	Permitted when have completed an approved educational program

Maryland Board of Nursing 201 West Preston Street Baltimore, MD 21201 301-764-4747	Examination: $60 Endorsement: $60 Renewal: $20/2 yr	Required to practice *Eligible:* 90 days for those awaiting endorsement	None required	Must be certified by the Board in order to practice
Massachusetts Board of Registered Nursing Room 1519 100 Cambridge Street Boston, MA 02202	Examination: $94 Endorsement: $50 Renewal: $25/2 yr	No temporary permits available	15 clock hr every 2 yr	Nurse Anesthetists, Nurse Midwives, and Primary Care Nurses permitted to practice with special authorization from Board
Michigan Board of Nursing P.O. Box 30018 611 W. Ottawa Lansing, MI 48909	Examination: $65 Endorsement: $25 Renewal: $20/2 yr	*Eligible:* New graduates for 16 weeks after exam; $10.00	Rules for CE being developed	Specialty certification required for practice
Minnesota Board of Nursing 2700 University Ave. W. #108 St. Paul, MN 55114	Examination: $75 Endorsement: $55 Renewal: $20/2 yr	Required to practice *Eligible:* New graduates awaiting exam results (6 mo for those awaiting endorsement)	30 contact hours/2 yr	Permitted to practice No special designation provided

(continued)

State Boards of Nursing* *(continued)*

State/Address	Licensure Fees†	Temporary Permit	Continuing Education	Nurse Practitioners
Mississippi Board of Nursing Suite 101 135 Bounds Street Jackson, MS 39206	Examination: $70 Endorsement: $50 Renewal: $25/2 yr	Required to practice *Eligible:* New graduates awaiting exam results (90 days for those awaiting endorsement)	None required	Permitted to practice Must have specialty certification and have 4 continuing education units every 2 yr
Missouri Board of Nursing P.O. Box 656 Jefferson City, MO 65102	Examination: $15 Endorsement: $25 Renewal: $12/yr	6 mo for those awaiting endorsement	None required	Permitted to practice under definition of registered professional nurse No special designation required
Montana Board of Nursing 1424 Ninth Avenue Helena, MT 59620-0407	Examination: $35 Endorsement: $35 Renewal: $10/yr ($5 late fee)	Required to practice *Eligible:* New graduates awaiting exam results (3 mo for those awaiting endorsement)	None required	Permitted to practice Must apply for special designation from board

State / Board	Fees	Temporary Permits	Continuing Education	Advanced Practice
Nebraska Department of Health Bureau of Examining Boards Board of Nursing Box 95007 Lincoln, NE 68509	Examination: $50 Endorsement: $50 Renewal: $30/2 yr	Required to practice *Eligible:* New graduates awaiting exam results (up to 1 yr for those awaiting endorsement)	200 hr of employment as an R.N. and 20 hr of continuing education in the last 5 yr or 75 contact hr per 5 yr	Designation by Board as Certified Nurse Anesthetist/Practitioner required
Nevada State Board of Nursing Suite 116 1281 Terminal Way Reno, NV 89502	Examination: $115 Endorsement: $65 Renewal: $50/2 yr	Required to practice *Eligible:* New graduates awaiting exam results and permanent licensures for 4 mo	30 contact hours/2 yr	Permitted to practice with certification by Board of Nursing
New Hampshire Board of Nursing Education and Nurse Registration Regional Blvd. Industrial Complex Concord, NH 03301	Examination: $70 Endorsement: $40 Renewal: $20/2 yr	No temporary permits issued (This is currently under consideration.)	None required for R.N.	Granted recognition as Advanced Registered Nurse Practitioner Must be approved by Board and must have 15 hr/yr contact of continuing education

(continued)

State Boards of Nursing* (continued)

State/Address	Licensure Fees†	Temporary Permit	Continuing Education	Nurse Practitioners
New Jersey Board of Nursing Room 319 1100 Raymond Building Newark, NJ 07102	Examination: $35 Endorsement: $30 Renewal: $18/2 yr	Required to practice *Eligible:* New graduates and those with licenses in other countries awaiting exam results; those awaiting endorsement	None required	Permitted to practice under the general law with no special designation required
New Mexico Board of Nursing 4125 Carlisle N.E. Albuquerque, NM 87107	Examination: $65 Endorsement: $62 Renewal: $30/2 yr	Required to practice *Eligible:* New graduates awaiting exam results (6 mo for those awaiting endorsement)	30 contact hr/2 yr	Permitted to practice after certification by Board as Nurse Practitioner
New York State Board of Nursing State Education Department Cultural Education Center Room 3013 Albany, NY 12230	Examination: $145 Endorsement: $60 Renewal: $45/3 yr	Required to practice *Eligible:* New graduates awaiting exam results (1 yr for those awaiting endorsement)	None required	Not permitted to practice

State	Address	Fees			
North Carolina	Board of Nursing Box 2129 Raleigh, NC 27602	Examination: $45 Endorsement: $45 Renewal: $25/2 yr	Required to practice *Eligible:* New graduates awaiting exam results (6 mo for those awaiting endorsement)	None required	Permitted to practice after approval by joint subcommittee of Board of Nursing of Medical Examiners
North Dakota	Board of Nursing Kirkwood Office Tower 7th and Arbor Ave. Suite 504 Bismarck, ND 58501	Examination: $65 Endorsement: $65 Renewal: $20/yr	Required to practice *Eligible:* New graduates awaiting exam results (90 days for those awaiting endorsement)	None required	Permitted to practice after approval as Nurse Practitioner by the Board
Ohio	Board of Nursing Education and Registration Suite 509 65 South Front Street Columbus, OH 43266-0316	Examination: $32 Endorsement: $32 Renewal: $10/2 yr	Required to practice *Eligible:* New graduates awaiting exam results (6 mo for those awaiting endorsement) Those in state for education or training with valid license in another state	None required	Permitted to practice, but not included in law

(continued)

State Boards of Nursing* (*continued*)

State/Address	Licensure Fees†		Temporary Permit	Continuing Education	Nurse Practitioners
Oklahoma					
Board of Nurse Registration and Nursing Education Suite 524 2915 N. Classen Blvd. Oklahoma City, OK 73106	Examination: Endorsement: Renewal:	$55 $55 $30/2 yr	Required to practice *Eligible:* 90 days for those awaiting endorsement	None required	Permitted to practice after recognition by the Board as Nurse Practitioner
Oregon					
Oregon State Board of Nursing 1400 SW 5th Avenue Room 904 Portland, OR 97201	Examination: Endorsement: Renewal:	$59 $41 $31/2 yr	New graduates allowed to practice while awaiting exam results	None required	Permitted to practice Must obtain a Nurse Practitioner certificate from the Board
Pennsylvania					
State Board of Nursing Department of State Box 2649 Harrisburg, PA 17105	Examination: Endorsement: Renewal:	$24 $24 $10/2 yr	Required to practice *Eligible:* 1 year for those awaiting endorsement	None required	Permitted to practice Must be certified by the board as Certified Registered Nurse Practitioner (CRNP)

	Fees			
Rhode Island Cannon Health Building 75 Davis Street Room 104 Providence, RI 02908	Examination: $75 Endorsement: $75 Renewal: $30/2 yr	Not required	None required	Permitted to practice No special designation required
South Carolina State Board of Nursing for South Carolina Suite 102 1777 St. Julian Place Columbia, SC 29204	Examination: $65 Endorsement: $50 Renewal: $12/yr	Required to practice *Eligible:* New graduates awaiting exam results; those awaiting endorsement; foreign nurse graduates awaiting exam results who have a certificate from the Commission on Graduate of Foreign Nursing Schools	None required	Permitted to practice Need Board approval to practice as a Private Independent Nurse
South Dakota Board of Nursing Suite 205 304 Phillips Avenue Sioux Falls, SD 57102	Examination: $50 Endorsement: $75 Renewal: $35/2 yr	Required to practice *Eligible:* New graduates awaiting exam results; those awaiting endorsement with current licensure in another state	None required	Permitted to practice Must have completed a certification program approved by the Board

(continued)

State Boards of Nursing* (continued)

State/Address	Licensure Fees†		Temporary Permit	Continuing Education	Nurse Practitioners
Tennessee					
Board of Nursing 283 Plus Park Blvd. Nashville, TN 37219-5407	Examination: Endorsement: Renewal:	$65 $60 $10/2 yr	Required to practice *Eligible:* New graduates awaiting exam results; those awaiting endorsement; foreign nurse graduates holding CGFNS Certificate and awaiting exam results	None required	Permitted to practice Must apply for a special designation in order to have prescriptive authority
Texas					
Board of Nurse Examiners 1300 East Anderson Lane, C-225 Austin, TX 78752	Examination: Endorsement: Renewal:	$60 $60 $16/2 yr	Required to practice *Eligible:* New graduates awaiting exam results; those awaiting endorsement	None required	Must be graduate of approved post-basic program and approved by board
Utah					
Board of Nursing 160 East 300 South P.O. Box 45802	Examination: Endorsement: Renewal:	$45 $45 $25/2 yr	Required to practice *Eligible:* New graduates awaiting	None required	Permitted to practice Must obtain special approval from the

Salt Lake City, UT 84145		exam results; those awaiting endorsement.	None required	Must be endorsed by board in order to practice board
Vermont Board of Nursing 26 Terrace St. Montpelier, VT 05602	Examination: $30 Endorsement: $25 Renewal: $10/2 yr	Required to practice *Eligible:* New graduates awaiting exam results (60 days for those awaiting endorsement) after application complete	None required	Must be endorsed by board in order to practice
Virginia Board of Nursing 1601 Rolling Hills Dr. Richmond, VA 23229	Examination: $40 Endorsement: $40 Renewal: $14/2 yr	Not required	None required	Permitted to practice Apply to Board for recognition as Certified Nurse Practitioner (CNP)
Washington Board of Nursing Division of Health Care Licensing Box 9649 Olympia, WA 98504	Examination: $30 Endorsement: $25 Renewal: $20/yr	Interim permit granted only to those new U.S. graduates awaiting exam results	None required at this time	Permitted to practice Apply for Board designation as an Advanced Registered Nurse Practitioner

(continued)

State Boards of Nursing* *(continued)*

State/Address	Licensure Fees†	Temporary Permit	Continuing Education	Nurse Practitioners
West Virginia Board of Nursing Examiners Room 309 Embleton Building 922 Quarrier Street Charleston, WV 25301	Examination: $51.50 Endorsement: $30 Renewal: $10/yr	Required to practice *Eligible:* New graduates awaiting results of exam	None required	Permitted to practice No special designation required
Wisconsin Board of Nursing P.O. Box 8935 Madison, WI 53708	Examination: $40 Endorsement: $50 Renewal: $32/2 yr	Required to practice *Eligible:* New graduates awaiting exam results ($10 fee)	None required	Those practicing must conform to guidelines of the Tri-Board (Nursing, Medicine, Pharmacy) regarding Nurse Specialists
Wyoming Board of Nursing Barrett Bldg. 4th Floor 2301 Central Ave. Cheyenne, WY 82002	Examination: $75 Endorsement: $80 Renewal: $50/2 yr	Required to practice *Eligible:* New graduates awaiting exam results (90 days for those awaiting endorsement)	None required	Permitted to practice Must apply for recognition status from the Board

Guam				
Board of Nurse Examiners P.O. Box 2816 Agana, Guam 96910	Examination: $56.50 Endorsement: $60.00 Renewal: $30.00	Required to practice *Eligible:* Qualify for exam or applicant for licensure by endorsement (90 days)	None required	Permitted to practice Titled: Certified Registered Nurse Practitioners
Virgin Islands				
Board of Nurse Licensure Knud Hansen Comples St. Thomas, VI 00801	Examination: $35.00	Required to practice *Eligible:* Valid license from U.S. and Canadian Graduates (1 yr for graduates, 3 mo for RNs seeking endorsement)	None	No

*Information in this table was obtained from the state boards in April–June of 1987.

†Fees are subject to change. An additional fee is paid to the NCLEX Examination Service by applicants to take the examination. This fee is $25.00. Some states collect an additional fee for processing and test administration.

Appendix B:
Nursing-Related
Organizations

Nursing-Related Organizations

	Year Established	Membership Eligibility	*Certification Available	Publications (monthly unless otherwise noted)
Overall Professional Organizations				
American Nurses Association (A.N.A.) 2420 Pershing Road Kansas City, MO 64108	1896	RNs only	Yes	American Journal of Nursing, The American Nurse (for others, write for list)
International Council of Nurses (I.C.N.) Box 42 1211 Geneva 20, Switzerland	1900	National professional nurse organizations	—	
National Student Nurse Assn. (N.S.N.A.) 55 West 57th St. New York, NY 10019	1953	Officially enrolled students of RN and RN baccalaureate programs	—	Imprint (5 times/yr)
National League For Nursing (N.L.N.) 10 Columbus Circle New York, NY 10019	1952	Individuals and agencies interested in the profession of nursing and delivery of nursing care	—	Nursing and Health Care (others; write for list)
Organizations Related to Scholarship and Leadership in Nursing				
American Academy of Nurses (A.A.N.) c/o American Nurses Association 2420 Pershing Road Kansas City, MO 64108	1973	Members elected by current members, based on contribution to nursing	Use title "Fellow" (F.A.A.N.)	Nursing Outlook (bimonthly)

Organization	Year	Membership		Publication
Alpha Tau Delta 14631 N. 2nd Dr. Phoenix, AZ 85023	1921	Students in baccalaureate programs in nursing	No	*Captions of Alpha Tau delta* (biennial)
Sigma Theta Tau 1200 Waterway Blvd. Indianapolis, IN 46202	1922	High achievers: Senior students in baccalaureate, master's, and doctoral programs Outstanding RN's with baccalaureate or higher degree	No	*Image, Reflections* (newsletters, both quarterly)

Groups Related to Ethnic/Racial Origin

Organization	Year	Membership		Publication
American Indian Nurses Association (A.I.N.A.) P.O. Box 1588 Norman, OK 73071	1972	Student nurses and RNs of American Indian ancestry	—	*Newsletter of the A.I.N.A.* (bimonthly)
National Black Nurses Association, Inc. P.O. Box 1835B Boston, MA 02118	1971	Black RNs	—	*Journal of National Black Nurses' Association* (twice yearly)
National Association of Hispanic Nurses 2018 Johnston St. Los Angeles, CA 90031	1976	Hispanic nurses, associate/all nurses	—	Newsletter (quarterly)

(continued)

Nursing-Related Organizations (continued)

	Year Established	Membership Eligibility	*Certification Available	Publication (monthly unless otherwise noted)
Educationally Oriented Associations				
American Association of Colleges of Nursing (A.A.C.N.) One Dupont Circle Suite 530 Washington, D.C. 20036	1969	Collegiate prgm with upper-division major in nursing	—	*Journal of Professional Nursing* (bimonthly) *ACCN Newsletter* (10 times/yr) (others: write) Write for list
Council on Collegiate Education for Nursing for the Southern Regional Education Board (S.R.E.B.) 1340 Spring St. NW Atlanta, GA 30309	1963	Colleges and universities in the southern states which have nursing programs	No	
Mid Atlantic Regional Nursing Association (M.A.R.N.A.) Columbus Circle New York, NY 10019	1981	Agencies preparing persons in health care and which deliver health care		*Marnagram* (Quarterly)
Midwest Alliance in Nursing, Inc. (M.A.I.N.) 1226 W. Michigan St., 108 BR Indianapolis, IN 46223	1979	Agencies engaged in providing direct nursing care or teaching persons to provide direct care		*MAINlines* (Bimonthly newsletter)
National Association for Practical Nurse Education and Service, Inc. (N.A.P.N.E.S.)	1941	All persons interested in LPN/LVN education	No	*Journal of Practical Nursing* (quarterly) *NAPNES Forum*

Address/Organization	Year	Membership		(newsletter)
10801 Pear Tree Lane Suite 151 St. Louis, MO 63074				
National Organization for the Advancement of Associate Degree Nursing (N.O.A.A.D.N.) Amarillo College P.O. Box 447 Amarillo, TX 79178	1985	Open	—	*AD Nurse* (bimonthly)
North American Nursing Diagnosis Association (N.A.N.D.A.) St. Louis University School of Nursing 3525 Caroline Street Room 439 St. Louis, MO 63104	1976	RNs	No	*Nursing Diagnoses* (three times yearly)
New England Organization for Nursing 55 Chapel St. Newton, MA 02160	1964	Colleges and universities in the New England states which have nursing programs	No	Write for list
Western Institute of Nursing (W.I.N.) P.O. Drawer P Boulder, CO 80302	1957	Colleges and universities in the western states which have nursing programs	No	Write for list

(continued)

Nursing-Related Organizations (continued)

	Year Established	Membership Eligibility	*Certification Available	Publications (monthly unless otherwise noted)
Occupational or Specialty-Related Nursing Organizations				
American Association of Critical Care Nurses (A.A.C.N.) One Civic Plaza Newport Beach, CA 92660	1969	RNs, LPNs, student nurses	Yes	*Heart and Lung Journal* (bimonthly) *Focus on Critical Care* (bimonthly)
American Association for the History of Nursing P.O. Box 90803 Washington, DC 20003	1980	Anyone interested in the history of nursing	No	*The Bulletin* (4 times per year)
American Nephrology Nurses Association (A.A.N.A.) North Woodbury Road Box 56 Pitman, NJ 08071	1969	RNs, LVNs employed in the field	Yes	*Journal of AANA* (6 times per year) *AANA Update* (Newsletter)
American Association of Neuroscience Nurses (A.A.N.N.) 218 North Jefferson Suite 204 Chicago, IL 60606	1968	RNs	No	*Journal of Neuroscience Nursing* (bimonthly)
American Association of Nurse Anesthetists (A.A.N.A.) 216 Higgins Road Park Ridge, IL 60068	1931	RNs who are certified Registered Nurse Anesthetists (CRNAs)	Yes	*American Association of Nurse Anesthetists Journal* (bimonthly) *A.A.N.A. Bulletin* (bimonthly)

Organization	Founded	Membership Eligibility	Journal/Official Publication	Publications
American Association of Occupational Health Nurses 50 Lenox Pointe Atlanta, GA 30324	1942	RNs practicing in an occupational health setting	Yes	*AAOHN Journal* *AAOH News*
American Burn Association c/o Dr. Charles E. Hartford Burn Treatment Center Crozier–Chester Medical Center 15th & Upland Avenue Chester, PA 19013		Professionals working with burn patients	No	
American College of Nurse Midwives (A.C.N.M.) 1522 K Street N.W. Suite 1120 Washington, D.C. 20005	1955	RNs who are certified Nurse Midwives or students in accredited programs	Yes	*Journal of Nurse Midwifery* *Quickening* (newsletter)
American Holistic Nurses Association 205 St. Louis St. Suite 506 Springfield, MO 65806	1981	Active: RN, LPN/LVN Contributing: All	In planning	*Journal of Holistic Nursing* (Annual) *Beginnings* (Newsletter)
American Organization of Nurse Executives 840 North Lake Shore Drive Chicago, IL 60611		RNs in administrative positions	No	
American Public Health Association Public Health Nursing Section 1015 15th Street N.W. Washington, D.C. 20005	APHA 1972	All persons interested in Public Health Various categories of membership available	All persons interested in Public Health Various categories of membership available	*American Journal of Public Health* *The Nation's Health*

(continued)

Nursing-Related Organizations (continued)

	Year Established	Membership Eligibility	*Certification Available	Publications (monthly unless otherwise noted)
American Radiological Nurses Association c/o E. Deutsch 502 Forest Court Carrboro, NC 27510	1981	*Active:* RNs employed in radiologic nursing *Associate:* Other RNs and LPNs in radiologic nursing	No	*ARNA Images* (4 times/yr)
American Society of Ophthalmic Registered Nurses (A.S.O.R.N.) P.O. Box 3030 San Francisco, CA 94119	1976	RNs working in ophthalmology	No	*Insight* (newsletter)
American Society of Plastic and Reconstructive Surgical Nurses Box 56, No. Woodbury Rd. Pitman, NJ 08071	1975	*Active:* RNs, LPNs working in the field *Assoc.:* RNs, LPNs interested in the field	No	*Journal of Plastic and Reconstructive Surgical Nursing*
American Society of Post-Anesthesia Nurses P.O. Box 11083 Richmond, VA 23230	1980	RNs, LPNs, Anesthiologists, CRNAs	Yes	*Breathline Journal of Post Anesthesia Nursing* (quarterly)
American Urological Association Allied 6845 Lake Shore Drive P.O. Box 9397 Raytown, MO 64133	1972	*Active:* RNs, LPNs, PAs, technicians *Assoc:* Industry, physicians	Yes	*AUAA Journal* (quarterly) *Urogram* (newsletter)
Association for Practitioners in Infection Control 505 E. Hawley St. Mundelein, IL 60060	1972	*Active:* Professionals in Infection Control *Associate:* Others	Yes	*AJIC* (bimonthly) (others: write)

Organization	Year	Membership	Nursing Specialty Certification	Publications
Association for the Care of Children's Health 3615 Wisconsin Ave. N.W. Washington, D.C. 20016	1965	All individuals interested in children's health	No	*Children's Health Care* (write for list of others)
Association of Operating Room Nurses (A.O.R.N.) 10170 East Mississippi Avenue Denver, CO 80231	1949	*Active:* RNs employed in OR or in a related educational program or in research	Yes	*A.O.R.N. Journal*
Association of Pediatric Oncology Nurses Suite 3A 1311 A Dolley Madison Blvd. McLean, VA 22001	1976	RNs	No	*APON Newsletter* (quarterly) (Write for list of others)
Association of Rehabilitation Nurses 2506 Gross Point Road Evanston, IL 60201	1974	*Regular:* RNs *Associate:* all interested persons	Yes	*Rehabilitation Nursing* (bimonthly journal) Pamphlets
Coalition of Nurse Practitioners, Inc. P.O. Box 123 East Greenbush, NY	1980	Nurse Practitioners and students in nurse practitioner programs	No	*Coalition Communique* (quarterly)
Department of School Nurses of the National Education Association (N.E.A.) 1201 Sixteenth Street N.W. Washington, D.C. 20036	1968	School nurse members of the N.E.A.	—	*The School Nurse*
Dermatology Nurses' Association North Woodbury Rd. Box 56 Pitman, NJ 08071	1981	*Active:* RNs, LPNs/LVNs involved in dermatology	No	*DNA Focus* (bimonthly newsletter)

(continued)

Nursing-Related Organizations *(continued)*

	Year Established	Membership Eligibility	*Certification Available	Publications (monthly unless otherwise noted)
Drug and Alcohol Nursing Association P.O. Box 6126 Annapolis, MD 21401	1979	*Active:* Nurses caring for clients with drug- and alcohol-related disorders *Associate:* all others	No	*DANA Newsletter* (quarterly)
Emergency Nurses Association (E.N.A.) 230 East Ohio Suite 600 Chicago, IL 60611	1970	RNs	Yes	*The Journal of Emergency Nursing* *Emergency Nursing Core Curriculum*
Flight Nurse Section Aerospace Medical Association Washington National Airport Washington, D.C. 20001	1964	Designated Flight Nurses and RNs who are members of Aerospace Medical Association	No	*Aviation, Space, and Environmental Medicine*
International Association for Enterostomal Therapy 2081 Business Center Drive Suite 290 Irvine, CA 92715	1968	*Active:* graduate of accredited I.A.E.T. program	Yes	*Journal of Enterostomal Therapy*
N.A.A.C.O.G.: The Organization for Obstetric, Gynecological and Neonatal Nurses 600 Maryland Ave. S.W.	1969	RNs and allied health individuals in OGN area	Yes	*Journal of Obstetric, Gynecologic and Neonatal Nursing* *(JOGN)* (bimonthly)

Organization	Year	Membership	Newsletter Column	Publication
Suite 200E Washington, D.C. 20024				NAACOG Newsletter
National Association for Health Care Retirement P.O. Box 93851 Cleveland, OH 44101-5851	1975	Active: health care recruiters	No	Recruitment Directions (10 times/yr)
National Association of Neonatal Nurses 35 Maria Drive, Suite 855 Petaluma, CA 94952	1984	Regular: RNs Associate: All	No	Neonatal Network: The Journal of Neonatal Nursing (Bi-monthly)
National Association of Orthopaedic Nurses North Woodbury Road Box 56 Pitman, NJ 08071	1980	RNs, LPNs, LVNs	In 1988	Orthopaedic Nursing (Write for others)
National Association of Pediatric Nurse Associates/Practitioners (N.A.P.N.A.P.) 1000 Maplewood Dr. Suite 104 Maple Shade, NJ 08052-1931	1973	RNs with advanced education who are primary care practitioners in pediatrics	Yes	The Pediatric Nurse Practitioner (newsletter) The Journal of Pediatric Health Care
National Association of School Nurses Lamplighter Lane, P.O. Box 1300 Scarborough, ME 04074	1969	Active: RNs employed by educational institutions; Other categories for students, retirees, organizations	Yes	School Nurse Journal NAS Newsletter (quarterly)
National Flight Nurses Association P.O. Box 8222 Rapid City, SD 57709	1981		In planning	Aeromedical Journal (bimonthly) Across the Board (quarterly)

(continued)

Nursing-Related Organizations (continued)

	Year Established	Membership Eligibility	*Certification Available	Publications (monthly unless otherwise noted)
National Intravenous Therapy Association Suite 4 87 Blanchard Rd. Cambridge, MA 02138	1973	Nurses interested in intravenous therapy	Yes	*NITA Journal* *NITA Update* (newsletter)
National Nurses Society on Addiction 2506 Gross Pointe Rd. Evanston, IL 60201	1983	*Regular:* RNs *Associate:* All	No (pending)	*Annual Review of Nursing and the Addictions* Quarterly newsletter
Nurse Consultants Association P.O. Box 25875 Colorado Springs, CO 80936	1979	RNs with 60% of income from consultant-type sources	No	Quarterly newsletter Annual membership directory
Oncology Nursing Society 1016 Greentree Rd. Pittsburgh, PA 15220	1975	Nurses with special interest in patients with cancer	Yes	*Oncology Nursing Forum* *ONS News*
Society for Peripheral Vascular Nursing P.O. Box 11356 Baltimore, MD 21239	1982	*Active:* Currently licensed nurses	No	*SPVN Journal* (quarterly)
Society of Gastrointestinal Assistants 1070 Sibley Tower Rochester, NY 14604	1974	Individuals employed as gastrointestinal assistants	Yes	*SGA Journal* (quarterly)

Organization	Year	Membership		Publication
Transcultural Nursing Society College of Nursing University of Utah 25 So. Medical Drive Salt Lake City, Utah 84112	1979	Nurses and non-nurses	No	Biannual newsletter
World Federation of Neurosurgical Nurses Avenue Appia 1211 Geneva 27 Switzerland		Professional nurses working in neurosurgery	—	

Miscellaneous

Organization	Year	Membership		Publication
American Assembly for Men in Nursing College of Nursing, Rush University 600 So. Paulina 474-H Chicago, IL 60612	1971	All men in nursing	No	Interaction
National Nurses for Life 1998 Menold Allison Park, PA 15104				
Nurses' Alliance for the Prevention of Nuclear War 225 Lafayette St. Room 207 New York, NY 10012	1981	RNs, Students, allied health, general public	No	Aegis (quarterly newsletter)
Nurses Christian Fellowship 6400 Schroeder Rd. P.O. Box 7895 Madison, WI 53707	1948	Christian students and R.N.'s		Journal of Christian Nursing (quarterly)

(continued)

Nursing-Related Organizations *(continued)*

	Year Established	Membership Eligibility	*Certification Available	Publications (monthly unless otherwise noted)
Nurses Educational Funds 555 West 57th St. New York, NY 10019	1911	Donors welcome	—	Semi-Annual Newsletter
Nurses Environmental Health Watch 33 Columbus Ave. Somerville, MA 02143				
Nurses' House, Inc. 10 Columbus Circle New York, NY 10019-1346	1925	Payment of annual contribution		

*Certification is frequently conducted by a legally separate though related organization. Information on the certification program is available from the specialty organizations.

434

Index

The letter *f* following a page number indicates a figure; the letter *t* following a page number indicates a table.

435